心血管内科会诊纪要

Essentials of Cardiovascular Consultations

郭素峡　主编

清華大學出版社
北　京

图书在版编目（CIP）数据

心血管内科会诊纪要 = Essentials of Cardiovascular Consultations / 郭素峡主编 . 北京 : 清华大学出版社, 2024. 11. -- ISBN 978-7-302-67655-3

Ⅰ. R54

中国国家版本馆 CIP 数据核字第 2024N1U042 号

责任编辑：孙　宇
封面设计：钟　达
责任校对：李建庄
责任印制：沈　露

出版发行：清华大学出版社
网　　址：https: // www.tup.com.cn, https: // www.wqxuetang.com
地　　址：北京清华大学学研大厦 A 座　　邮　　编：100084
社 总 机：010-83470000　　邮　　购：010-62786544
投稿与读者服务：010-62776969, c-service@tup.tsinghua.edu.cn
质量反馈：010-62772015, zhiliang@tup.tsinghua.edu.cn
印 装 者：三河市龙大印装有限公司
经　　销：全国新华书店
开　　本：185mm×260mm　　印　　张：24　　字　　数：550 千字
版　　次：2024 年 11 月第 1 版　　印　　次：2024 年 11 月第 1 次印刷
定　　价：128.00 元

产品编号：107718-01

编委会

主　　审：周建平

主　　编：郭素峡

英文审校：廖敏琪　王亦泷

编　　者（按姓氏汉语拼音排序）：

陈国栋　陈丽华　陈子龙　何如平

黄志超　简政威　李　盛　李志聪

梁广柱　列镇邦　林玉萍　卢炯斌

沈利汉　苏少辉　卫展扬　吴泽奎

吴智豪　熊　斌　杨燕华　姚永钊

叶继亮　叶嘉华　尹海贤　尹俊文

袁志明　张　斌　张海林　张晓明

周国祥　周伟良　周永巧

Editorial Board

Preface

Cardiovascular diseases, malignant tumors, and cerebrovascular diseases are the three major diseases that threaten human health. Among them, cardiovascular disease is considered "the number one killer". Due to its rapid changing in condition and high risk of mortality, attending physicians in cardiovascular medicine face a large volume of emergency consultations and routine consultations daily. In the consultation cases, there are patients with other medical conditions combined with cardiovascular diseases, surgical patients requiring preoperative cardiovascular risk assessment, obstetrics and gynecology patients with concomitant cardiovascular diseases requiring preoperative or delivery risk assessment, and patients with heart failure caused by various reasons (such as chronic atrial fibrillation). Cases like coronary artery stenting patients with gastrointestinal bleeding, cerebral hemorrhage, or the need for non-cardiac surgery involve consultations on cardiac function assessment, anticoagulation, and antiplatelet therapy management. These cases have a high level of specialization, and the attending physicians may not fully explain the situation when consulting other departments, leading to repeated inquiries to senior physicians or even repeated consultations from clinical departments. For these reasons, we conceived the idea of inviting experienced clinicians who have been working on the front lines to compile a book entitled *Cardiovascular Consultation Summary* to address common difficulties encountered during clinical consultations, thereby meeting the needs of both the consulting departments and the cardiovascular physicians providing consultations. Inevitably, due to our limited capabilities, there may be oversights and shortcomings, and we would like to welcome readers' critiques and suggestions.

This book is divided into seven chapters that introduce the most common questions faced by cardiovascular physicians during consultations. Chapter 1 covers coronary artery disease, which has the highest incidence and broadest scope among critical cardiovascular diseases, including differential diagnosis of acute chest pain, treatment procedures for ACS, diagnosis and treatment of sudden death, risk stratification, treatment strategies, management of complications, and medication management. Chapter 2 discusses the management of heart failure, which is the "final battleground" of cardiovascular diseases, with not only a high incidence but also complex clinical situations for some patients. In addition to introducing basic knowledge about heart failure, this book also includes the differential diagnosis of dyspnea and edema, which are frequently encountered during consultations. Chapter 3 covers arrhythmias, a challenging topic that most physicians are hesitant to address. From the perspective of identifying and providing emergency treatment for various high-risk arrhythmias, this book aims to help less experienced physicians quickly grasp the principles of rapid identification and management. Chapters 4 and 5 discuss various clinical situations related to hypertension, pericardial diseases, and valvular diseases, including refractory hypertension, secondary hypertension, and pulmonary hypertension, which are frequently encountered during consultations. Chapter 6 introduces the management principles for various cardiovascular diseases during pregnancy. With the implementation of the two-child policy and the increase in women's educational level, the number of older and medically complicated pregnancies has surged, necessitating greater knowledge in this area for consulting physicians. Chapter 7 covers cardiovascular risk assessment for non-cardiac surgeries, which is a significant consultation request from surgical departments. This book discusses preoperative assessment, surgical risk classification, perioperative cardiovascular evaluation methods, the management of concomitant cardiovascular diseases, and perioperative examinations.

We believe that the issues faced by cardiovascular physicians during consultations are not limited to the above content. This book aims to familiarize consulting physicians with the most common clinical scenarios and effective management strategies to meet the majority of clinical needs.

Editors

Contents

Chapter 1

Coronary Artery Disease

Section 1 Differential Diagnosis of Chest Pain

Chest pain ranks among the most common clinical conditions, with patients frequently presenting to departments such as pulmonology, cardiology, and thoracic surgery. Acute chest pain cases typically seek emergency department care, while patients exhibiting atypical chest pain symptoms may consult various specialized departments, with gastroenterology being the most common. This situation often leads to cardiology consultations requested by other departments. Cross-sectional studies in the Beijing area of China indicate that chest pain patients account for 4.7% of emergency department visits. According to international registry data, acute chest pain constitutes 5%-20% of internal medicine emergency cases. Acute chest pain encompasses conditions such as Acute Coronary Syndrome (ACS), aortic dissection, pulmonary embolism, pneumothorax, pericarditis, cardiac tamponade, and esophageal rupture. Among these, Acute Coronary Syndrome represents the highest proportion of life-threatening diseases, with a misdiagnosis rate for myocardial infarction between 3% and 5%. The incidence rate of aortic dissection aneurysms is (0.5-1) / 100,000 people, with a misdiagnosis leading to a mortality rate exceeding 90%. Pulmonary embolism has an incidence rate of approximately 70 / 100,000 people, spontaneous pneumothorax (2.5-18) / 100,000 people, and esophageal rupture 12.5 / 100,000 people. In clinical practice, due to the multitude of causes for chest pain and the atypical clinical presentations of cardiogenic chest pain combined with other diseases or symptoms, there is a higher risk of misdiagnosis and missed diagnosis. The primary objectives of consultations include, on one hand, performing a risk assessment on all chest pain patients to determine whether the pain is cardiogenic or life-threatening, such as in cases of acute myocardial infarction, aortic dissection, and pulmonary embolism, thereby deciding if there is a need for immediate resuscitation, department transfer, or hospital transfer. On the other hand, consultations aim to identify the majority of patients with low to moderate risk of chest pain, to provide necessary further diagnostic tests for a definitive diagnosis, to reduce unnecessary hospital admissions, and to prevent the wastage of medical resources.

I Causes and Characteristics of Chest Pain

The classification of chest pain is multifaceted, categorized by its origin as deriving from the chest wall, pleuropulmonary, and mediastinal organs. These pains are often induced by inflammation, ischemia, mechanical compression, or neural stimulation within these organs.

According to the *Standardized Assessment and Diagnosis of Chest Pain—Chinese Expert Consensus* issued in 2014, chest pain is divided by severity into life-threatening and non-life-threatening, and by cause into cardiogenic and non-cardiogenic. Table 1-1 presents a classification of chest pain and its common causes. It is crucial to note that symptoms of chest pain may not be solely attributed to anomalies in chest organs; abdominal disorders and psychiatric diseases can also manifest as chest pain. A thorough medical history, particularly an accurate description of the characteristics of the chest pain episodes, is vital for analyzing and differentiating the cause. During consultations, a comprehensive understanding of each patient's chest pain, including location, nature, radiation, triggering and alleviating factors, duration, and accompanying symptoms, should be achieved, adhering to the OPQRST principle (Onset, Provocation / Palliation, Quality, Radiation, Severity / Scale, Timing).

1. Location of Chest Pain. Onset Pain originating from the chest wall, such as left intercostal neuralgia, costochondritis, and herpes zoster, often presents with precise localization. Conversely, pain stemming from intrathoracic visceral organ abnormalities is typically difficult to pinpoint accurately. Although angina pectoris commonly manifests as pain in the precordial region, its diffuse nature makes precise localization challenging, and it is frequently accompanied by radiating pain. If a patient can pinpoint the pain location with a finger and the area is relatively small ($<$3 cm), it is usually not indicative of angina pectoris. The typical location of angina pectoris is behind the sternum, radiating to the left shoulder, left upper limb, scapular area, teeth, and upper abdomen. In less common instances, it may radiate to the area below the navel, the back of the neck, or the occiput. If the pain is localized to the skin or superficial tissues and becomes evident upon palpation, this type of pain generally originates from the chest wall; lateral chest pain often occurs in acute pleuritis, acute pulmonary embolism, and intercostal myositis. It is important to note that liver or subphrenic abnormalities can also manifest as right-sided chest pain. Chest pain localized to the precordial area or below the left nipple is often caused by cardiac neurosis and other functional pains. Moreover, chest pain radiating to the back can be seen in aortic dissection and acute myocardial infarction. Pain radiating to the right shoulder often suggests liver, gallbladder, or subdiaphragmatic abnormalities.

Table 1-1 Classification and Common Causes of Chest Pain

Classification	Causes
Life-threatening Chest Pain	
Cardiac	Acute coronary syndromes, aortic dissection, cardiac tamponade, cardiac contusion (traumatic injury)
Non-cardiac	Acute pulmonary embolism, tension pneumothorax
Non-life-threatening Chest Pain	
Cardiac	Stable angina, acute pericarditis, myocarditis, hypertrophic obstructive cardiomyopathy, stress cardiomyopathy, aortic valve disease, mitral valve prolapse
Non-cardiac	
Chest wall diseases	Costochondritis, intercostal neuritis, herpes zoster, acute dermatitis, cellulitis, myositis, rib fractures, bone metastases or infiltration from tumors or hematologic malignancies

(Continued)

Classification	Causes
Respiratory diseases	Pulmonary hypertension, pleuritis, spontaneous pneumothorax, pneumonia, acute bronchitis, pleural tumor, lung cancer
Gastrointestinal diseases	Gastroesophageal reflux (reflux esophagitis), esophageal spasm, hiatal hernia, esophageal cancer, acute pancreatitis, cholecystitis, peptic ulcers and perforation
Psychiatric / Other depression	Anxiety, panic attacks, perimenopausal syndrome, etc. Hyperventilation syndrome, gout, cervical spondylosis, etc.

2. Characteristics of Chest Pain. When patients describe their chest discomfort as a squeezing sensation, a feeling of heaviness, or as if a stone were pressing down, the actual intensity of the pain may not be severe, but the discomfort is significant, often accompanied by a sense of impending doom. This is typically indicative of ischemic myocardial pain. Aortic dissection is commonly characterized by a tearing pain, continuous and severe, due to stimulation of the nerves in the arterial adventitia, considered a form of "true pain". Knife-like sharp pains are frequently associated with pericarditis, pleuritis, and pulmonary embolism. Pathologies within the lung affecting the parietal pleura often result in hidden or dull pain; esophagitis usually presents as a burning pain, intercostal neuralgia as episodic burning or stabbing pain, and muscular pain manifests as soreness.

3. Provoking and Alleviating Factors. Angina pectoris often occurs or intensifies with physical exertion or emotional stress, especially when walking against the wind, after a full meal, in a hurry, or uphill, and can be relieved by rest or the administration of nitroglycerin. Unstable angina may occur at rest. Generally, chest pain that occurs after physical activity does not fall under the category of angina pectoris. Esophageal pain commonly occurs or worsens upon swallowing food; hiatal hernia can also present as pain behind the sternum, which typically worsens in a lying position. Acute pleuritic chest pain is often associated with respiration and movement, can be induced or aggravated by deep breathing, and alleviated by holding one's breath. Musculoskeletal or neuralgic chest pain often worsens with touch or chest movement. Most functional pains are associated with emotional distress, and the chest pain caused by cardiac neurosis often decreases with physical activity.

4. Duration of Pain. The duration of chest pain is of significant diagnostic value, particularly in distinguishing between ischemic and non-ischemic chest pain. Pain that lasts only momentarily or does not exceed 1 minute is unlikely to be indicative of ischemic pain but may rather be attributed to musculoskeletal or neuralgic pain, esophageal or hiatal hernia discomfort, or functional pain. Conversely, chest pain lasting 2-10 minutes is often indicative of stable angina, while pain persisting for 10-30 minutes is commonly associated with unstable angina. Pain that lasts for over 30 minutes, and even several hours, can be indicative of acute myocardial infarction, pericarditis, aortic dissection, herpes zoster, or skeletal pain.

5. Accompanying Symptoms. Chest pain accompanied by pallor, profuse sweating, hypotension, or shock may be observed in acute myocardial infarction, aortic dissection, aortic sinus aneurysm rupture, or acute pulmonary embolism. Severe chest pain with nausea and

vomiting is often caused by acute myocardial infarction; chest pain accompanied by hemoptysis suggests respiratory system diseases such as pulmonary embolism, bronchogenic carcinoma, or bronchiectasis. When chest pain is accompanied by significant dyspnea, it often indicates severe involvement of cardiopulmonary function, as seen in acute myocardial infarction, pulmonary embolism, lobar pneumonia, spontaneous pneumothorax, mediastinal emphysema, among others. Chest pain with fever can be seen in conditions like lobar pneumonia, acute pleuritis, and acute pericarditis, which are acute infectious diseases. Pain in the chest accompanied by dysphagia suggests the presence of esophageal diseases. The occurrence of significant anxiety, depression, and similar symptoms in patients with chest pain should prompt consideration of functional chest pain, such as cardiac neurosis.

Ⅱ Physical Examination

Physical examination is not the primary method for differentiating chest pain, as many patients with chest pain often present with normal findings during the examination. However, specific conditions like herpes zoster and pneumothorax can provide important diagnostic clues through physical examination. The examination should be targeted and purposeful, focusing on the patient's history and individual clinical reasoning. Vital signs, including blood pressure, pulse, respiration, and body temperature, should be the initial focus. When suspecting aortic dissection, measuring blood pressure in all four limbs is essential, and the neck should be examined for any abnormal pulsations, as sometimes the dissection of the aortic arch can cause abnormal pulsations above the sternum. Jugular venous distension or pulsation can be observed in acute right heart failure caused by conditions such as cardiac tamponade and pulmonary embolism. The presence or absence of tracheal deviation is a simple sign for diagnosing spontaneous pneumothorax. Examination of the chest is naturally a focus, paying attention to any unilateral bulging of the thorax, local skin abnormalities, and the presence of tenderness or pain on palpation; changes in pulmonary breath sounds and the presence of pleural friction rubs should be noted. The size of the cardiac silhouette, the strength of heart sounds, murmurs, and pericardial friction rubs are components of the cardiac examination. Additionally, abdominal examination should not be overlooked, with attention to any abdominal tenderness, especially in the epigastric and gallbladder regions. In patients suspected of having pulmonary embolism, examination for swelling in the lower limbs and the presence of deep vein thrombosis is required.

Ⅲ Auxiliary Examinations for Chest Pain

Due to the diverse etiologies of chest pain, there is no specific "package" of auxiliary examinations. The choice of diagnostic tests is based on the patient's history and the results of the physical examination to confirm or exclude causes of chest pain.

1. Complete blood count is crucial for confirming the presence or absence of infection.

2. Electrocardiogram (ECG), troponins, and myocardial enzymes are essential for diagnosing angina and confirming acute myocardial infarction.

3. D-dimer has good supportive value in diagnosing acute pulmonary embolism, though its specificity is low. A negative result is significant for excluding pulmonary embolism.

4. Arterial blood gas analysis and chest X-ray are helpful in assessing the presence of respiratory failure and pneumothorax; large pulmonary embolisms can lead to refractory hypoxemia.

5. Fecal occult blood test aids in excluding atypical peptic ulcers.

6. Abdominal ultrasonography can assist in diagnosing liver, gallbladder, and subdiaphragmatic diseases.

7. Gastroscopy is beneficial for diagnosing gastroesophageal diseases.

8. Echocardiography has diagnostic value for chest pain caused by mitral valve prolapse, aortic valve diseases, hypertrophic cardiomyopathy, and pericardial diseases.

9. Multidetector computed tomography (MDCT) has a high detection rate for aortic dissection, pulmonary embolism, and coronary artery diseases.

10. Coronary angiography is the most valuable diagnostic procedure for patients with recurrent chest pain but normal ECG, suspected of having coronary artery disease.

11. Exercise stress testing or other cardiac stress tests are useful for determining if chest pain is related to myocardial ischemia, suitable for the differential diagnosis of patients with medium or low-risk chest pain.

Ⅳ Differential Diagnosis Approach for Chest Pain

The most commonly utilized method of thought is the focused exclusion approach, which entails gathering information through routine inquiry, physical examination, and necessary auxiliary tests to establish case characteristics and consider the most probable spectrum of serious diseases. Subsequently, diseases are excluded one by one from most to least serious until a definitive diagnosis is made. If the patient's characteristics are highly typical and the physician is well-acquainted with the disease, a clear diagnosis can be made through confirmatory testing and necessary exclusionary tests. In the emergency department setting, given the multitude of causes of chest pain covering diseases across various systems and the large volume of information, especially when chest pain symptoms lack specificity, a simplified diagnostic process or tool is often required for risk stratification of chest pain. The HEART scoring system is an essential tool for the risk stratification of all patients with chest pain in the emergency setting (Table 1-2). Patients with a HEART score of 0-3, indicating low-risk chest pain, are unlikely to experience acute cardiovascular events within the following three months and can, in principle, be discharged. Figure 1-1 presents a flowchart for the differential diagnosis of acute chest pain.

Table 1-2 HEART Score for Risk Stratification of Acute Chest Pain

HEART Score Criteria for Chest Pain Patients		Score
History	Highly suspicious	2
	Moderately suspicious	1
	Slightly suspicious	0
ECG	Typical ST segment elevation	2
	Nonspecific negative pole anomaly	1

(Continued)

HEART Score Criteria for Chest Pain Patients		Score
ECG	Bundle branch block	1
	Left ventricular hypertrophy	1
	Normal	0
Age (years)	>65	2
	45-65	1
	45	0
Risk Factors	≥3 risk factors, or history of coronary revascularization, myocardial infarction, stroke or peripheral arterial disease	2
	1-2	1
	None	0
Troponin	>2x the standard value	2
	1-2x the standard value	1
	Standard value	0

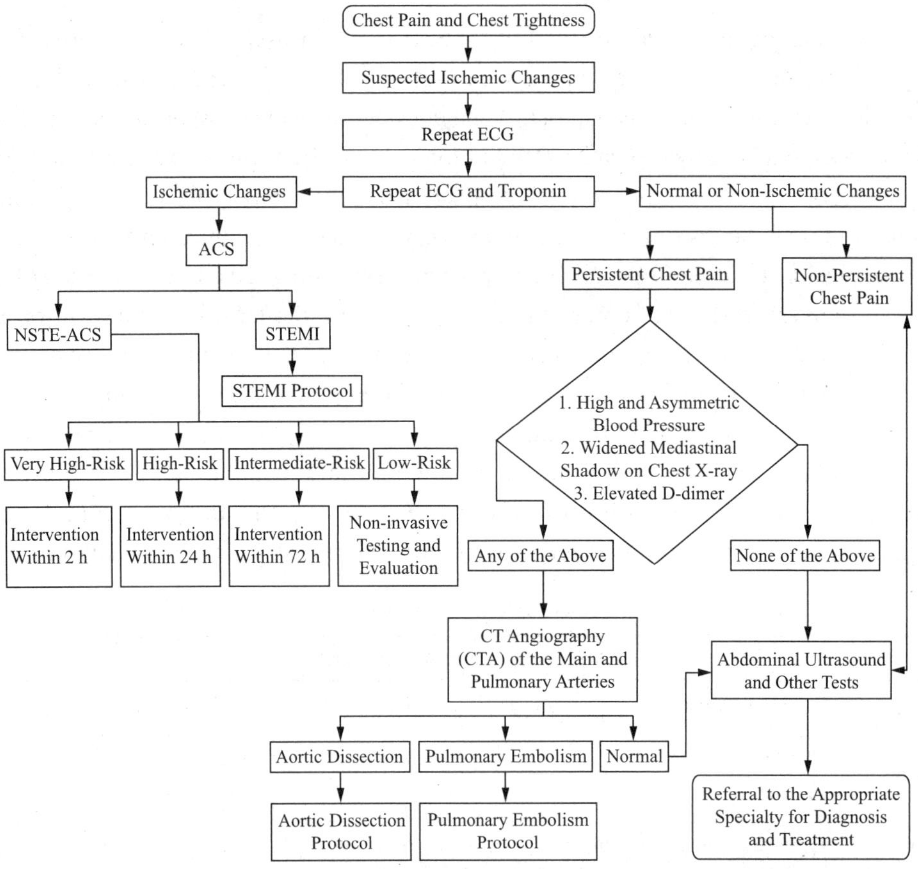

Figure 1-1 Differential Diagnosis Flowchart for Acute Chest Pain

V Considerations During Chest Pain Consultation

The most crucial step during the consultation of a patient with chest pain is to rapidly differentiate or conclusively exclude the presence of acute coronary syndrome (ACS) or other high-risk, life-threatening causes of chest pain, including aortic dissection, pulmonary embolism, etc. As long as the possibility of these conditions is considered during the consultation, they can be diagnosed without difficulty through specific tests.

1. Chest Pain and Chest Pain Centers. Acute Coronary Syndrome (ACS), which includes acute myocardial infarction and unstable angina, is the primary cause of cardiogenic chest pain. For patients with acute myocardial infarction, time is of the essence. Electrocardiographic ischemic changes during an ACS episode are of utmost diagnostic importance; thus, a 12-lead or 18-lead ECG should be obtained as soon as possible (within 10 minutes) after the onset of chest pain symptoms. In recent years, the construction of STEMI treatment chest pain centers in China has been rapidly advancing. Through the establishment of chest pain centers, most hospitals have gradually developed a regional collaborative treatment network for acute myocardial infarction, facilitating the seamless integration of pre-hospital and in-hospital care for patients with acute chest pain. Pre-hospital or external hospital ECGs can be transmitted to the consulting physician via WeChat or other information transmission methods, enabling the consulting physician to possess and apply rapid identification skills for acute myocardial infarction ECGs, thereby initiating the hospital's green channel for chest pain treatment and implementing rescue according to the hospital's chest pain treatment standard procedures. Cardiac biomarkers, particularly troponins, are highly sensitive and specific for myocardial necrosis. It is recommended that blood tests be conducted as early as possible for patients suspected of ACS, aiming to obtain results within 20 minutes to help achieve a timely definitive diagnosis and risk stratification for patients with ACS chest pain. For some patients with typical symptoms of angina but negative ECG and troponin results, the diagnosis of ACS should not be easily dismissed. Close observation and timely reevaluation of ECG and troponins according to guidelines are advised. Some patients may require urgent coronary angiography and interventional treatment.

2. The Chest Pain Triad: One-stop CTA for Differentiating ACS and Aortic Dissection. The chest pain triad refers to three life-threatening conditions manifested primarily by chest pain: Acute Coronary Syndrome (ACS), pulmonary embolism, and aortic dissection. Early diagnosis and differentiation of the chest pain triad are crucial for improving patient survival rates. Occasionally, ACS and some aortic dissection cases present with ST-T changes on the ECG and varying degrees of troponin elevation, as well as acute myocardial infarction due to the involvement of the aortic dissection extending to the coronary artery ostia, which complicates clinical diagnosis. Previously, the chest pain triad exhibited distinctive characteristics under different examination methods such as X-ray imaging, ultrasound, CT, and MRI, each with its limitations. Currently, with advancements in multidetector computed tomography (MDCT) scanner detector systems and improvements in both hardware and software, utilizing advanced scanning modes, optimized scanning conditions, and new iterative algorithms, it is possible to

image the pulmonary arteries, aorta, and coronary arteries in a single CT enhancement scan. This equipment, known for its non-invasive, rapid, and accurate features, is an essential tool for the differential diagnosis of patients with suspected high-risk chest pain during consultation.

3. Distinguishing Between Angina and Digestive System Diseases. Atypical angina can be easily confused with chest pain caused by gastrointestinal diseases. Sometimes, clinicians may attribute relief of symptoms to the administration of nitroglycerin, calcium channel blockers, or fast-acting heart-saving pills during a chest pain episode, presuming it to be an angina attack. In fact, these medications can also be effective for chest pain caused by certain esophageal conditions, such as esophageal spasms and gastroesophageal reflux disease. During consultation, in addition to repeatedly inquiring about the patient's history and closely monitoring for dynamic changes in the ECG during chest pain episodes, it may be necessary to perform coronary angiography for differentiation.

Approximately 10% of the patients with cardiogenic chest pain present with typical acute myocardial infarction ST-segment elevation on electrocardiogram and a certain degree of elevation in troponin levels. However, coronary angiography does not reveal significant coronary artery obstruction. Such cases of chest pain are attributed to myocardial infarction without coronary artery obstruction and require differentiation. Conditions such as stress cardiomyopathy and acute myocarditis fall into this category. These patients generally do not need coronary angiography, and even if performed, it may sometimes be challenging to differentiate. Magnetic resonance imaging plays a significant role in diagnosing myocardial infarction without coronary artery obstruction.

Ⅵ Consultation Process

1. The Initial Step Involves Assessing Whether the Patient's Vital Signs Are Stable. If there is a decline in oxygen saturation, rapid shallow breathing, hypotension, or malignant arrhythmias indicating instability of vital signs, immediate intervention with non-invasive or mechanical ventilation, vasoactive drugs to maintain blood pressure, electrical cardioversion or temporary pacing, and anti-arrhythmic therapy is warranted.

2. Identification of Preliminary Breakthroughs or Differentiating Points Based on Five Aspects of Chest Pain. Identification of preliminary breakthroughs or differentiation points for chest pain involves analysis across five dimensions: The location of onset, characteristics, provoking and alleviating factors, duration, and accompanying symptoms. ① Location of Onset: Whether the location is precisely identified; the size of the affected area; presence of tenderness, radiating pain. ② Characteristics: Presence of a squeezing or impending doom sensation; continuous tearing pain; knife-like pain; dull or sharp (stabbing) pain; burning pain, etc. ③ Provoking and Alleviating Factors: Whether the pain occurs or intensifies with physical exertion, emotional stress, cold exposure, facing wind, or after a full meal; whether rest or taking nitroglycerin relieves the pain; relation to swallowing; relation to changes in body position (or specific positions), breathing; occurrence under emotional distress or specific environments (noisy, enclosed spaces). ④ Duration: Less than 10 minutes, 10-30 minutes, more than 30 minutes. ⑤ Accompanying Symptoms: Whether accompanied by pallor, profuse sweating, hypotension, or shock; presence of hemoptysis or

significant respiratory distress; fever; dysphagia; notable anxiety, depression, etc.

3. Attention to Key Physical Examinations. Key physical examinations include measuring blood pressure in all limbs; observing the neck for any abnormal pulsations; assessing jugular vein for distension or pulsation; checking for tracheal deviation; examining the thorax for unilateral bulging, local skin abnormalities, and the presence of tenderness or pain on palpation; evaluating changes in pulmonary breath sounds and the presence of pleural friction rubs; assessing the size of the cardiac silhouette, the strength of heart sounds, murmurs, and pericardial friction rubs; checking for abdominal tenderness (especially in the epigastric and gallbladder regions); and looking for swelling in the lower limbs.

4. Rapid Auxiliary Examinations Required. Rapid auxiliary examinations that are often necessary include complete blood count, electrocardiogram (ECG), troponins (cardiac enzymes), chest X-ray, arterial blood gas analysis, D-dimer, B-type natriuretic peptide (BNP or NT-proBNP), fecal occult blood test, abdominal ultrasonography, gastroscopy (or gastroduodenal ultrasonography), echocardiography, multidetector computed tomography (MDCT), exercise stress test (or cardiac stress testing), and coronary angiography.

5. Etiological Treatment After Definitive Diagnosis. Following a definitive diagnosis, etiological treatment is tailored based on the underlying cause. For symptoms, ECG findings, and myocardial enzyme levels indicative of ACS, immediate dual antiplatelet therapy and statins are administered. Based on the onset time, vital signs (including hemodynamics), and type of ACS (ST-segment elevation or non-elevation), the timing for revascularization therapy is promptly assessed. For cases suggested by chest X-ray or CT to have pneumothorax or significant pleural effusion, a thoracic surgery consultation is requested for possible drainage. In patients with pulmonary embolism, risk stratification is evaluated, and consultations with respiratory and critical care are sought to assess the choice between thrombolytic or anticoagulant therapy. Aortic dissection patients require blood pressure and heart rate control; a cardiothoracic surgery consultation is advised to evaluate the need for endovascular aortic repair or surgical aortic replacement. Patients with heart failure are administered diuretics and vasodilators, and when necessary, inotropic agents or mechanical therapy. After symptom relief, comprehensive cardiac echocardiography and coronary angiography are performed to clarify the underlying cause. Patients with severe pneumonia receive antimicrobial and symptomatic treatment. Those with acute exacerbation of chronic lung disease are treated with bronchodilators or mechanical ventilation. Conditions such as ketoacidosis, uremia, intracranial lesions, poisoning, airway compression, or obstruction are managed with appropriate cause-specific and symptomatic treatments.

Section 2 Diagnosis and Early Treatment of Acute Coronary Syndrome

Acute Coronary Syndrome (ACS) refers to the acute ischemic syndrome of the heart caused by the formation of thrombus due to the rupture or erosion of unstable atherosclerotic plaques within the coronary arteries. It includes ST-segment Elevation Myocardial Infarction (STEMI),

Non-ST-segment Elevation Myocardial Infarction (NSTEMI), and Unstable Angina (UA), with NSTEMI and UA collectively termed as Non-ST-segment Elevation Acute Coronary Syndrome (NSTE-ACS). The incidence and mortality rates of ACS have shown a rapid upward trend in recent years. According to the *Report of China Cardiovascular Disease* (2015), the rural acute myocardial infarction mortality rate in China is 68.6 per 100,000, and the urban rate is 55.32 per 100,000. The early detection, diagnosis, and treatment of ACS are essential. Chest pain is a common complaint among hospitalized patients; in non-cardiology departments, the primary task in treating patients with chest pain is to identify its cause and provide early, standardized treatment.

I Diagnosis of ACS

The diagnostic criteria for Acute Coronary Syndrome (ACS) include symptoms, electrocardiographic changes, and cardiac enzyme levels. The timing of treatment is a crucial factor affecting the prognosis of ACS patients. Additionally, other serious conditions that may present with chest pain, such as aortic dissection and pulmonary embolism, also have strict requirements regarding the timing of treatment. Therefore, a rapid diagnosis should be made based on the following elements.

1. Important Medical History. Chest pain is often the initial symptom of Acute Coronary Syndrome (ACS), and the nature of the chest pain can preliminarily determine its cause. The following medical history in patients with chest pain should raise a high suspicion of ACS:

(1) A past medical history of coronary artery disease, cerebrovascular disease, or peripheral vascular disease.

(2) The presence of high-risk factors for coronary artery disease, such as advanced age, male gender, smoking history, hypertension, diabetes, and hyperli-pidemia.

2. Physical Examination. Physical examination plays a crucial role in assessing the severity of the condition and guiding the choice of subsequent treatments. Key aspects include:

(1) Hemodynamic stability, respiratory rate, and airway patency.

(2) Presence of heart failure symptoms, such as jugular venous distension, pulmonary rales, and the third heart sound gallop rhythm.

(3) Signs of systemic hypoperfusion, such as hypotension, cold and clammy limbs, pallor, and altered consciousness.

(4) If thrombolytic therapy is considered, a neurological examination is required to exclude contraindications.

3. Lead Electrocardiogram. Electrocardiography (ECG) is of paramount importance for the early diagnosis of Acute Coronary Syndrome (ACS), and all patients suspected of ACS should immediately undergo an ECG examination. The ECG characteristics of STEMI and NSTE-ACS are as follows:

(1) STEMI

1) New ST-segment elevation at the J point in at least two adjacent leads (≥0.25 mV in leads V2-V3 for men under 40, ≥0.2 mV for men aged 40 and above, or ≥0.15 mV for women; ≥0.1 mV in the other contiguous chest or limb leads).

2) With or without the presence of pathological Q waves, reduction in R-wave amplitude.

3) New onset of complete Left Bundle Branch Block (LBBB).

4) Hyperacute T-wave changes.

5) The diagnosis via ECG becomes challenging when a myocardial infarction occurs in a patient with pre-existing LBBB or when MI causes LBBB, necessitating careful correlation with clinical findings.

(2) NSTE-ACS

1) New onset of ST-segment depression≥0.05 mV in two or more contiguous leads.

2) T-wave inversion≥0.1 mV in two or more contiguous leads with a prominent *R* wave or an *R* / *S* ratio>1.

If the initial ECG does not yield diagnostic value, dynamic observation should be performed, with the ECG repeated every 20-30 minutes. If there is a dynamic evolution of ST-segment or T-waves, ACS should be highly suspected. ECG may produce false-negative results; studies suggest that conducting two consecutive ECG examinations in patients with ACS, 45% of the ECG results may not diagnose ACS, and 20% of patients may show no abnormalities. Early in myocardial infarction, peaked T-waves may be the sole ECG manifestation, warranting close attention.

4. Cardiac Enzymology Examination. Cardiac Troponin I / T (cTnI / T) is a biomarker with high specificity and sensitivity for the diagnosis of acute myocardial infarction. When detected through high-sensitivity methods, cTnI / T is referred to as high-sensitivity cardiac troponin (hs-cTn). The use of hs-cTn is recommended as the first choice. If the initial results are not elevated (negative), blood sampling should be repeated after 1-2 hours and compared with the initial results. An increase of more than 30% should prompt consideration of an acute myocardial injury diagnosis. If the initial two tests still do not provide a clear diagnosis and clinical indicators suggest the possibility of ACS, a repeat examination should be conducted after 3-6 hours. Additional considerations for cardiac enzymology examination include:

(1) The absence of elevated cardiac enzyme markers at the time of symptom onset does not exclude the diagnosis of acute myocardial infarction; dynamic observation every 20-30 minutes is advised.

(2) In most patients with acute myocardial infarction, hs-cTn can show a meaningful increase within 2-3 hours of symptom onset.

(3) If there is no significant increase in hs-cTn 6 hours after symptom onset, acute myocardial infarction can be largely excluded; however, if ACS is highly suspected, cardiac enzyme markers should be retested 12 hours after symptom onset.

5. Imaging Examination. Imaging examinations are helpful in assessing the patient's condition and excluding other related diseases, including:

(1) Echocardiography is recommended to assess cardiac structure, motion, and function, which can also have diagnostic or differential diagnostic significance.

(2) For patients without recurrent chest pain, normal ECG results, and normal cardiac enzyme levels but still suspected of ACS, a non-invasive stress test to induce ischemic episodes is suggested, with further invasive examination considered based on the results.

(3) If cardiac enzyme and / / or ECG results are normal but ACS is still suspected, multidetector computed tomography (MDCT) coronary angiography is recommended.

Ⅱ Risk Assessment in Patients with ACS

STEMI: High-risk factors include advanced age, hypotension, tachycardia, heart failure, anterior wall myocardial infarction, among others. The TIMI score provides an objective standard for risk stratification in STEMI, with high-risk patients recommended for early reperfusion therapy.

NSTE-ACS: The risk of ischemic events in patients with NSTE-ACS significantly influences their treatment strategy. Therefore, early risk stratification of NSTE-ACS patients is crucial for estimating ischemic risk and deciding on aggressive reperfusion therapy. In recent years, multiple clinical studies have assessed the ischemic risk in NSTE-ACS, resulting in various risk prediction models, including the GRACE score, TIMI score, PURSUIT score, etc., among which the GRACE score has been proven to have superior predictive ability. Risk factors in the GRACE score include age, heart rate, systolic blood pressure, Killip class, serum creatinine, presence of ST-segment depression, elevation in cTn, and cardiac arrest. If Killip classification and serum creatinine are not available, the use of diuretics and the presence of renal insufficiency can be used as substitutes.

For patients with a GRACE score>140 combined with multiple other high-risk factors, an early (<24 hours) invasive assessment strategy is recommended. For intermediate-risk patients (GRACE score 109-140), non-invasive myocardial ischemia assessment should be conducted, and the decision for invasive reperfusion therapy should be based on clinical symptoms, lesion characteristics, and bleeding risk. Routine invasive assessment is not advocated for low-risk patients.

Ⅲ Early Treatment of Patients with ACS

For any patient suspected of having Acute Coronary Syndrome (ACS), early initiation of treatment is imperative. During the diagnostic process, it is essential to maintain airway patency, administer oxygen, establish venous access, connect to bedside monitoring equipment, prepare resuscitation devices, and administer 300 mg of aspirin and sublingual nitroglycerin. Other therapeutic measures include the following.

1. Symptom Relief Treatment

(1) Oxygen Therapy: Patients with oxygen saturation below 90%, respiratory distress, or other high-risk factors for hypoxemia should receive oxygen therapy. Currently, there is no evidence to support the administration of oxygen to patients with normal blood oxygen levels, as excessive oxygen could potentially increase vasoconstriction. Studies indicate that oxygen therapy for ACS patients does not affect long-term prognosis, though some research shows that hyperbaric oxygen therapy can benefit prognosis.

(2) Nitroglycerin: Sublingual administration of nitroglycerin can improve symptoms of angina. If continuous angina symptoms persist after taking 3 tablets, intravenous use may be considered. However, in patients with right ventricular myocardial infarction, aortic stenosis, or

hypotension, nitroglycerin may cause severe hemodynamic disturbances and should be used with caution or avoided.

(3) Morphine: Can rapidly relieve symptoms of angina. However, a large retrospective study has shown that morphine increases the mortality rate in patients with acute myocardial infarction. Other studies have indicated that morphine might interact with P2Y12 receptor inhibitors, reducing their antiplatelet effects. Therefore, if patients can tolerate the pain, the use of morphine should be minimized or kept at the lowest dose possible.

(4) Beta-blockers: Have been proven to significantly improve the prognosis of patients with ACS and effectively relieve symptoms of chest pain. If there are no contraindications, intravenous administration of beta-blockers within 24 hours of symptom onset is particularly necessary for patients with continuous chest pain, hypertension, and tachycardia not caused by heart failure. In patients with hemodynamic instability, the use of beta-blockers should be appropriately delayed until hemodynamic stability is achieved.

2. Antithrombotic Therapy

(1) Antiplatelet Drugs: Dual antiplatelet therapy should be initiated imme-diately after ACS is diagnosed unless there are absolute contraindications. Ticagrelor has been proven to significantly reduce mortality in ACS patients compared to clopidogrel; therefore, a loading dose of aspirin (300 mg) and ticagrelor (180 mg) is recommended.

(2) Anticoagulants: The benefit of non-oral anticoagulants in both STEMI and NSTE-ACS has been established, and they should be used early after a definitive diagnosis. However, the choice of specific anticoagulant drugs lacks clear guidance and should be based on the patient's specific circumstances.

3. Statin Therapy. All patients diagnosed with Acute Coronary Syndrome (ACS) should immediately start on a loading dose of statin therapy (Atorvastatin 40-80 mg or Rosuvastatin 20 mg) without consideration of baseline cholesterol and low-density lipoprotein levels.

4. Other Treatments

(1) Maintaining Electrolyte Balance: Studies indicate that patients with blood potassium levels between 3.5 and 4.5 mmol / L have the best long-term prognosis. Blood magnesium levels should be maintained above 2 mmol / L.

(2) Discontinuation of Non-Steroidal Anti-Inflammatory Drugs (NSAIDs) Other Than Aspirin: Non-selective NSAIDs have been shown to increase the incidence of cardiovascular events. Therefore, upon definitive diagnosis, NSAIDs other than aspirin should be discontinued.

(3) Glucose-Insulin-Potassium (GIK) Infusion: Although previous studies suggested that metabolic support for ischemic myocardium could improve myocardial injury, recent large clinical trials have not proven that glucose-insulin-potassium can improve the prognosis for patients with ACS. Therefore, its use is not recommended.

Ⅳ Summary

Chest pain can be caused by various life-threatening conditions, including Acute Coronary Syndrome (ACS), aortic dissection, pulmonary embolism, pneumothorax, etc. Primary care physicians should exclude causes other than ACS before proceeding with treatment.

1. If a patient is suspected of having ACS, the primary care physician should follow these steps for assessment and preliminary treatment:

(1) Evaluate respiratory and circulatory functions.

(2) Collect medical history and perform a physical examination.

(3) Conduct a 12-lead ECG and cardiac enzyme tests.

(4) Connect to cardiac monitoring and prepare resuscitation equipment.

(5) Establish venous access.

(6) Administer oral aspirin and nitroglycerin.

2. If initial ECG and cardiac enzyme tests do not show positive results, dynamic observation should be conducted.

3. Upon diagnosis, immediate administration of a loading dose of aspirin, ticagrelor, and atorvastatin is recommended, and beta-blockers should be used as soon as hemodynamic stability is achieved.

V Consultation Process

1. The primary assessment should focus on the stability of the patient's vital signs. If abnormalities are present, such as a decrease in blood oxygen levels, rapid and shallow breathing, a drop in blood pressure, or malignant arrhythmias, immediate emergency treatment should be provided. This includes non-invasive or mechanical ventilation, vasopressor agents to maintain blood pressure, electrical cardioversion or temporary pacing, and anti-arrhythmic therapy.

2. Gathering critical medical history is essential, focusing on the location, nature, triggers, and alleviation methods of chest pain, its duration, and accompanying symptoms. These elements serve as preliminary indicators for differential diagnosis, aiming to exclude conditions other than ACS (with particular emphasis on ruling out aortic dissection, pulmonary embolism, pneumothorax, acute abdomen, etc.): ①Location: Is the location precise? What is the extent of the area affected? Are there tenderness and radiating pain? ②Nature: Is there a sensation of squeezing or impending doom? Is it a continuous, tearing pain? Is it a sharp pain like being cut, a dull pain, or a stabbing pain? Is there a burning sensation? ③Triggers and Alleviation Methods: Does it occur with exertion, emotional stress, cold exposure, after a full meal, and can it be relieved by rest or sublingual nitroglycerin? Is it related to swallowing? Is it related to changes in posture (or specific positions), breathing, or does it occur in emotional states or specific environments (noisy, confined spaces)? ④Duration: Is it less than 10 minutes, 10 to 30 minutes, or more than 30 minutes? ⑤Accompanying Symptoms: Is it accompanied by pallor, sweating, a drop in blood pressure, or shock? Is there expectoration of blood or significant respiratory difficulty? Is there a fever? Is there difficulty swallowing? Are there significant symptoms of anxiety or depression?

3. Attention to Essential and Necessary Physical Examinations. To exclude non-cardiac causes of acute chest pain, important and necessary physical examinations should be conducted, including:

Blood pressure in the limbs: Noting any discrepancies.

Neck: Observing for any abnormal pulsations.

Jugular veins: Checking for distention or engorgement.

Trachea: Assessing for any deviation.

Thorax: Looking for unilateral swelling, any localized skin abnormalities, or tenderness and palpation pain.

Lungs: Evaluating for changes in respiratory sounds or the presence of pleural friction rub.

Cardiac examination: Assessing heart size, heart sounds intensity, murmurs, and pericardial friction rub.

Abdomen: Checking for tenderness, especially in the subxiphoid and gallbladder areas.

Lower limbs: Observing for any swelling.

These examinations aid in distinguishing between cardiac and non-cardiac causes of chest pain.

4. Rapid Diagnostic Tests Required. Rapid diagnostic tests that need to be conducted include complete blood count (CBC), electrocardiogram (ECG), cardiac troponins (cardiac enzymes), chest radiography, blood gas analysis, D-dimer, BNP (or NT-proBNP), fecal occult blood test, abdominal ultrasound, gastroscopy (with gastric-duodenal ultrasonography preferred before excluding Acute Coronary Syndrome), echocardiography, multidetector computed tomography (MDCT), coronary angiography, among others.

5. Treatment after Excluding Non-Cardiac Causes of Acute Chest Pain and Confirming Diagnosis of ACS. Initial Management: Informing the patient about the seriousness of their condition, cardiac monitoring, oxygen therapy, and establishing venous access.

Assessment: Evaluating whether the patient's current vital signs and hemo-dynamics are stable.

Pharmacotherapy: Anticoagulation (low molecular weight heparin, unless thrombolysis or emergency interventional treatment is needed), dual antiplatelet therapy (aspirin + clopidogrel or ticagrelor, initially requiring oral loading doses), statins (atorvastatin or rosuvastatin), prognosis-improving medications [beta-blockers, angiotensin-converting enzyme inhibitors (ACEI) or angiotensin receptor blockers (ARB)], and medications for symptom relief (morphine, nitrates).

Revascularization: Evaluating indications for thrombolysis, emergency interventional surgery, or scheduled interventional surgery.

Section 3 The Management of ST-Segment Elevation Myocardial Infarction

I Definition

Myocardial infarction (MI) refers to ischemic necrosis of the myocardium, resulting from a rapid decrease or cessation of coronary artery blood supply on a basis of coronary artery disease, causing severe and sustained acute ischemia leading to myocardial death. Acute myocardial infarction (AMI) clinically manifests as persistent severe retrosternal pain, fever, elevated white blood cell counts and serum myocardial necrosis markers, and progressive changes on the electrocardiogram; it can lead to arrhythmias, shock, or heart failure, representing a severe type of Acute Coronary Syndrome (ACS).

Ⅱ Classification

Type 1: Spontaneous myocardial infarction;

Type 2: Myocardial infarction secondary to an imbalance between myocardial oxygen supply and demand;

Type 3: Cardiac sudden death;

Type 4a: Myocardial infarction related to percutaneous coronary intervention (PCI);

Type 4b: Myocardial infarction caused by stent thrombosis;

Type 5: Myocardial infarction associated with coronary artery bypass grafting (CABG).

This section primarily discusses the diagnosis and treatment of Type 1 myocardial infarction (i.e., ischemia-related spontaneous acute ST-segment elevation myocardial infarction).

Ⅲ Diagnosis

1. Clinical Presentation

(1) Retrosternal or precordial squeezing pain, not relieved by rest or sublingual nitroglycerin, often accompanied by restlessness, sweating, and a sense of impending doom.

(2) A minority of patients present with no pain, initially manifesting as shock or acute heart failure.

(3) Some patients experience pain in the upper abdomen, potentially misdiagnosed as gastric perforation, acute pancreatitis, or other acute abdominal conditions.

(4) A few patients present with neck, lower jaw, pharyngeal, and dental pain, which can lead to misdiagnosis.

(5) Confusion, particularly in elderly patients.

(6) General symptoms, indescribable discomfort, and fever.

(7) Gastrointestinal symptoms such as nausea, vomiting, and bloating, more common in patients with inferior wall myocardial infarction.

(8) Arrhythmias, with ventricular arrhythmias more likely in anterior wall infarctions and bradycardia or atrioventricular block more common in inferior wall infarctions.

(9) Heart failure, mainly acute left heart failure.

(10) Hypotension, and shock.

2. Laboratory Tests

(1) Blood indicators: ① Increased creatine kinase-MB (CK-MB); ② Elevated troponins.

(2) ECG findings: ① ST-segment elevation in anterior leads (V_1-V_6); ② Inferior leads (Ⅱ, Ⅲ, aVF); ③ lateral leads (I, aVL, V_4-V_6); ④ Right ventricular leads (V_3R-V_6R); ⑤ New-onset left bundle branch block, and some non-typical ECG patterns.

(3) Imaging / Special Examinations: ①Echocardiography showing segmental wall motion abnormalities or absence; ②Coronary angiography (CT, angiography, CTA) revealing coronary artery occlusion.

3. Diagnosis and Differential Diagnosis

(1) 2012 Global Consensus for Diagnosis: In the presence of clinical conditions consistent with acute myocardial ischemia, detection of elevated and / or decreased cardiac biomarker values [preferably cardiac troponin (cTc)] at least once above the 99 th percentile of the upper reference limit (URL) and at least one of the following: ① New or presumed new significant ST-T changes or new left bundle branch block; ② Pathological Q waves on ECG; ③ Evidence of new loss of viable myocardium or new regional wall motion abnormality on imaging.

(2) Differential Diagnosis: ① Aortic dissection; ② Acute pericarditis; ③ Acute pulmonary embolism; ④ Pneumothorax; ⑤ Gastrointestinal diseases (such as reflux esophagitis); ⑥ Others such as acute cholecystitis, herpes zoster.

Ⅳ Principles of Treatment

1. The emergency management process for STEMI patients is outlined in Figure 1-2. Early, rapid, and complete reperfusion of the infarct-related artery is crucial for improving the prognosis of STEMI patients.

(1) Reducing the time from symptom onset to the arrival of the patient at the hospital or emergency personnel at the scene.

(2) Minimizing the time from First Medical Contact (FMC) to the reperfusion of the infarct-related artery.

(3) Bypassing the emergency room and coronary care unit whenever possible.

(4) For hospitals without direct PCI capabilities, transferring the patient to a facility where PCI is feasible to perform direct PCI (Class Ⅰ, Level B).

(5) If possible, qualified physicians could be requested to perform direct PCI at hospitals unable to independently conduct PCI (Class Ⅱb, Level B).

Class Ⅰ: Procedures or treatments that have been proven and / or universally recognized as beneficial, useful, and effective.

Class Ⅱ: Procedures or treatments for which there is conflicting evidence or divergent opinions on utility and / or effectiveness.

Class Ⅱa: The evidence / opinion leans towards being useful and / or effective; it is reasonable to perform these procedures or treatments.

Class Ⅱb: The evidence / opinion is not sufficiently demonstrated to be useful and / or effective; consideration may be given to their use.

Class Ⅲ: Procedures or treatments that have been proven and / or universally recognized as not useful and / or ineffective and may be harmful in some cases; not recommended.

2. Antithrombotic Therapy. The primary cause of STEMI is thrombotic occlusion due to plaque rupture within the coronary artery. Therefore, antithrombotic therapy (including antiplatelet and anticoagulant therapy) is essential (Class Ⅰ, Level A).

(1) Antiplatelet Therapy: Taking a loading dose of aspirin 300 mg, followed by a maintenance dose of 100 mg daily (Class Ⅰ, Level A). All STEMI patients should add one P2Y12 receptor antagonist to low-dose aspirin for at least 12 months, unless contraindications exist (e.g., high bleeding risk) (Class Ⅰ, Level A). Ticagrelor 180 mg can be used, followed by 90 mg twice

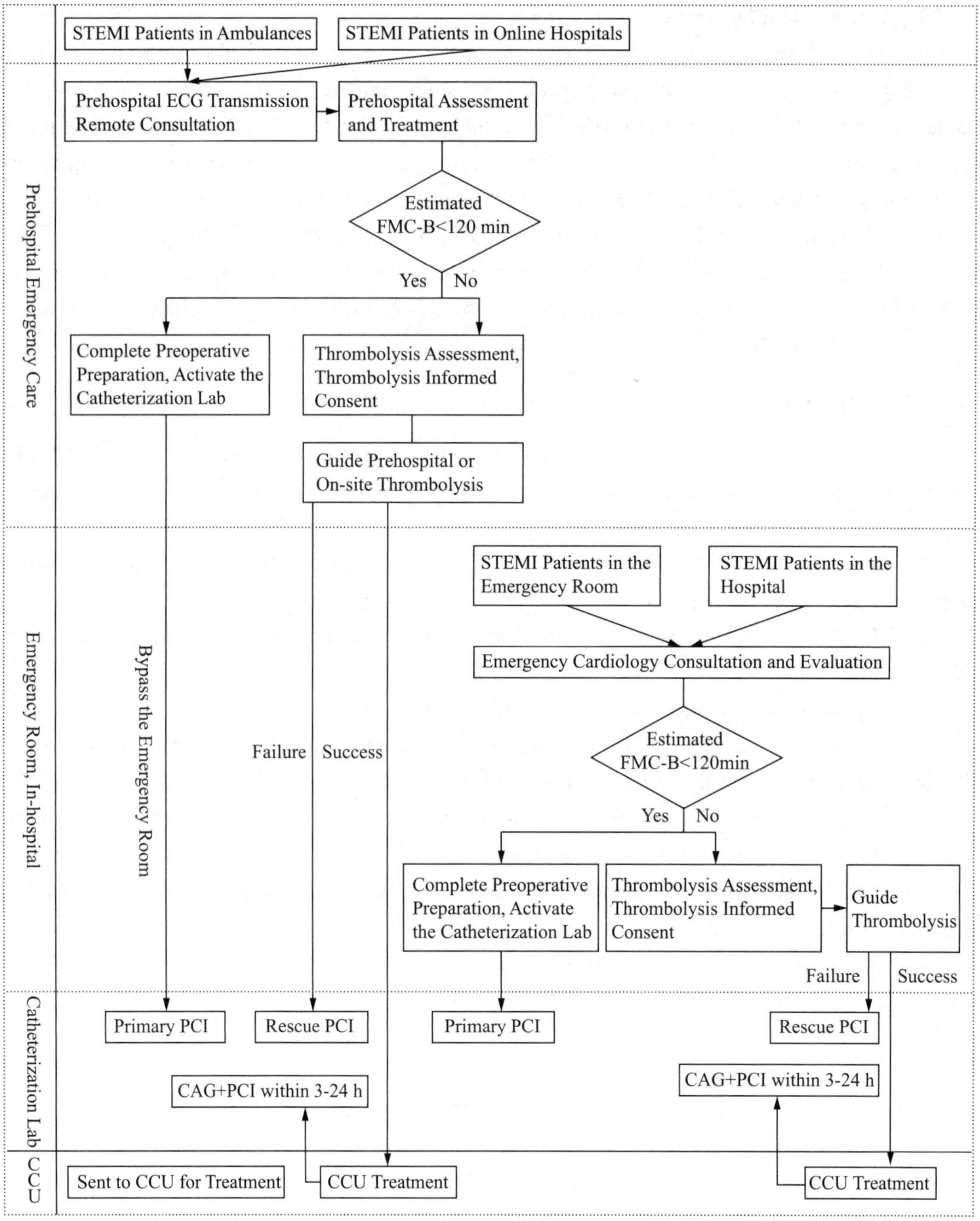

Figure 1-2 Differential Diagnosis Flowchart for Acute Chest Pain

daily for at least 12 months (Class Ⅰ, Level B); if ticagrelor is not available or contraindicated, clopidogrel 600 mg loading dose, followed by 75 mg once daily for at least 12 months (Class Ⅰ, Level B).

(2) Heparin (70-100 U / kg) maintaining an activated clotting time (ACT) of 250-300 seconds.

(3) Bivalirudin 0.75 mg / kg followed by 1.75 mg / (kg·h) Ⅳ infusion, mainta-ined for 3-4 hours post-PCI (Class Ⅰ, Level A).

3. Thrombolytic Therapy. For hospitals without the capacity for Percut-aneous Coronary Intervention (PCI), intravenous thrombolysis remains a preferable option for eligible STEMI patients, with pre-hospital thrombolysis being superior to in-hospital. For patients within 3 hours of symptom onset, the immediate effectiveness of thrombolytic therapy is fundamentally similar to direct PCI; conditions permitting, thrombolysis can commence in the ambulance (Class Ⅱa, Level A).

(1) Indications and Contraindications for Thrombolytic Therapy

1) Within 12 hours of onset, if the expected delay from First Medical Contact (FMC) to PCI exceeds 120 minutes, without contraindications for thrombolysis (Class Ⅰ, Level A).

2) For patients presenting within 12-24 hours, still experiencing progressive ischemic chest pain and at least two contiguous chest or limb leads showing ST-segment elevation $>$0.1 mV, or in cases of hemodynamic instability, if direct PCI is not an option, thrombolysis is considered reasonable (Class Ⅱa, Level C).

3) Thrombolytic therapy is not recommended prior to a planned direct PCI (Class Ⅲ, Level A).

4) Patients with ST-segment depression (excluding true posterior myocardial infarction or concurrent ST-segment elevation in lead aVR) should not undergo thrombolytic therapy (Class Ⅲ, Level B).

5) Thrombolytic therapy should not be administered to STEMI patients presenting more than 12 hours after symptom onset with symptoms that have resolved or disappeared (Class Ⅲ, Level C).

(2) Absolute Contraindications for Thrombolytic Therapy

1) Previous cerebral hemorrhage or stroke of unknown origin.

2) Known structural cerebral vascular lesion.

3) Intracranial neoplasm.

4) Ischemic stroke within the past 3 months, excluding acute ischemic stroke within 4.5 hours.

5) Suspected aortic dissection.

6) Active bleeding or bleeding diathesis, excluding menstruation.

7) Significant closed-head or facial trauma within the past 3 months.

8) Intracranial or spinal surgery within the last 2 months.

9) Severe uncontrolled hypertension (systolic $>$180 mmHg and / or diastolic $>$110 mmHg) unresponsive to emergency treatment.

(3) Relative Contraindications for Thrombolytic Therapy

1) Age $\geq$75 years.

2) Ischemic stroke more than 3 months prior.

3) Recent trauma or prolonged CPR $>$10 minutes within 3 weeks.

4) Recent major surgery within 3 weeks.

5) Recent internal bleeding within 4 weeks.

6) Recent (within 2 weeks) non-compressible vascular punctures.

7) Pregnancy.

8) Known intracranial pathology not covered by absolute contraindications.

9) Active peptic ulcer disease.

10) Current anticoagulant use, where higher international normalized ratio (INR) levels indicate greater bleeding risk.

(4) Selection of Thrombolytic Agents

1) Alteplase: ①Full-dose 90-minute accelerated infusion protocol, beginning with a 15 mg Ⅳ bolus, followed by 0.75 mg / kg over 30 minutes (not to exceed 50 mg), then 0.5 mg / kg over 60 minutes (not to exceed 35 mg). ②Half-dose regimen, 50 mg dissolved in 50 mL of diluent, initially an 8 mg Ⅳ push, with the remaining 42 mg infused over 90 minutes.

2) Streptokinase: 1.5 million units dissolved in 100 mL saline, Ⅳ infused over 30 minutes. Post-thrombolysis, subcutaneous administration of standard heparin 7,500 U or low-molecular-weight heparin for 3-5 days is recommended.

(5) Indirect Indicators of Thrombolytic Revascularization

1) At least a 50% reduction in ST-segment elevation on the ECG within 60-90 minutes.

2) cTn peak levels advance to within 12 hours of onset, CK-MB enzyme peak within 14 hours.

3) Significant alleviation of chest pain symptoms within 2 hours.

4) Reperfusion arrhythmias occurring within 2-3 hours.

Among these, ECG changes and early peaking of myocardial injury markers are the most significant.

(6) Direct Indicators of Thrombolytic Revascularization

4. Interventional Treatment. Direct Percutaneous Coronary Intervention (PCI) is conducted based on patient-specific conditions or in consultation with the cardiology department.

(1) Class Ⅰ Recommendations

1) Patients within 12 hours of onset (including true posterior myocardial infarction) (Evidence Level A).

2) Patients with cardiogenic shock or heart failure, even if the onset is beyond 12 hours (Evidence Level B).

3) Routine stent implantation (Evidence Level A).

4) Radial artery access is preferred for general patients (Evidence Level B), while femoral artery access may be considered for critically ill patients.

(2) Class Ⅱa Recommendations

1) Patients presenting 12-24 hours with clinical and / or electrocardiographic evidence of ongoing ischemia (Evidence Level B).

2) Direct PCI should be limited to the infarct-related artery unless there is ongoing ischemia after PCI or cardiogenic shock (Evidence Level B).

3) Thrombus aspiration is suggested in cases of significant intracoronary thrombus burden (Evidence Level B).

4) Drug-eluting stents (DES) are preferred for direct PCI (Evidence Level A).

(3) Class Ⅲ Recommendations

1) Emergency PCI should not be performed on non-infarct-related vessels in patients without

hemodynamic instability (Evidence Level C).

2) Patients presenting more than 24 hours after onset without myocardial ischemia, stable hemodynamics, and electrical stability are not suitable for direct PCI (Evidence Level C).

3) Routine use of intra-aortic balloon pump (IABP) is not recommended (Evidence Level A).

4) Routine use of distal protection devices is not advocated (Evidence Level C).

(4) Post-Thrombolysis PCI

Patients successfully treated with thrombolysis should be transported as soon as possible to a facility capable of PCI, to undergo coronary angiography and revascularization treatment within 3-24 hours (Class IIa, Level B); early rescue PCI is advised for thrombolysis failures (Class IIa, Level B).

Emergency PCI is not recommended for patients without symptoms of myocardial ischemia or stable hemodynamics after thrombolysis (Class III, Level C).

(5) PCI for STEMI Patients not Undergoing Early Reperfusion Therapy (Symptom Onset> 24 h)

PCI is recommended for lesions suitable for PCI in patients with recurrent myocardial infarction, spontaneous or induced myocardial ischemia, cardiogenic shock, or hemodynamic instability (Class I, Level B).

This translation adheres to the scientific and objective tone typical of research papers, ensuring logical coherence, professional vocabulary accuracy, and clear, concise expression that aligns with native English scientific writing standards.

5. Additional Pharmacological Treatments

(1) Beta-Blockers

1) STEMI patients without contraindications should commence oral beta-blockers within 24 hours post-onset (Class I, Level B).

2) Patients with early contraindications to beta-blockers should be reassessed and commenced on beta-blockers as soon as possible after 24 hours (Class I, Level C).

3) For STEMI patients presenting with sustained atrial fibrillation or flutter accompanied by angina but stable hemodynamics, beta-blockers can be employed (Class I, Level C).

4) In cases of STEMI with refractory polymorphic ventricular tachycardia and signs of sympathetic storm, intravenous beta-blockers are advised (Class I, Level B).

(2) Nitrates

1) Intravenous nitrate infusion is indicated for relief of ischemic chest pain, control of hypertension, or alleviation of pulmonary edema (Class I, Level B).

2) Nitrates should not be used in STEMI patients suspected of right ventricular myocardial infarction (Class III, Level C).

3) Intravenous nitroglycerin should be initiated at a low dosage (5-10 μg / min).

(3) Calcium Channel Blockers

1) Short-acting dihydropyridine calcium channel blockers are not recommended for STEMI patients.

2) Non-dihydropyridine calcium channel blockers may be utilized if beta-blockers are ineffective or contraindicated (Class IIa, Level C).

(4) ACE Inhibitors and ARBs

1) All STEMI patients without contraindications should be placed on long-term ACE inhibitor therapy (Class Ⅰ, Level A).

2) ARBs should be substituted in patients who cannot tolerate ACE inhibitors (Class Ⅰ, Level B).

(5) Statins

Statin therapy should be initiated early in all STEMI patients without contraindications, regardless of cholesterol levels (Class Ⅰ, Level A).

This translation adheres to the logical and coherent structure required in scien-tific publications, with attention to accuracy in the use of professional terminology and maintaining readability and precision in content.

V Common Questions in Consultation

1. Right Ventricular Myocardial Infarction

(1) Right ventricular myocardial infarction often occurs concurrently with inferior wall myocardial infarction but can also present independently.

(2) An ST-segment elevation≥0.1 mV in right precordial leads, especially V4R, is highly indicative of right ventricular myocardial infarction.

(3) Right precordial leads should be recorded for all patients with inferior wall STEMI.

(4) Echocardiographic examination may aid in diagnosis.

(5) Right ventricular myocardial infarction commonly results in hypotension but seldom leads to cardiogenic shock.

(6) The prevention and treatment principle involves maintaining effective right ventricular preload and avoiding the use of diuretics and vasodilators.

2. Heart Failure

(1) Administer oxygen, continuously monitor oxygen saturation and conduct periodic blood gas analysis and electrocardiographic monitoring. Chest X-ray can estimate pulmonary congestion. Echocardiography not only assists in diagnosis but also in understanding the extent of myocardial damage and potential mechanical complications such as mitral valve regurgitation or ventricular septal perforation.

(2) For mild heart failure (Killip class Ⅱ), diuretic therapy usually elicits a rapid response. For instance, furosemide 20-40 mg slow Ⅳ injection, repeated once if necessary after 1-4 hours. Ⅳ nitrate drugs can be applied. ACE inhibitors should be initiated within 24 hours for patients without hypotension, hypovolemia, or significant renal failure, switching to ARBs if intolerant.

(3) Severe heart failure (Killip class Ⅲ) or acute pulmonary edema patients should promptly utilize mechanical ventilation support. Apply diuretics judiciously.

(4) STEMI patients should not be administered digitalis within 24 hours of onset to avoid the risk of ventricular arrhythmias. Amiodarone may be used in cases of rapid atrial fibrillation with chest pain but stable hemodynamics.

3. Cardiogenic Shock

(1) Clinically presents as a low perfusion state including cold extremities, reduced urine

output, and / or altered mental status.

(2) Inotropic agents can stabilize the patient's hemodynamics. Severe hypotension may require intravenous infusion of dopamine at a dose of 5-15 μg / (kg·min), possibly in conjunction with dobutamine [3-10 μg / (kg·min)].

(3) Pre-revascularization placement of an intra-aortic balloon pump (IABP) can stabilize hemodynamic status, though its long-term mortality impact remains debated.

4. Arrhythmias

(1) Ventricular Arrhythmias: Immediate unsynchronized direct current defibrillation for ventricular fibrillation or persistent polymorphic ventricular tachycardia. Early synchronized cardioversion for stable monomorphic ventricular tachycardia. Asymptomatic ventricular premature beats, non-sustained ventricular tachycardia (duration $<$30 s), and accelerated idioventricular rhythm do not necessitate prophylactic anti-arrhythmic drug use.

(2) Atrial Fibrillation: STEMI can induce or exacerbate heart failure. Thus, rapid control of ventricular rate or restoration of sinus rhythm is imperative. Use of Class Ic anti-arrhythmic drugs to convert atrial fibrillation is contraindicated.

(3) Atrioventricular Block: Occurs in about 7% of STEMI patients, with sustained bundle branch block in 5.3%. Immediate temporary pacing is recom-mended for any hemodynamically significant AV block during acute STEMI.

5. Mechanical Complications

(1) Left Ventricular Free Wall Rupture: Accounts for 15% of in-hospital mortality following myocardial infarction. Echocardiography can detect this complication.

(2) Ventricular Septal Rupture: Surgical repair or interventional closure offers a survival opportunity for patients with ventricular septal rupture accompanied by cardiogenic shock. Percutaneous catheter septal defect closure may be considered for selected patients.

(3) Papillary Muscle Dysfunction or Rupture: Requires specific attention for diagnosis and treatment.

Ⅵ Consultation Process

1. Diagnosis of Acute ST-Elevation Myocardial Infarction (Type 1 MI, i.e., spontaneous myocardial infarction related to ischemia)

(1) Clinical Presentation: Typical symptoms include retrosternal or precordial crushing chest pain that is not relieved by rest or nitroglycerin administration, often accompanied by restlessness, sweating, and a sense of impending doom. Atypical symptoms may include abdominal discomfort, toothache, or hand numbness. Another subset of patients may present with generalized symptoms or an altered mental status. In severe cases, the initial or subsequent symptoms may be arrhythmias, heart failure, or shock.

(2) Auxiliary Examinations

1) Blood Markers (Necessary Condition): Elevated CK-MB or cardiac troponin levels.

2) Electrocardiogram (Necessary Condition): ST-segment elevation in the anterior leads (V1-V6); ST-segment elevation in the inferior leads (Ⅱ, Ⅲ, aVF); ST-segment elevation in the lateral leads (Ⅰ, aVL, V4-V6); ST-segment elevation in the right ventricular leads (V3R-V6R);

new left bundle branch block; some atypical ECG findings.

3) Imaging / Special Examinations (Not Necessary): Echocardiography showing segmental wall motion abnormalities or akinesis; coronary CTA revealing coronary artery occlusion.

(3) Differential Diagnosis: Aortic dissection, acute pericarditis, acute pulmonary embolism, pneumothorax, gastrointestinal diseases (e.g., reflux esophagitis), acute cholecystitis, herpes zoster, etc.

2. Management of Acute ST-Elevation Myocardial Infarction

(1) Notify severity, initiate cardiac monitoring, provide oxygen, and establish intravenous access.

(2) Evaluate the patient's current vital signs and hemodynamic stability.

(3) Pharmacological Treatment: Anticoagulation (low molecular weight heparin, unless thrombolysis or urgent intervention is required), dual antiplatelet therapy (aspirin + clopidogrel or ticagrelor, with loading doses for initial use), statins (atorvastatin or rosuvastatin), medications for improving prognosis (β-blockers, ACEIs, or ARBs if blood pressure and heart rate permit), and medications for relieving chest pain (morphine, nitrates if no contraindications).

(4) Reperfusion Strategies

1) Thrombolytic Therapy: In hospitals without PCI capabilities, intravenous thrombolysis remains a reasonable option for eligible STEMI patients. Pre-hospital thrombolysis is preferred over in-hospital thrombolysis. For patients presenting within 3 hours of symptom onset, the immediate efficacy of thrombolytic therapy is similar to that of direct PCI. If possible, thrombolytic therapy can be initiated in the ambulance (Class Ⅱa, Level A).

A. Evaluate the indications and contraindications (including absolute and relative) for thrombolytic therapy.

B. Choice of Thrombolytic Agent: Alteplase (higher recanalization rate, lower risk of cerebral hemorrhage); Urokinase (lacks fibrin specificity, lower recanalization rate, cost-effective).

C. Indirect indicators of successful thrombolysis and vessel recanalization include: ≥50% ST-segment resolution within 60-90 minutes; earlier peak levels of cardiac troponin (within 12 hours) and CK-MB (within 14 hours); significant relief of chest pain within 2 hours; and reperfusion arrhythmias within 2-3 hours. Of these, ECG changes and earlier peaking of cardiac biomarkers are most important. Direct indicators include an angiographic assessment of coronary artery patency.

2) Interventional Treatment: Direct PCI, with the decision made based on patient characteristics, guideline recommendations, and evidence, or in consultation with the cardiology department.

Section 4 Diagnosis and Treatment of Sudden Cardiac Death

I Definition of Sudden Death

Sudden death (SD) refers to an unexpected natural death. The World Health Organization defines sudden death as the unexpected death of an apparently healthy person, a person with a stable condition, or a person recovering from illness within 6 hours. However, many scholars suggest defining it as death within 1 hour, while others include deaths within 24 hours of symptom onset. Thus, sudden death is a rapidly progressing, unexpected death caused by an underlying condition, potentially occurring without warning.

Sudden death can be classified as sudden cardiac death (SCD) or non-cardiac sudden death. In adults, SCD accounts for more than 80% of all sudden death cases. The out-of-hospital resuscitation success rate for SCD is only 4%-9%, while the in-hospital resuscitation success rate is 15%-40%. These rates vary significantly across regions and hospitals, but most estimate an in-hospital resuscitation success rate of around 20%, which is higher than out-of-hospital SCD but still relatively low, with a certain proportion of neurological disability.

Sudden death is not untreatable; timely and effective cardiopulmonary resuscitation (CPR) and rapid use of external defibrillators can improve the resuscitation success rate for SCD. In cardiology consultations, a considerable portion involves emergency consultations related to sudden death and CPR. Therefore, consulting cardiologists must master CPR and related considerations.

Ⅱ Diagnosis of Cardiac Arrest and Precautions

Cardiac arrest (CA) refers to the sudden cessation of effective cardiac contractions due to various causes, resulting in the abrupt termination of the pumping function, disruption of systemic circulation, respiratory arrest, and loss of consciousness. Early, timely, and accurate detection of cardiac arrest is crucial for improving resuscitation success rates.

1. Diagnostic Criteria for Cardiac Arrest

(1) Sudden loss of consciousness, or loss of consciousness following a brief seizure.

(2) Agonal breathing, quickly followed by respiratory arrest.

(3) Absence of a carotid or femoral pulse.

(4) Dilated and non-reactive pupils bilaterally.

(5) Absence of heart sounds.

(6) Electrocardiographic findings: ① Ventricular fibrillation or ventricular tachycardia; ② Pulseless ventricular tachycardia; ③ Pulseless electrical activity (PEA): Organized electrical activity without effective mechanical contraction. Three scenarios: Electromechanical dissociation with baseline contractility; pseudo-PEA with extremely weak contractions detectable by ultrasound but no palpable pulse; true PEA with complete electromechanical dissociation; ④ Asystole: A flat line or only P waves without QRS complexes.

2. Precautions in Diagnosing Cardiac Arrest

(1) The earlier a cardiac arrest is diagnosed, the better. A prompt diagnosis should be made if the first 1-3 diagnostic criteria are met without waiting for respiratory arrest, dilated pupils, or ECG confirmation. Delaying the diagnosis may miss the optimal resuscitation window, potentially leading to hypoxic brain injury or death.

(2) For comatose patients, cardiac arrest should be confirmed by repeatedly checking for the presence of respiration and a central pulse. Do not assume cardiac arrest based solely on coma,

and do not immediately initiate CPR and defibrillation without excluding other causes of coma, such as cerebrovascular accidents, hypoglycemia, seizures, or hepatic encephalopathy.

(3) Some less experienced physicians may rush to initiate CPR and defibrillation upon seeing a flat line or suspected ventricular fibrillation on the cardiac monitor. In such cases, remain calm and reconfirm the presence of respiration and a central pulse, while checking for potential electrode displacement.

Ⅲ Cardiopulmonary Resuscitation

Once cardiac arrest is confirmed, do not dwell on the underlying cause but immediately initiate on-site resuscitation. The keys to successful resuscitation are timely intervention and effective resuscitation measures.

1. Calling for Help and Seeking Assistance for In-Hospital Cardiac Arrest: Cardiac arrest can occur anywhere within a hospital setting. Upon confirming cardiac arrest (check if the patient is unresponsive, whether there is absent or abnormal breathing, and if there is no major arterial pulse within 10 seconds), the immediate steps are to call for help and seek assistance. The first responder should instruct others present to dial emergency services, retrieve an automated external defibrillator (AED) as quickly as possible, and commence cardiopulmonary resuscitation (CPR) immediately. If alone, one should first make the emergency call and, if an AED is readily available, bring it to the patient's side before starting CPR.

2. Manual Circulation (Chest Compressions) Technique Standards: During CPR, effective chest compressions are essential to ensure organ perfusion. Effective compressions must be rapid and forceful. Place the patient supine on a firm surface, with the rescuer standing or kneeling beside them. Position the heel of one hand on the lower third of the sternum, place the other hand on top, interlock fingers, straighten elbows, and use body weight to depress the sternum. Compress at a rate of 100-120 compressions per minute, with a depth of at least 5 cm but not exceeding 6 cm in adults. Allow full chest recoil after each compression, with equal compression and relaxation times. Minimize interruptions and maintain a compression fraction (percentage of total CPR time spent compressing) of $\geqslant$60%. Before establishing an advanced airway, compression-to-ventilation ratio is 30 ∶ 2 for both single and two-rescuer adult CPR. After establishing an advanced airway (e.g., endotracheal intubation), compressions and ventilations may be asynchronous, with a ventilation rate of 10 breaths / minute.

3. Airway: If the patient is not breathing or has agonal respirations, provide rescue breaths after 30 chest compressions. Ensuring a patent airway is a prerequisite for effective ventilation. First, clear any airway obstructions (dentures or vomitus). Position the patient supine, and if no cervical spine injury is suspected, use the head-tilt, chin-lift, or jaw-thrust maneuver. For suspected cervical spine injuries, avoid excessive head / neck extension and use the jaw-thrust technique.

(1) Head-Tilt / Chin-Lift: Place one hand on the patient's forehead and apply firm backward pressure to tilt the head back. Use the fingers of the other hand to lift the chin upward, close the mouth, and lift the jaw forward without compressing the soft tissues underneath to avoid airway obstruction. Do not use the thumb to lift the chin. An open airway facilitates spontaneous

breathing and mouth-to-mouth ventilation during CPR.

(2) Jaw-Thrust: Position your hands on either side of the patient's head, supporting your elbows on the surface. Grasp the angles of the jaw and lift upward, opening the mouth with your thumbs if necessary. If mouth-to-mouth ventilation is required, maintain jaw-thrust while sealing the patient's nose with your cheek. This maneuver is effective but effortful and technically challenging. It is safer for patients with suspected head or neck trauma, as it avoids exacerbating injuries from neck movement.

4. Rescue Breathing: During rescue breaths, each ventilation must achieve adequate chest rise. After establishing an advanced airway, provide continuous ventilation at a rate of one breath every 6 seconds (10 breaths / minute). In a hospital setting, a bag-valve-mask device is commonly available for ventilation, with techniques for both single and two-rescuer CPR. Single-rescuer ventilation is often complicated by air leaks, leading to inadequate ventilation, so two-rescuer CPR is generally more effective. If the airway is patent without leaks, compressing a 1 L adult bag by 1 / 2 to 2 / 3 or a 2 L adult bag by 1 / 3 can achieve an adequate tidal volume. If a bag-valve mask is not immediately available, initiate mouth-to-mouth ventilation.

5. Defibrillation: As most cardiac arrests are caused by ventricular fibrillation, so defibrillation is the most effective treatment. Research has shown that for every minute of delay in defibrillation, the success rate of resuscitation decreases by 7%-10% in patients with ventricular fibrillation. Therefore, early defibrillation is crucial for successful resuscitation in cardiac arrest. For in-hospital cardiac arrests with ECG monitoring, the time from the onset of ventricular fibrillation to defibrillation should be less than 3 minutes. CPR should be initiated while awaiting the defibrillator, and defibrillation should be performed as soon as the device is ready. Defibrillators can deliver either monophasic or biphasic waveforms. For monophasic defibrillators, the initial shock energy is 360 J, while for biphasic defibrillators, it is typically 150-200 J. After defibrillation, CPR should be continued until the patient exhibits clear signs of restored circulation (e.g., coughing, speaking, or spontaneous limb movement).

6. Drugs in CPR: Drug administration should be considered after initiating basic CPR and early defibrillation. Establish intravenous (Ⅳ) access as soon as possible and consider pharmacological interventions. Medications can be administered through Ⅳ or intraosseous (IO) routes.

(1) Epinephrine: The drug of choice in CPR, with key pharmacological effects including enhanced myocardial contractility, increased coronary and cerebral blood flow, increased myocardial automaticity, and facilitation of defibrillation from ventricular fibrillation. It can be used for refractory ventricular fibrillation / pulseless ventricular tachycardia, asystole, or pulseless electrical activity (PEA). Epinephrine Dosing: 1 mg Ⅳ bolus, repeated every 3-5 minutes. After each peripheral Ⅳ dose, flush the line with 20 mL of normal saline to ensure delivery to the central circulation.

(2) Amiodarone: A Class Ⅲ anti-arrhythmic agent, can be considered for patients with ventricular fibrillation / pulseless ventricular tachycardia refractory to CPR, two defibrillation attempts, and vasopressors. Amiodarone Dosing: An initial dose of 300 mg diluted in 20-30 mL dextrose and rapidly injected, followed by a 150 mg bolus in 3-5 minutes, and then a maintenance

infusion of 1 mg / min for 6 hours. The maximum daily dose generally should not exceed 2 g. Due to its negative inotropic and vasodilatory effects, amiodarone can cause hypotension and bradycardia, often related to the rate of administration. Slower infusion rates, particularly in patients with impaired cardiac function or cardiomegaly, and blood pressure monitoring can mitigate these effects. Additionally, amiodarone prolongs the QT interval, so it should be avoided in torsades de pointes ventricular tachycardia, severe hypokalemia, and bradycardia.

(3) Lidocaine: Studies have not demonstrated long-term or short-term benefits in cardiac arrest, so it is considered an alternative to amiodarone. Lidocaine Dosing: Initial dose of 1.0-1.5 mg / kg Ⅳ bolus. If ventricular fibrillation or pulseless ventricular tachycardia persists, additional doses of 0.50-0.75 mg / kg may be given every 5-10 minutes, up to a maximum of 3 mg / kg.

(4) Magnesium Sulfate: Used only for torsades de pointes ventricular tachycardia caused by prolonged QT interval. Magnesium Sulfate Dosing: 1-2 g diluted in a 10% dextrose solution and administered intravenously over 5-20 minutes, or 1-2 g added to 50-100 mL of fluid for a slow intravenous infusion.

(5) Norepinephrine: a potent α-adrenergic agonist that causes intense vasoconstriction, increased blood pressure, and augmented coronary blood flow. It also stimulates β-receptors, enhancing myocardial contractility and cardiac output. It can be considered for severe hypotension (systolic blood pressure＜70 mmHg) and low peripheral resistance states.

Norepinephrine Dosing: Typically, 4 mg or 8 mg of norepinephrine bitartrate (1 mg norepinephrine＝2 mg norepinephrine bitartrate) is diluted in 250 mL of 5% dextrose or 5% dextrose in normal saline (not in normal saline alone), yielding concentrations of 16 μg / mL norepinephrine or 32 μg / mL norepinephrine bitartrate. The initial infusion rate is 0.5-1 μg / min, titrated to achieve the desired effect.

(6) Sodium Bicarbonate: During cardiac arrest and CPR, the lack of or diminished blood flow can lead to metabolic acidosis and acidemia. However, current evidence does not strongly support the use of alkalizing agents early in CPR to improve defibrillation success or survival rates. Therefore, sodium bicarbonate administration is only beneficial in cases of pre-existing metabolic acidosis, hyperkalemia, or tricyclic antidepressant overdose. Additionally, bicarbonate therapy may be beneficial for patients with prolonged cardiac arrest when defibrillation, chest compressions, intubation, mechanical ventilation, and vasopressor therapy have been ineffective. The dose should be guided by the patient's clinical status, with 1 mmol / kg as the initial dose, without necessarily correcting the entire alkali deficit. To prevent iatrogenic alkalosis, it is preferable to adjust the dose based on blood gas analysis results.

7. Special Circumstances in CPR

(1) Abdominal Compression CPR: For patients with thoracic trauma, chest wall deformities, tension pneumothorax, or cardiac tamponade, where conventional CPR is contraindicated or high-quality CPR cannot be ensured, abdominal compression CPR can be performed. A mechanical abdominal compression-decompression device applies alternating downward compression (approximately 50 kg force) and upward decompression (approximately 30 kg force) to the abdomen at a rate of 100 compressions per minute, causing diaphragmatic motion and subsequent changes in intrathoracic pressure, thereby establishing effective circulation and ventilation.

(2) Open-Chest Direct Cardiac Compression: Direct cardiac compression is a specialized form of CPR that may provide near-normal cerebral and myocardial blood flow. However, it should not be employed as a last resort during prolonged resuscitation efforts, but rather reserved for specific situations, such as during cardiac surgical procedures.

(3) Mechanical Chest Compression Devices: Currently, there is no evidence that mechanical chest compression devices provide superior hemodynamic support or survival rates compared to manual CPR. Therefore, their routine use is not recommended. However, they may be considered in special circumstances, such as during in-hospital transport, prolonged CPR, CT scanning, or emergency coronary angiography.

(4) CPR in Pregnancy: For pregnant women in cardiac arrest, the location for chest compressions should be slightly higher than the standard position. If the fundal height exceeds the umbilical level, manual left uterine displacement may facilitate relief of aortocaval compression during compressions. Furthermore, for pregnant women with severe trauma and confirmed non-survivability, resuscitative efforts should be terminated, and an immediate cesarean delivery performed. It is recommended to consider cesarean delivery upon the onset of cardiac arrest or after 4 minutes of unsuccessful resuscitation. However, the decision for emergent cesarean delivery is often complex, depending on patient factors (cause of arrest, gestational age), team capabilities, and other considerations.

(5) Prolonged CPR: Generally, if there are no signs of return of spontaneous circulation after 30 minutes of CPR, with evidence of irreversible neurological impairment, resuscitation efforts may be terminated. However, with advancements in medical knowledge and technology, prolonged CPR duration can still prove lifesaving for certain cardiac arrest patients. There are no strict guidelines on CPR duration, and decisions should be made based on the patient's overall condition, reversibility of the underlying cause, time of CPR initiation, quality of CPR, and the potential use of extracorporeal membrane oxygenation (ECMO). Favorable prognostic features that may warrant prolonged CPR include younger age, acute myocardial infarction as the primary etiology, and the ability to address reversible causes (e.g., hypothermia, pulmonary embolism).

Ⅳ Post-Resuscitation Care

1. Maintaining Effective Ventilation and Circulation: For in-hospital cardiac arrests without prompt recovery of spontaneous respiration or persistent coma, advanced airway management (e.g., endotracheal intubation) should be promptly established, followed by bag-valve-mask ventilation or mechanical ventilation. Hemodynamic status should be closely monitored, with consideration for invasive hemodynamic monitoring if necessary, and efforts made to maintain stability through fluid resuscitation and vasopressor administration. Electrolyte disturbances should be corrected, and anti-arrhythmic drugs should be used to stabilize dysrhythmias. Temporary pacing may be required for bradyarrhythmias. For cardiogenic shock due to coronary artery disease, intra-aortic balloon pump (IABP) counterpulsation can be considered to support blood pressure, although the benefit of IABP in post-resuscitation patients remains controversial. Additionally, extracorporeal membrane oxygenation (ECMO) is now a well-established therapeutic modality for critical cardiovascular and respiratory conditions. In cardiac arrest

management, ECMO can also provide circulatory support. Experimental and clinical evidence has demonstrated that ECMO can improve hemodynamics, survival, and neurological outcomes in cases of prolonged cardiac arrest. However, due to the complexity and high costs associated with this technology, ECMO should not be considered a routine resuscitation measure but rather reserved for specific situations, such as fulminant myocarditis, acute myocardial infarction with cardiogenic shock, massive pulmonary embolism, profound hypothermia, or as a bridge to cardiac or lung transplantation.

2. Identifying the Cause of Cardiac Arrest: After successful resuscitation, the patient's clinical data should be promptly obtained and completed, including electrocardiography and other necessary laboratory and diagnostic tests. Patients with recurrent malignant arrhythmias must undergo electrocardiography during periods of sinus rhythm to identify the underlying cause of cardiac arrest. Among the numerous etiologies of cardiac arrest, over 80% are of cardiac origin, while some are due to non-cardiac causes.

(1) Cardiogenic Factors

① Coronary Artery Disease: Among the multitude of cardiovascular diseases, Coronary Artery Disease (CAD) accounts for approximately 80% of cardiac arrests, especially in the early phases of acute myocardial infarction. Furthermore, old myocardial infarctions and ischemic cardiomyopathy often lead to ventricular tachycardia and ventricular fibrillation, while coronary artery spasms are also a common cause of cardiac arrest. ② Other Organic Heart Diseases: Beyond CAD, other common organic heart diseases include hypertrophic cardiomyopathy, dilated cardiomyopathy, aortic stenosis, pulmonary stenosis, pulmonary hypertension, pulmonary embolism, acute myocarditis, hypertensive heart disease, congenital heart disease, and cardiac tumors. ③ Non-organic Heart Disease: These commonly involve sick sinus syndrome, third-degree atrioventricular block, long QT syndrome, pre-excitation syndromes, idiopathic ventricular tachycardia, and Brugada syndrome.

(2) Non-Cardiogenic Factors

① Electrolyte Imbalances and Acid-Base Disorders: Severe hyperkalemia, hypokalemia, hypernatremia, hypercalcemia, hypermagnesemia, and acidosis. ② Various Causes of Severe Shock: Septic shock, anaphylactic shock, and hemorrhagic shock. ③ Acute Poisoning: Various pesticide poisonings, drug overdoses. ④ Sudden Accidental Events: Severe trauma, drowning, electric shock, asphyxiation, and complications related to surgeries, diagnostic procedures, or anesthesia. ⑤ Cerebrovascular Accidents. ⑥ Reflex Cardiac Arrest Induced by Vagal Nerve Stimulation: Common reflexes include biliary-cardiac reflex, pharyngeal-cardiac reflex triggered by laryngeal stimulation, and corneal-cardiac reflex or sinus arch reflex triggered by compression of both eyeballs or bilateral carotid sinuses, as well as reflexes during thoracoabdominal surgeries involving traction on the pulmonary hilum or mesentery.

3. Emergency Coronary Angiography: Treatment targeted at the underlying causes of cardiac arrest after CPR is critical to improving patient survival rates. If the root causes of cardiac arrest are not addressed, there could be a recurrence. Among the various causes leading to cardiac arrest, Acute Coronary Syndromes (ACS) within the context of CAD are the most common. Therefore, if ST-segment elevation is observed after a comprehensive 12- or 18-lead ECG, or if there is

a suspicion of coronary artery disease, emergency coronary angiography should be performed as soon as possible, regardless of whether the patient is conscious or in a coma. Studies have shown that emergency coronary angiography can improve survival rates in adult patients who are comatose and suspected of having a cardiac etiology for arrest, even without evident ST-segment elevation.

4. Targeted Temperature Management (TTM): TTM is currently regarded as an effective method to improve outcomes in patients who experience cardiac arrest. It should be applied to comatose adults who regain spontaneous circulation after resuscitation, with initiation as early as possible. The target temperature should be set between 32°C and 36°C and maintained for at least 24 hours. The rate of rewarming should be controlled at 0.25°C to 0.5°C per hour, with proactive measures taken to prevent hyperthermia post-rewarming.

5. Neurological Monitoring and Protection: Neurological damage follo-wing CPR is a major cause of disability and death after cardiac arrest. Actively protecting neurological function to ensure that patients regain a healthy brain and neurological function post-recovery is critical. Recommended assessment methods include clinical symptom signs (pupil responses, level of coma, myoclonus), neurophysiological tests (bedside EEG, somatosensory evoked potentials), imaging studies (CT, MRI), and biomarkers. Appropriate methods should be selected based on the patient's recovery status to monitor neurological functions and perform prognostic assessments.

V Prevention of In-Hospital Cardiac Arrest

Preventing in-hospital cardiac arrest is crucial yet challenging, with sub-optimal outcomes in domestic settings. Identifying high-risk individuals and implementing effective measures to reduce the incidence of cardiac arrest is key. Studies have shown that in-hospital rapid response teams (RRT) or medical emergency teams (MET) significantly reduce the incidence and mortality of in-hospital cardiac arrests, especially in general wards. RRT and MET are composed of ICU or emergency physicians, nurses, and respiratory therapists. They are equipped with monitoring and resuscitation equipment and medications. When other medical staff, especially those in general wards, notice a patient's condition deteriorating, they must immediately notify the RRT or MET to attend to the situation. Since most cardiac arrest cases are related to cardiological conditions, hospitals that are able should consider including cardiologists in their RRT and MET. Cardiologists' expertise in diagnosing cardiac conditions post-cardiopulmonary resuscitation can be more accurate and quicker compared to doctors from other specialties, potentially enhancing the success rate of resuscitations and survival rates of cardiac arrest patients.

VI Consultation Process

1. Diagnosis and Considerations for Cardiac Arrest

(1) Key Points for Diagnosing Cardiac Arrest: Sudden loss of consciousness, occasionally preceded by brief convulsions. Gasping breaths, followed by a cessation of breathing. Absence of major arterial (carotid, femoral) pulses. Bilateral pupil dilation with a reduced or absent response to light. Absence of heart sounds. The ECG shows ventricular fibrillation or flutter, pulseless ventricular tachycardia, pulseless electrical activity (PEA), or asystole.

(2) Considerations for Diagnosing Cardiac Arrest: The earlier the diagnosis of cardiac arrest, the better the chances for rapid intervention. For unconscious patients, confirm cardiac arrest by assessing breathing and major arterial pulses; exclude other causes of unconsciousness such as cerebrovascular accidents, hypoglycemic coma, epileptic seizures, hepatic encephalopathy, etc. Repeat the above diagnostic checks, ensuring electrode patches are secure and functional.

2. Cardiopulmonary Resuscitation (CPR): Once Cardiopulmonary Resuscita-tion is confirmed, do not delay by attempting to identify the cause. Immediate on-site resuscitation is crucial, and success hinges on rapid action and effective measures: ① Call for help, quickly access an Automated External Defibrillator (AED), and start CPR immediately. ② Perform chest compressions to establish artificial circulation. ③ Open the airway and clear any obstructions (such as dentures or vomit); position the patient supine. ④ Provide artificial respiration to ensure full expansion of the lungs with each ventilation, which is more effectively performed by two responders. ⑤ Defibrillation should be carried out since most cardiac arrests are caused by ventricular fibrillation, making electrical defibrillation the most effective treatment. Before obtaining an AED, begin CPR and use the AED as soon as it is ready.

Common drugs used in CPR: Establish an intravenous line as soon as basic CPR and early defibrillation are initiated and consider the administration of resuscitative drugs. The route of administration can be intravenous or intraosseous. ① Epinephrine: the first-choice drug in CPR. ② Amiodarone: a Class Ⅲ anti-arrhythmic useful for CPR, especially after two defibrillation attempts and if vasopressors have had no response in cases of ventricular fibrillation / pulseless ventricular tachycardia. Avoid in patients with prolonged QT causing torsades de pointes, severe hypokalemia, or bradycardia. ③ Lidocaine: an alternative to amiodarone. ④ Magnesium sulfate: only for torsades de pointes caused by prolonged QT. ⑤ Norepinephrine: a potent α-adrenergic agonist that causes strong vasoconstriction, increased blood pressure, enhanced coronary blood flow, and β-adrenergic stimulation, increasing myocardial contractility and cardiac output. Consider severe hypotension (systolic blood pressure$<$70 mmHg) and low peripheral resistance. ⑥ Sodium bicarbonate: beneficial in existing metabolic acidosis, hyperkalemia, or tricyclic antidepressant overdose.

3. Post-CPR Management

(1) Maintain effective breathing and circulation: ① Quickly establish advanced airways using intubation, then assist ventilation with a bag-valve mask or mechanical ventilation. ② Monitor hemodynamic status closely, using invasive hemodynamic monitoring if necessary. ③ Correct electrolyte imbalances and stabilize rhythm with anti-arrhythmic drugs; use a temporary pacemaker if required. ④ Consider intra-aortic balloon pump (IABP) insertion for cardiogenic shock caused by Coronary Artery Disease. ⑤ Extracorporeal membrane oxygenation (ECMO) as a circulatory support measure in cardiac arrest treatment scenarios such as severe myocarditis, acute myocardial infarction with cardiogenic shock, massive pulmonary embolism, profound hypothermia, or while awaiting heart or lung transplantation.

(2) Actively search for the cause of cardiac arrest: Over 80% are cardiogenic, with other causes also leading to cardiac arrest.

(3) Emergency coronary angiography: Among the many factors causing cardiac arrest,

CAD, particularly acute coronary syndromes, is the most common. Thus, emergency coronary angiography should be performed promptly after completing a 12- or 18-lead ECG showing ST-segment elevation, or if CAD is suspected, regardless of the patient's consciousness state. Research indicates that emergency coronary angiography can improve survival rates in adult patients with suspected cardiogenic causes of arrest who are comatose, even if no ST-segment elevation is seen.

(4) Targeted Temperature Management (TTM): Currently considered an effective method to improve prognosis after cardiac arrest.

(5) Neurological Monitoring and Protection.

Section 5 Analysis of Causes for Abnormal Cardiac Injury Markers

The elevation of cardiac injury markers has become the primary diagnostic criterion for acute myocardial infarction (AMI). Currently, the most commonly used cardiac injury markers in clinical practice include myoglobin, creatine kinase (CK) and its isoenzyme CK-MB, as well as cardiac troponins (cTn), including cardiac troponin I (cTnI) and cardiac troponin T (cTnT).

I Evolution of Cardiac Markers in AMI

The evolution of cardiac markers in AMI is shown in Tables 1-3.

Tables 1-3 Cardiac Markers and Their Evolution in AMI

	Myoglobin	CK	CK-MB	cTnI	cTnT
Appearing Time (h)	1 2	6	3 4	2 4	2 4
Peak Time (h)	4-8	24	10-24	10-24	10-24
Duration (d)	0.5-1.0	3-4	2-4	5-10	5-14

1. Myoglobin: It appears earliest in serum, with high sensitivity but low specificity. Its negative result helps rule out AMI. Its short half-life is helpful for observing reinfarction or infarct extension during AMI.

2. CK and CK-MB

(1) Composition of CK: CK is a dimer composed of M and / or B subunits, forming 3 isoenzymes.

CK-MM: Accounts for 95%-100% of serum CK, mainly present in skeletal muscle.

CK-MB: Accounts for 5%, mainly in myocardium, and a and a small amount in skeletal muscle.

CK-BB: Almost zero in serum, mainly in brain, lung, and skeletal muscle.

(2) CK-MB / CK ratio: Normal<5%, elevated CK-MB suggests myocardial injury possibility but can also be seen in acute rhabdomyolysis.<6% mostly skeletal muscle damage; 6%-25% highly suspicious of AMI;>25% or CK-MB / CK ratio reversal may indicate autoimmune diseases or tumors.

The CK-MB / CK percentage is more predictive of macro CK immunoglobulin complexes (macro CK) associated with proliferative and autoimmune pathologies than absolute CK-MB values.

When the CK-MB / CK ratio is reversed, qualitative CK-MB assays like imm-unochemiluminometric or agarose gel electrophoresis should be performed.

(3) Current common CK-MB assay—immunoinhibition: Measures CK-MB activity, ignoring CK-BB in serum and considering only CK-MM and CK-MB release. Anti-CK-M antibody inhibits M subunit (all CK-MM and 50% CK-MB) but not B subunit activity. CK-MM loses all activity, CK-MB loses half, so the residual B activity measured represents twice the CK-MB activity.

Normally, CK-BB is nearly zero in serum, not affecting CK-MB measurement. However, when CK-BB is markedly elevated for various reasons, the instrument misidentifies it as CK-MB, reporting CK-MB=2 (CK-BB+CK-B), leading to falsely elevated CK-MB, even exceeding total CK. This should not be considered for an AMI diagnosis.

This method gives falsely elevated CK-MB in conditions like macro CK, central nervous system injury, various organ malignancies like prostate and adenocarcinomas, and labor.

(4) Causes of elevated CK

1) Physiological CK elevation: Influenced by age, gender, race, and exercise status. Mild elevation in newborns, males, blacks, and after exercise.

2) Pathological CK elevation: Any factor causing changes in muscle cell membrane permeability and / or cell injury can lead to CK leakage and increased serum CK.

A. Primary skeletal muscle diseases

a. Myositis: infectious, autoimmune disorders.

b. Myopathies: congenital, hereditary, and metabolic diseases.

B. Secondary factors

a. Physical factors: excessive exercise, trauma, burns, surgery, intramuscular injections, electromyography, etc.

b. Chemical factors: drugs like statins, antipsychotics like chlorpromazine, and toxins like alcohol, organophosphates, carbon monoxide, and morphine can cause muscle injury.

c. Biological factors: Eating fish / shrimp including small lobsters, can trigger acute rhabdomyolysis within 24 hours.

d. Systemic diseases: Ischemia, hypoxia, and shock; electrolyte imbalances like hyponatremia, hypokalemia, and hypophosphatemia; endocrine disorders like hyperthyroidism, hypothyroidism, and hyperparathyroidism; central, peripheral, and neuromuscular junction diseases like status epilepticus, Guillain-Barre syndrome, and myasthenia gravis can cause denervation atrophy or damage to the supplied skeletal muscles with mild CK elevation; heart, kidney diseases, and malignancies can also elevate CK.

(5) Causes of elevated CK-MB

1) Macro CK: includes macro CK1 and macro CK2, both unaffected by anti-CK-M antibody inhibition, potentially causing overestimation.

A. Macro CK1: More common in unhealthy populations like the elderly and females.

Detected by enzyme electrophoresis.

B. Macro CK2: Bound to mitochondrial membranes in muscle, brain, and liver, possibly mitochondrial membrane fragments. Absent in normal serum and AMI unless extreme tissue damage releases mitochondria and cell debris into circulation. Seen in malignancies, cirrhosis, myocarditis, etc.

2) Elevated CK-BB: Mainly present in smooth muscle, nerves, and brain tissue; low levels in other organs.

Elevated in acute brain injury, epilepsy, malignancies, hepatitis B, leading to primary hepatic cancer, and hematological diseases. In some studies, CK-MB / total CK levels were higher than 50% by immunoinhibition assay, and CK-BB levels were higher on isoenzyme electrophoresis, which wasn't the case in the control group. For patients with a clear brain injury history, a direct CK-MB mass assay is preferred.

3) CK-MB elevation in non-regenerating states: Like Duchenne muscular dystrophy and other neuromuscular disorders, possibly due to high CK-MB content in abnormally regenerating skeletal muscle fibers. Additionally, immunoglobulin cofactor effects in some cancer patients with immune dysregulation may influence CK-MB results.

3. cTn. When CK and CK-MB produce abnormal results, cTn can be tested. Currently, cTn has higher sensitivity and specificity than cardiac enzymes for AMI diagnosis. cTn is a muscle contraction regulatory protein with 3 subtypes: cTnC, cTnI, and cTnT. cTnI and cTnT are more cardiac-specific. Compared to cTnT, cTnI has higher initial sensitivity and specificity, but cTnT has a longer diagnostic window.

cTn elevation, besides AMI, is seen in various diseases:

(1) Cardiac causes: Coronary artery spasm; stress cardiomyopathy; acute heart failure; viral myocarditis, pericarditis; cardiac procedures (PCI, RF ablation, CABG, etc.); malignancy; arrhythmias; tachycardia, etc.

(2) Non-cardiac causes: Acute pulmonary embolism; renal failure and end-stage renal disease; cerebrovascular diseases including ischemic stroke, hemorrhagic stroke, and subarachnoid hemorrhage; severe infections like sepsis and septic shock; blunt chest trauma; strenuous exercise (cTn elevation is transient, normalizing within 24-48 hours).

(3) Other causes: Assay performance issues, the presence of heterophilic antibodies or interfering substances in the sample, etc.

II Common Questions in Consultation

How to approach elevated cardiac injury markers in consultation?

(1) First, determine the tissue source of CK based on the CK-MB / CK ratio. If less than 6%, it is often from skeletal muscle damage. If between 6% and 25%, consider cardiac origin. If greater than 25%, consider the possibility of autoimmune diseases and tumors.

(2) If CK-MB is disproportionately elevated, even exceeding total CK, use immunoassays or agarose gel electrophoresis for qualitative CK-MB analysis along with cTn testing.

(3) cTn elevation suggests myocardial injury but is not specific for AMI—it can occur in other conditions. Do not diagnose AMI based solely on elevated cardiac markers—correlate with

clinical history, ECG changes, marker kinetics, etc.

(4) Ensure proper quality control for cardiac marker assays—rule out systematic and random errors, exclusion of samples outside the analytical measurement range, hemolysis, lipemia, etc.

Section 6 Diagnosis and Treatment of Myocardial Bridges

I Overview

A myocardial bridge (MB) is a congenital anatomical anomaly of the coronary arteries. Normally, the main coronary artery trunks and branches course along the subepicardial surface within the connective tissue. However, sometimes a segment of a coronary artery takes an intramuscular course, covered by overlying myocardial fibers, forming the "myocardial bridge". The tunneled coronary artery segment is referred to as the "mural coronary artery".

The prevalence of myocardial bridges ranges from 15%-85% on autopsy and 3.5%-58% on coronary CT angiography, but it is lower (0.5%-16%) on invasive coronary angiography. The vast majority (67%-98%) involve the left anterior descending artery, commonly in its proximal or mid-third segments. They are occasionally seen in the circumflex or right coronary arteries. Usually, a single coronary artery is affected, but two or more bridges in the same or different arteries can occur.

II Classification

There are two main classification systems for myocardial bridges:

Type 1. Based on autopsy findings, there are superficial and deep / intramuscular types. The superficial type has a myocardial thickness generally $<$2 mm, while the deep type lies deeper within the myocardium with a thickness$>$2 mm and is less common. Due to their superficial location and thin muscle cover, superficial bridges are often asymptomatic clinically. In contrast, deep intramuscular bridges frequently cause angina and other symptoms, and are associated with major adverse cardiovascular events like acute MI, sudden death, and malignant arrhythmias.

Type 2. The Schwarz angiographic classification is more commonly used clinically, with 3 types: Type A—incidentally detected without objective evidence of ischemia, usually superficial; Type B—with objective evidence of inducible ischemia on stress testing; Type C—with a definite hemodynamic milking effect on quantitative coronary angiography, fractional flow reserve, or Doppler flow measurements, irrespective of ischemic changes. Types B and C tend to have deep intramuscular bridges.

III Clinical Presentation and Pathogenic Mechanisms

The clinical manifestations of myocardial bridges are highly variable. Many patients remain asymptomatic long-term. Some develop symptoms of myocardial ischemia like atypical chest pain, exertional angina with poor response, or even worsening with nitrates. A small subset may present with severe ischemic events like ACS, acute LV dysfunction, malignant arrhythmias, syncope, or sudden death, often precipitated by exertion, intense exercise, or emotional stress. The severity generally correlates with the degree of systolic coronary compression, with angina symptoms expected when the muscle bridge causes>40% systolic narrowing. Concomitant proximal atherosclerotic disease worsens symptoms. Coexisting CAD, cardiomyopathy, or valvular heart disease can further complicate the clinical picture.

The mechanism of myocardial ischemia caused by myocardial bridges is partly intuitive; by definition, during systole, the tunneled or mural segment of the coronary artery gets compressed by the overlying myocardial fibers, resulting in lumen narrowing, reduced regional blood flow, and myocardial underperfusion, akin to coronary artery spasm. However, two other key points must be emphasized:

(1) The compression is not limited to systole but can persist into mid- and late-diastole, leading to markedly delayed restoration of distal coronary flow and pressure gradients, further exacerbating ischemia.

(2) Myocardial bridges promote accelerated proximal atherosclerosis. The proximal mural segment is exposed to high wall stress, flow disturbances, and low shear forces, which disrupt endothelial function—a pivotal initiator of atherosclerosis. Autopsy and intravascular ultrasound studies confirm increased susceptibility to atherosclerotic plaque formation in these proximal segments, while the tunneled and distal portions are relatively spared. Dislodgment of unstable proximal plaque with acute thrombus formation is an important mechanism underlying acute myocardial infarction in some patients, explaining their propensity for severe ischemic events.

IV Diagnosis

As the clinical manifestations of myocardial bridges are diverse and non-specific, diagnosis relies heavily on imaging modalities-primarily non-invasive multislice CT (MSCT)and invasive coronary angiography (CAG)with intravascular ultrasound (IVUS).

1. MSCT is currently the most widely used clinical diagnostic tool for myocardial bridges and the most commonly employed in consultation. 16-, 64-, 128- and 256-slice MSCT scanners are routinely utilized to measure bridge length, thickness, and overall morphology. MSCT defines a myocardial bridge as a segment of coronary artery completely>50% circumferentially surrounded by myocardial fibers, with proximal and distal segments coursing in the epicardial fat; this tunneled segment represents the "mural" artery overlaid by the "myocardial bridge". MSCT has high sensitivity, specificity, and accuracy for bridge diagnosis.

2. CAG was the initial imaging modality for myocardial bridge detection and remains the clinical gold standard. Diagnosis relies on identifying a "milking effect", i.e. systolic lumen narrowing / complete obliteration with partial or complete normalization in mid-late diastole, in at least two projections. The degree of systolic narrowing can be semi-quantified using the Noble grading: Grade 1<50%, Grade 2 50%-75%, Grade 3>75%, with Grade≥2 associated with a higher risk of ischemia and symptoms. However, it is worth noting that CAG can miss myocardial bridges, depending on factors like bridge length, width, use of vasodilators / constrictors, angiographic technique, projections, and operator experience.

3. Intravascular ultrasound (IVUS) has emerged as a significant diagnostic tool for

myocardial bridging in recent years. Compared to coronary angiography (CAG), IVUS allows for real-time, cross-sectional imaging to display conditions within the lumen and the vascular wall. Under IVUS, myocardial bridging can exhibit the classic "half-moon sign", characterized by an anechoic, crescent-shaped space between the coronary artery within the myocardial bridge and the epicardial tissue during both systole and diastole. Additionally, IVUS can identify atherosclerotic plaque features near the proximal end of the coronary artery under the bridge. Doppler flow measurements reveal the "fingertip phenomenon" associated with myocardial bridging, which involves a rapid acceleration of blood flow in early diastole followed by a deceleration in mid-diastole, and a steady flow in late diastole, which then rapidly decreases or even stops during systole.

V Treatment

Current clinical management is primarily guided by the Schwarz classification. Type A patients generally require no treatment, while Type B and C are initially managed with medical therapy, proceeding to intervention or surgery if medications fail.

1. Pharmacotherapy is the cornerstone, aimed at reducing myocardial contractility, heart rate, and oxygen demand. Beta-blockers are first-line, slowing the ventricular rate, alleviating systolic compression, improving coronary flow reserve, reducing ischemic symptoms, and enhancing exercise tolerance. Non-dihydropyridine calcium channel blockers are an alternative to beta-blocker contraindications / intolerance, providing vasodilation and relief of vasospasm to improve myocardial perfusion. The two can be combined. Given the increased atherosclerotic risk, antiplatelet agents and statins may be individualized. Nitrates are generally avoided, as they can reflexively increase heart rate and contractility, worsening compression.

2. Percutaneous intervention with intracoronary stenting can be considered, though associated with higher restenosis rates and risks like stent displacement, fracture, or vessel perforation in myocardial bridges. It is reserved for symptomatic patients' refractory to medical therapy, with IVUS guidance recommended to optimize stent sizing and deployment across the tunneled segment.

3. Surgical options include surgical myotomy (unroofing) or coronary artery bypass grafting (CABG). Unroofing may be preferred for superficial bridges with severe (Grade Ⅲ) systolic compression causing refractory angina or adverse events. CABG is indicated for deep bridges (> 5 mm depth, > 25 mm length) causing complete systolic obliteration without diastolic re-opening. However, both are major open surgical procedures with potential serious complications like ventricular aneurysm or rupture, and resultant scarring can worsen extrinsic compression. Thus, indications must be carefully assessed.

Ⅵ Common Questions in Consultation

1. Does a myocardial bridge mandate surgery? Theoretically, as a structural coronary anomaly, definitive treatment requires surgical unroofing.

However, most myocardial bridges are relatively benign clinically, while surgery is high-risk with potentially catastrophic complications like vessel rupture or ventricular perforation that may outweigh the benefits. Medical management is generally recommended first-line unless symptoms are truly refractory. It is important to exclude other causes of atypical chest pain like gastroesophageal reflux, pleuritis, costochondritis, or cardiac neuropathy before considering higher-risk interventions if ischemia is definitively attributable to the bridge after such an evaluation. Risks and benefits must be carefully weighed in a shared decision-making process.

2. Are activities restricted after discharge? For incidentally detected Type A bridges without objective ischemia, no activity restrictions are required. For other types, recommendations are based on the individual's functional status, as strenuous exertion can potentially precipitate acute ischemic events in myocardial bridges.

3. Lifestyle modifications? Myocardial bridges predispose to accelerated proximal atherosclerosis. Therefore, patients are advised a heart-healthy lifestyle: a low-salt, low-fat diet, smoking cessation, regular exercise, weight optimization, blood pressure and glycemic control, stress management, and anxiety reduction strategies.

4. Prognosis? While major adverse events like acute MI, heart failure, syncope, and sudden death have been reported, most myocardial bridges follow a benign course, with many remaining asymptomatic lifelong. Longer, deeper bridges, especially with coexisting CAD, valvular, or myocardial disease, are at higher risk of severe ischemic complications impacting long-term survival.

Section 7 Key Points for the Diagnosis and Treatment of Coronary Artery Disease

I Definition and Classification

CAD, also known as ischemic heart disease, refers to cardiac disorders caused by myocardial ischemia, hypoxia, or necrosis secondary to organic stenosis or obstruction of the coronary arteries due to atherosclerosis or vasospastic functional changes. Along with conditions like coronary spasm, inflammation (Kawasaki disease, SLE, polyarteritis nodosa, syphilitic aortitis, drug abuse), emboli, and congenital anomalies (coronary artery fistulas, abnormal origins), it is collectively termed coronary artery heart disease (CHD), of which atherosclerosis accounts for over 95% of cases.

CAD is typically diagnosed when at least one major coronary artery has>50% luminal stenosis. During exertion or stress, this causes an imbalance between myocardial oxygen supply and demand, resulting in ischemia manifesting as angina, which is relieved by rest or nitroglycerin. Unstable plaque rupture with platelet aggregation and thrombosis can also precipitate anginal symptoms.

Clinically, CAD is categorized into five types: ① Asymptomatic (silent); ② Angina pectoris; ③ Myocardial infarction; ④ Ischemic cardiomyopathy; ⑤ Sudden death. Among these, angina pectoris is the most common, while myocardial infarction and sudden death are the most severe. These five types may coexist.

Coronary artery disease (CAD) is broadly classified into two categories: Stable coronary artery disease (SCAD) and acute coronary syndromes (ACS).

II Clinical Presentation and Risk Factors

1. Clinical Presentation includes symptoms and signs. Angina pectoris is the principal manifestation of CAD. The location, quality, precipitating factors, duration, and relieving factors of typical anginal episodes, along with associated symptoms, aid in the preliminary diagnosis of CAD. Physical examination findings have limited diagnostic value.

(1) Typical Symptoms: Angina is a syndrome caused by acute, transient myocardial ischemia and hypoxia.

1) Location: Retrosternal or left precordial chest pain, often radiating to the left shoulder or arm. Sometimes extending to the throat.

2) Distribution: Handprint or fist-sized area.

3) Quality: Dull, constricting, crushing, burning, suffocating, or heavy sensation. It may be accompanied by diaphoresis, dyspnea, anxiety, palpitations, nausea, or dizziness.

4) Duration: Generally 2-5 minutes, occasionally $>$15 minutes, with spontaneous relief.

5) Precipitated by increased cardiac demand (exertion, emotional stress, cold exposure) and relieved by rest or sublingual nitroglycerin within minutes.

(2) Atypical Symptoms: Atypical location and quality, often more concerning.

1) Atypical location: Jaw, teeth, back, left shoulder, or epigastrium. May mimic gastrointestinal symptoms like epigastric discomfort, especially with nausea / vomiting, prompting misdiagnosis as gastritis, cholecystitis, or pancreatitis. Dental, throat, or shoulder pain requires differentiation from respective organ pathologies. Some patients present with arrhythmias like atrial fibrillation, premature ventricular contractions, AV block, or heart failure symptoms like dyspnea instead of chest pain—the "arrhythmic" and "heart failure" variants of angina.

2) Atypical quality: Described as mild discomfort or chest heaviness. Often reported as exertional dyspnea relieved by rest. Some may be asymptomatic until precipitated by exertion, alcohol, stress, excessive smoking, insomnia, exposure, travel, or coitus—unmasking vasospastic angina.

2. Risk Factors

(1) Non-modifiable

1) Age and Gender: Incidence rises in men $>$40 years; pre-menopausal women have a lower risk than age-matched men.

2) Family history: 1.5-2 folds higher risk with a positive family history.

(2) Lifestyle factors

1) Dyslipidemia: After age, the most important predictor of CAD risk.

2) Hypertension: Doubles MI risk compared to normotensives. Every 2 mmHg rise in SBP increases CAD mortality by 7%. Over 70% of Indian CAD patients are hypertensive. Hypertension accelerates atherosclerosis and CAD progression. SBP is a better predictor than DBP to predict CAD.

3) Smoking: A major risk factor, with a dose-dependent relationship between smoking duration / intensity and CAD mortality. Passive smoking also confers risks.

4) Diabetes: 2-3 folds higher CAD risk than non-diabetics. Diabetic CAD tends to be more severe, with higher prevalence, mortality, premature onset, and MI rates. Complications like painless MI, cardiogenic shock, and heart failure are more frequent.

5) Obesity: An increasing global pandemic and an established CAD risk factor associated with higher mortality.

6) Sedentary lifestyle: Doubles CAD risk compared to active individuals.

Ⅲ Diagnosis

With increasing research into CAD, the diagnostic modalities have evolved considerably. Initially, the diagnosis relied on typical clinical presentation, cardiac enzyme changes, and ECG findings. More recently, newer techniques like radionuclide imaging, multi-slice CT (MSCT), and invasive coronary angiography (CAG) have emerged.

1. The ECG is the earliest, most widely used, and most basic diagnostic test for CAD. Compared to other modalities, it is convenient, inexpensive, widely available, and can capture real-time changes serially or with provocative testing to enhance sensitivity. However, its limitations include that some patients have a normal ECG and difficulty capturing transient ischemic changes. ST-T changes are the most reliable ECG manifestation of unstable angina / non-ST elevation MI (NSTEMI). Unstable angina may show ≥0.1 mV ST depression in ≥2 contiguous leads on the resting ECG. Transient ST shift or T-wave inversion / pseudo-normalization during symptoms, with resolution after relief, strongly suggests acute ischemia and severe CAD. Variant angina typically shows transient ST elevation. A normal ECG during severe pain suggests a non-cardiac etiology.

In NSTEMI, ST depression and T inversion are more marked and persistent than unstable angina, evolving with deepening and then resolving T inversions.

2. Ambulatory (Holter) ECG monitoring allows continuous ECG recording over extended durations, enhancing the detection of transient arrhythmias and silent ischemic episodes compared to a resting ECG. It can capture over 100,000 cardiac cycles over 24 hours, temporally correlating symptoms / activities with ECG changes. This expands the clinical utility, particularly for detecting asymptomatic ischemia in CAD.

3. Exercise electrocardiogram (ECG) stress tests primarily include treadmill exercise tests and bicycle ergometer tests. Without myocardial ischemia, many patients with CAD can maintain normal coronary blood flow and have normal ECGs at rest. However, during exercise, the limited coronary artery flow reserve due to stenosis can induce myocardial ischemia and angina symptoms. Exercise stress testing provides cardiac stress to provoke myocardial ischemia and confirm the presence of angina. It is also important for evaluating ischemic arrhythmias and post-infarction cardiac function.

4. Echocardiography can examine cardiac morphology, wall motion, and left ventricular function. It is one of the most commonly used cardiac diagnostic tools, with important diagnostic values for ventricular aneurysms, intracardiac thrombi, cardiac rupture, and papillary muscle

function. With the increasing clinical applications of multi-slice CT angiography and coronary angiography, stress echocardiography is currently less frequently used for CAD diagnosis.

5. Myocardial perfusion imaging can reveal ischemic regions and delineate the location and extent of ischemia. The two commonly used radioactive tracers are technetium-99 m (99 mTc) and thallium-201 (201Tl). 201Tl is a cationic myocardial imaging agent that is easily taken up by normal myocardial cells. However, ischemic areas have less or no uptake, which shows up as perfusion defects. For patients with atypical angina, ST-T changes without confirmed early CAD, segmental perfusion defects along coronary artery distributions, or delayed 201Tl imaging (3-4 hours) suggest a high likelihood of myocardial ischemia due to CAD. This sensitive, safe, non-invasive technique with good reproducibility is widely used for diagnosing early CAD, myocardial infarction, and assessing cardiac function. Myocardial perfusion imaging is internationally recognized as the most reliable non-invasive test for diagnosing CAD, determining ischemia location, extent, and severity. Its average sensitivity and specificity for CAD diagnosis are 84% and 77% respectively. However, with the increasing clinical use of multi-slice CT and coronary angiography, myocardial perfusion imaging is less frequently used for CAD diagnosis.

6. Multi-slice CT coronary angiography is a non-invasive method for visualizing coronary artery lesions and morphology, with important implications for prognostic evaluation and treatment guidance in CAD patients. It has a high negative predictive value; patients without obstructive CAD on CT have an extremely low risk of future coronary events on follow-up. Therefore, invasive testing is generally unnecessary if CT shows no significant stenosis. However, CT has limitations in evaluating stenosis severity, particularly in the presence of calcification. Its assessment of in-stent restenosis (especially for stents$\leqslant$3.0 mm) is also limited. Currently, 16-slice, 64-slice, 128-slice, and 256-slice multi-detector CT scanners are widely used clinically.

7. Coronary angiography remains the "gold standard" for CAD diagnosis, definitively revealing the presence, location, extent, and severity of coronary stenoses to guide further treatment strategies. Concurrent left ventriculography enables functional assessment. For patients with angina or suspected angina, coronary angiography can confirm the diagnosis, delineate vascular lesions, and determine treatment strategies and prognosis. It remains the most accurate clinical test for evaluating coronary atherosclerosis and the less common non-atherosclerotic causes of angina. An angiographic evaluation of coronary anatomy and left ventricular function provides the most important prognostic information. Coronary lesion severity is commonly graded based on the number of vessels involved (1, 2, 3 vessels or left main disease).

Ⅳ Treatment

1. Non-Pharmacological Treatment

(1) Smoking Cessation: One of the most effective ways to prevent disease progression. Quitting smoking can reduce angina episodes, enhance medication efficacy, and decrease adverse events, including myocardial infarction and mortality. Patients should make efforts to completely stop smoking, aided by medical interventions if needed. Exposure to second-hand smoke should also be eliminated. For CAD patients who quit smoking, cardiovascular risk declines to non-smoker levels within 2-3 years.

(2) Dietary and Lifestyle Modifications: Dietary control to maintain appropriate body weight, lower elevated lipids, and improve other unhealthy dietary patterns, such as limiting salt intake. Specific measures include controlling total caloric intake; reducing fat, especially cholesterol and saturated fatty acid intake; and appropriately increasing protein and carbohydrate proportions. Reducing alcohol consumption and quitting hard liquor. Other non-pharmacological measures include exercise: at least 3-4 sessions per week for 30-60 minutes each. Daily exercise and appropriate physical activity are preferable; patients with severe disease should exercise under medical guidance.

2. Pharmacological Treatment

(1) Drugs Improving Prognosis

1) Antiplatelet Agents: Platelet activation and aggregation play a key role in coronary plaque rupture and thrombus formation; thus, aggressive antiplatelet therapy clearly benefits CAD patients. Currently, the classical antiplatelet drugs are aspirin and clopidogrel. The emergence of new agents such as prasugrel and ticagrelor also provides additional options for CAD treatment.

A. Aspirin: All stable CAD patients without contraindications should take aspirin. The optimal dosage range is 75-150 mg / day. Major adverse effects are gastrointestinal bleeding and aspirin allergy. For aspirin-intolerant patients, clopidogrel can be used as an alternative.

B. Clopidogrel: Selectively and irreversibly inhibits the platelet ADP receptor, blocking ADP-dependent activation of the GPIIb / Ⅲa complex and effectively reducing ADP-mediated platelet activation and aggregation. Its antiplatelet effect is superior to that of aspirin, and it can be used in combination for ACS and PCI patients. The typical maintenance dose is 75 mg / day orally.

C. Ticagrelor: A non-thienopyridine ADP receptor antagonist approved by the FDA in 2011, It selectively and reversibly inhibits the P2Y12 receptor on platelets. It is already in an active form, not requiring hepatic biotransformation and acting faster with reversible effects. Reversibly binding P2Y12, platelet function is comparable to clopidogrel after 5 days off therapy versus 72 hours for ticagrelor, thus reducing bleeding risk. It has an average absolute bioavailability of 36%. Typical dosing: 180 mg loading, 90 mg maintenance twice daily. Common adverse effects in clinical trials include dyspnea and bleeding events.

D. Prasugrel: A new thienopyridine platelet ADP receptor antagonist approved by the FDA in 2009. It has the same mechanism as clopidogrel but higher efficiency as the active metabolite. A 60 mg loading dose achieves faster and more persistent antiplatelet effects than 300 mg clopidogrel. Typical dosing: 60 mg loading, 10 mg / day maintenance.

2) Beta-Blockers: The discovery of beta-blockers is considered one of the most important contributions to CAD treatment. Unless contraindicated, CAD patients should receive long-term beta-blocker therapy. Recent pooled data analyses on the mortality effects of various beta-blockers show that long-term secondary prevention with beta-blockers after myocardial infarction reduces relative mortality by 24%. Beta-blockers with intrinsic sympathomimetic activity have poorer cardioprotective effects; those without such activity are recommended. Beta-blocker dosing should be individualized, starting low and titrating up to relieve symptoms while keeping a heart rate of≥50 bpm. Commonly used oral beta-blockers include metoprolol 25-200 mg / day in 2-3

divided doses; extended-release metoprolol 47.5-190 mg / day once daily; atenolol 25-50 mg / day twice daily; bisoprolol 5-10 mg / day once daily; and carvedilol 5-10 mg / day twice daily.

3) Lipid-Lowering Therapy: The relationship between TC levels and CAD event risk is continuous, starting from TC<4.68 mmol / L (180 mg / dL), with low-density lipoprotein cholesterol (LDL-C) being the most important risk factor. Numerous randomized, double-blind primary and secondary prevention clinical trials have shown that statins can effectively lower TC and LDL-C levels, thereby reducing cardiovascular events. Statin therapy also has the beneficial effects of delaying plaque progression, stabilizing plaques, and having anti-inflammatory actions. The LDL-C target for CAD patients should be<2.60 mmol / L (100 mg / dL); for very high-risk patients (diagnosed CAD with diabetes or acute coronary syndromes), an LDL-C goal< 2.07 mmol / L (80 mg / dL) is also reasonable. This lower target can be extended to very high-risk patients with baseline LDL-C<2.60 mmol / L (100 mg / dL). To achieve greater lipid-lowering, the cholesterol absorption inhibitor ezetimibe (10 mg / day) can be added to statin therapy. For high-risk patients with high triglycerides or low HDL-C, a combination of statin and fibrate (non-gemfibrozil) or niacin can be considered. For high- or moderate-risk patients receiving LDL-C-lowering drugs, treatment intensity should be sufficient to reduce LDL-C by at least 30%-40%.

When using statins, closely monitor liver transaminases, creatine kinase, and other biochemical indices to promptly detect potential hepatic and muscle toxicities. Careful safety monitoring is even more critical with intensive lipid-lowering therapy. Commonly used statins include: rosuvastatin 10-20 mg / day orally; atorvastatin 10-20 mg / day orally; simvastatin 20-40 mg / day orally; fluvastatin 40-80 mg / day orally; pravastatin 20-40 mg / day orally; and lovastatin 20-40 mg / day orally. For CAD patients, the potent statins rosuvastatin and atorvastatin are recommended.

(2) Drugs for Symptomatic Relief and Improving Ischemia: Should be used in combination with drugs preventing myocardial infarction and death. Some drugs, like beta-blockers, have both effects. The main current drug classes for symptom relief and improving ischemia are beta-blockers, nitrates, and calcium channel blockers.

1) Beta-Blockers: By inhibiting cardiac β-adrenergic receptors, beta-blockers reduce heart rate, myocardial contractility, and blood pressure, thereby decreasing myocardial oxygen demand and reducing angina episodes while increasing exercise tolerance. Therapy aims to lower the resting heart rate to 55-60 bpm, or 50 bpm for severe angina, if no bradycardia symptoms occur. Unless contraindicated, beta-blockers should be initiated for stable angina. They reduce mortality and reinfarction risk in post-MI stable angina patients. When dosed properly, many beta-blockers are available for angina treatment and are effective in preventing episodes. Preference is given to selective β1 agents such as metoprolol, atenolol, and bisoprolol. Beta-blockers are contraindicated with severe bradycardia, high-degree AV block, sinus node dysfunction, significant bronchospasm, or asthma. Relative contraindications include peripheral vascular disease and severe depression; highly selective β1 agents can be used cautiously in chronic obstructive pulmonary disease. For vasospastic angina without fixed stenosis, such as variant angina, calcium channel blockers are preferred over beta-blockers.

2) Nitrates: As endothelium-dependent vasodilators, nitrates reduce myocardial oxygen demand and improve perfusion, relieving angina symptoms. However, they reflexively increase sympathetic tone and heart rate, so they are often combined with negative chronotropic agents like beta-blockers or non-dihydropyridine calcium channel blockers for chronic stable angina treatment. Combination therapy provides superior anti-anginal effects compared to monotherapy. Adequate nitrate-free intervals should be observed daily to minimize tolerance development. For effort angina, nitroglycerin can be dosed during the day with a nitrate-free period overnight, or transdermal patches applied in the morning and removed at bedtime.

Common nitrate adverse effects include headache, flushing, reflex tachycardia, and hypotension, more pronounced with short-acting nitroglycerin. Commonly used nitrate formulations include sublingual nitroglycerin 0.5 mg per dose; oral isosorbide mononitrate 40 mg once or twice daily; and oral isosorbide dinitrate 20-40 mg three to four times daily.

3) Calcium Channel Blockers: By improving coronary blood flow and reducing myocardial oxygen demand, calcium channel blockers relieve angina. For variant angina or angina primarily due to coronary vasospasm, they are first-line agents. Diltiazem and verapamil can slow AV conduction and are useful for angina patients with atrial fibrillation or flutter, but should be avoided with severe bradycardia, high-degree AV block, or sick sinus syndrome.

Common adverse effects of all calcium channel blockers include peripheral edema, constipation, palpitations, and flushing. Hypotension can also occur. Other side effects like headaches, dizziness, and fatigue may be seen. For stable angina with heart failure requiring long-acting calcium channel blockers, amlodipine or felodipine can be used.

Combination therapy with a beta-blocker and a long-acting calcium channel blocker is more effective than monotherapy. Additionally, beta-blockers can mitigate reflex tachycardia caused by dihydropyridine calcium channel blockers. Non-dihydropyridines like diltiazem or verapamil can be alternative options when beta-blockers are contraindicated, but caution is needed with this combination due to the increased risk of conduction disturbances and negative inotropy. It should be avoided in the elderly, especially those with bradycardia or LV dysfunction.

Commonly used calcium channel blockers include extended-release diltiazem 90-180 mg once daily; regular diltiazem 30-90 mg three times daily; amlodipine 5-10 mg once daily; felodipine 5-10 mg once daily; extended-release nifedipine 30-60 mg once daily; extended-release verapamil 120-240 mg once daily; and regular verapamil 40-80 mg three times daily.

(3) Other Therapeutic Agents

1) Trimetazidine: By modulating myocardial energy substrate utilization, inhibiting fatty acid oxidation, and optimizing myocardial energy metabolism, trimetazidine can improve myocardial ischemia, left-ventricular function, and relieve angina. It can be combined with anti-ischemic agents like beta-blockers to further relieve symptoms and increase exercise tolerance. The typical dose is 60 mg / day in three divided doses.

2) Nicorandil is a potassium channel opener with pharmacological properties similar to those of nitrates and may be effective for stable angina treatment. The typical dose is 6 mg / day in three divided doses.

V Common Questions in Consultation

1. Does Typical Angina Necessarily Indicate CAD? Angina is not unique to CAD; any diseases causing myocardial ischemia and hypoxia can induce angina. For example, aortic valve lesions (severe stenosis or regurgitation) and hypertrophic cardiomyopathy can reduce coronary blood flow and cause angina. Moreover, inflammatory small vessel lesions from conditions like rheumatic myocarditis, systemic lupus erythematosus, and polyarteritis nodosa may lead to angina. Therefore, during consultation, a thorough history (including family history) and physical examination are crucial. If auscultation reveals significant murmurs at the aortic area or left sternal border, aortic valve disease or hypertrophic cardiomyopathy should be considered as potential causes of angina.

2. Understanding the Value of ECG in CAD Diagnosis. Clinically, it is common for other departments to rule out CAD solely based on an ECG report of ST-T changes. However, disputes over postoperative deaths from acute myocardial infarction are not uncommon. As a result, preoperative consultations are increasingly requested to exclude CAD based on routine ECG ST-T abnormalities. Interpreting the value of ECG in CAD diagnosis is a frequent question we need to address. A single ECG cannot definitively evaluate CAD, whereas a normal ECG does not exclude its presence. ECG is not a highly sensitive diagnostic method for CAD; during the non-acute phase, only 30%-50% of cases show abnormalities, while over 50% have normal ECGs. Horizontal or downsloping ST-segment depression is often considered indicative of myocardial ischemia, but its sensitivity for diagnosing CAD is only around 50%. Conditions like hypertensive heart disease, cardiomyopathy, rheumatic heart disease, pericarditis, and autonomic dysfunction can also cause ST-T changes. "False positive" ECG changes are commonly seen in cardiovascular neurosis (due to sympathetic overactivity, more frequent in females). Therefore, a careful history, consideration of risk factors, age, and analysis of any atypical ischemic symptoms are necessary.

Evaluate for dynamic ST-T changes and localized abnormalities, and then decide if further testing with coronary CT or angiography is needed to establish the CAD diagnosis.

3. Stable vs. Unstable CAD. The terms "stable" and "unstable" are not permanent states, although their pathophysiological mechanisms differ. Stable CAD results from a supply-demand mismatch due to stenosis, causing relatively stable ischemic symptoms and a higher safety profile. In contrast, unstable CAD (acute coronary syndrome, ACS) is caused by plaque disruption and thrombosis, which lead to ischemia and an unstable clinical course that may progress to acute ST-elevation myocardial infarction. Therefore, in terms of antiplatelet therapy, intensified dual antiplatelet treatment is required for unstable CAD. Statin therapy should also be intensified.

If stable CAD is considered in consultation, a single antiplatelet agent like aspirin, along with statin therapy, is generally sufficient. For unstable CAD, dual antiplatelet therapy and intensive statin treatment are indicated. If unstable CAD is suspected, inpatient cardiology management is typically recommended. A common consultation question is the rationale for dual antiplatelet therapy, which aims to enhance antiplatelet effects and overcome potential drug resistance (e.g., aspirin or clopidogrel resistance).

4. Role of Antiplatelets and Statins in CAD Treatment. These are the two most important therapies for CAD. Antiplatelets are one of the most effective drugs for preventing the progression to acute myocardial infarction, as platelet activation and white thrombus formation are the initiating mechanisms in unstable CAD. If this progresses to a red / mixed thrombus, it represents the most severe stage: acute ST-elevation myocardial infarction. Statin therapy is currently the best treatment for atherosclerosis, with its main action being plaque stabilization and even regression, reducing stenosis. By converting unstable to stable CAD, statins are mechanistically the most important therapy for stable CAD from a pathophysiological perspective.

Ⅵ Consultation Process

1. Inquire about the patient's symptoms and signs. Details on chest pain location, quality, precipitating factors, duration, relieving factors, and associated symptoms can aid in the preliminary diagnosis of CAD. Physical examination findings are not particularly valuable for CAD diagnosis.

2. Assess the presence of risk factors

(1) Non-modifiable risks: age, gender, family history.

(2) Unhealthy lifestyle factors: hyperlipidemia, hypertension, smoking, diabetes, obesity, and sedentary behavior.

3. Diagnosis is based on clinical presentation, cardiac enzyme tests, and ECG changes. Recently, new diagnostic methods like radionuclide imaging, multi-slice CT (MSCT), and coronary angiography (CAG) have emerged for CAD evaluation.

4. Treatment

(1) Non-pharmacological: smoking cessation, dietary, and lifestyle modifica-tions.

(2) Pharmacological.

1) Drugs improving prognosis

A. Antiplatelets: aspirin, clopidogrel, ticagrelor, and prasugrel

B. Beta-blockers: Unless contraindicated, long-term use in CAD patients. Dosing is individualized, starting low and titrating to relieve symptoms while maintaining a heart rate of ≥50 bpm.

C. Lipid-lowering: Statins effectively reduce TC and LDL-C, decreasing cardiovascular events. They also slow plaque progression, stabilize plaques, and have anti-inflammatory effects. Potent statins, like rosuvastatin and atorvastatin, are recommended for CAD.

2) Drugs for symptom relief and improving ischemia

A. Beta-blockers: Unless contraindicated, first-line for stable angina. Reduce mortality and reinfarction risk in post-MI stable angina. Not preferred for vasospastic angina without fixed stenosis like variant angina; calcium channel blockers preferred.

B. Nitrates: Often combined with negative chronotropes like beta-blockers or non-dihydropyridine calcium channel blockers for chronic stable angina. Combination therapy is superior to monotherapy for symptom relief but does not improve the prognosis.

C. Calcium channel blockers: Relieve angina by improving coronary flow and reducing oxygen demand. First-line for variant angina or angina primarily due to vasospasm.

Combination beta-blockers and long-acting calcium channel blockers are more effective than monotherapy and can mitigate reflex tachycardia from dihydropyridines.

3) Other therapeutic agents

A. Trimetazidine optimizes myocardial energy metabolism by inhibiting fatty acid oxidation, improving ischemia and LV function, and relieving angina. It can be combined with anti-ischemic agents like beta-blockers to further relieve symptoms and increase exercise tolerance. Typical dose: 60 mg / day in 3 divided doses.

B. Nicorandil is a potassium channel opener with similar properties to nitrates and may be effective for stable angina treatment. Typical dose: 6 mg / day in 3 divided doses.

4) If medical therapy is suboptimal for recurrent angina, coronary angiography can evaluate the need for percutaneous or surgical revascularization.

Section 8 Strategies for CAD Myocardial Revascularization

I Revascularization Methods and Appropriateness

Coronary artery disease (CAD) is a leading global cause of disability and death. Myocardial revascularization, including percutaneous coronary intervention (PCI) and coronary artery bypass grafting (CABG), is an important CAD treatment. The main goals are to relieve symptoms and improve quality of life, as well as prolong survival.

Revascularization appropriateness refers to whether the anticipated benefits outweigh the expected negative impacts of the procedure, based on the patient's survival or health outcomes (symptoms, functional status, and / or quality of life). Determining revascularization appropriateness requires individualized consideration of multiple factors, primarily: ① Clinical presentation, such as acute coronary syndrome (ACS) or stable angina; ② Angina severity by Canadian Cardiovascular Society (CCS) class; ③ Degree of non-invasive ischemia testing; and presence of other prognostic factors, such as congestive heart failure, LV dysfunction, or diabetes; ④ Medical therapy status; ⑤ Anatomical extent of disease (1, 2 or 3-vessel, proximal LAD or left main involvement); In general, revascularization is appropriate for ACS and patients with severe symptoms and / or ischemia. Conversely, it may not be appropriate for asymptomatic patients or those at low risk for non-invasive testing receiving minimal medical therapy.

Ⅱ Risk Assessment

Risk-benefit assessment is fundamental to revascularization decision-making. Risk scoring systems can predict operative mortality or post-procedural major adverse cardiac and cerebrovascular events (MACCE), guiding risk stratification to inform the appropriate revascularization strategy. Common risk scores include:

1. The European System for Cardiac Operative Risk Evaluation Ⅱ (EuroSCORE Ⅱ) uses 18 clinical variables to estimate in-hospital mortality, replacing the original EuroSCORE, which overestimated procedural risk.

2. The SYNTAX score quantifies anatomical complexity based on 11 angiographic characteristics. For patients suitable for either PCI or CABG with low predicted surgical mortality, the SYNTAX score can guide revascularization strategy and remains widely used clinically.

3. The SYNTAX Ⅱ score incorporates the presence of unprotected left main disease into the original SYNTAX score, along with six clinical factors (age, creatinine clearance, LVEF, gender, COPD, and peripheral vascular disease) to enhance long-term mortality prediction after left main or complex 3-vessel revascularization compared to the SYNTAX score alone.

Ⅲ CAD Myocardial Revascularization Strategies

The choice of revascularization strategy for CAD is influenced by multiple factors, including patient characteristics, comorbidities, clinical presentation, coronary anatomy and lesion complexity, ischemic burden, left ventricular function, and patient preferences. For complex coronary disease, especially left main disease, a dedicated Heart Team of interventional and surgical specialists should comprehensively assess the risks and weigh the pros and cons of PCI versus CABG to individualize treatment selection. In principle, revascularization should be built upon optimal medical therapy to improve symptoms or prolong survival. While both PCI and CABG are important revascularization modalities with well-established techniques, their application should be guided by practice guidelines, integrating clinical expertise, technical proficiency, and thorough evaluation of patient risks and benefits to select the appropriate treatment strategy and devices that maximize benefit while minimizing harm.

1. Revascularization Strategy for Stable CAD. According to the 2016 Chinese Guidelines for Percutaneous Coronary Intervention, the decision for revascularization in stable coronary artery disease (SCAD) is based on the degree of coronary diameter stenosis. For $\geq 90\%$ diameter stenosis, revascularization can proceed directly. For $<90\%$ stenosis, intervention is recommended only if there is corresponding ischemic evidence or a fractional flow reserve (FFR) ≤ 0.8. In recent years, the widespread adoption of drug-eluting stents (DES) has significantly reduced long-term adverse event rates after PCI.

The indications for percutaneous coronary intervention (PCI) in stable coronary artery disease (SCAD) have gradually expanded. For patients with concomitant left main coronary artery (LMCA) and / or proximal left anterior descending (LAD) lesions, or multi-vessel disease, the guidelines recommend that for single or double vessel disease involving the proximal LAD, or LMCA or triple vessel disease with a SYNTAX score ≤ 22, revascularization strategy with either CABG or PCI is a Class Ⅰ recommendation. PCI for LMCA disease with a SYNTAX score of 23-32 is no longer contraindicated (Class Ⅱa, Level B evidence). However, for LMCA disease with a SYNTAX score >32 or triple vessel disease with a SYNTAX score >23, CABG remains the recommended revascularization strategy (Class Ⅰ) while PCI is considered inappropriate (Class Ⅲ, Level B).

Compared to PCI, CABG has the notable advantage that its benefit is consistent regardless of disease complexity, whereas for PCI, the rates of major adverse cardiovascular and cerebrovascular events and mortality gradually increase with greater complexity. Therefore, for complex multi-vessel coronary disease, current European and American guidelines still give a preferential Class Ⅰ recommendation for CABG over PCI (Clas Ⅱb, benefit uncertain) for improving survival. However, with advances in interventional devices and techniques, this advantage of CABG may diminish over time. For instance, optimal drug-eluting stent selection can impact the long-term efficacy and safety of PCI revascularization.

2. For non-ST-elevation acute coronary syndromes (NSTE-ACS). In the absence of ST-elevation on ECG, the 2016 Chinese guidelines first recommended using high-sensitivity cardiac troponin (hs-cTn) as an early diagnostic tool (Class Ⅰ, Level A). The guidelines recommend urgent (<2 hours) coronary angiography for very high-risk NSTE-ACS patients (Class Ⅰ, Level C), where very high-risk factors include: ①hemodynamic instability or cardiogenic shock; ②refractory angina; ③life-threatening arrhythmias or cardiac arrest; ④mechanical complications of myocardial infarction; ⑤acute heart failure with refractory angina and ST deviation; ⑥recurrent dynamic ST-T changes, especially intermittent ST-elevation. For high-risk patients, early (<24 hours) angiography is recommended to guide an invasive strategy according to findings (Class Ⅰ, Level A), with high-risk features including: ①elevated cardiac biomarkers; ②dynamic ECG ST-segment or T-wave changes (symptomatic or asymptomatic); ③GRACE risk score>140. Patients must have at least one intermediate-risk criterion: diabetes mellitus; renal dysfunction [eGFR<60 mL / (min1.73 m^2)]; LV ejection fraction<40% or congestive heart failure; post-infarction angina; recent PCI; prior CABG; or GRACE score 109-140, with a Class Ⅰ, Level A recommendation for invasive evaluation within 72 hours if there is recurrent angina or ischemia on non-invasive testing. For patients without high-risk features or recurrent symptoms, non-invasive testing (preferably imaging) is recommended before invasive evaluation (Class Ⅰ, Level A).

Ⅳ Common Questions and Considerations in Consultations

Common questions during consultation often include: whether to pursue PCI or CABG?

While the guidelines provide relatively clear indications, several important considerations must be weighed. Firstly, there is an imbalance in the development of interventional and surgical revascularization capabilities in China, especially at regional / municipal level hospitals. Secondly, the risks and success rates of redo CABG surgery must be considered. Age is another key factor—very young patients raise concerns about the long-term patency of bypass grafts, while advanced age increases surgical risks. In general, PCI may be preferred for: Moderate or larger areas of myocardial ischemia or viable myocardium, with single / double vessel disease involving the proximal LAD amenable to complete revascularization; Lesions with high angiographic PCI success rates, low surgical risk, and low restenosis rates (e.g. short lesions in vessels>2.5 mm diameter); Multi-vessel disease allowing complete revascularization by PCI; Surgical contraindications or need for major non-cardiac surgery; Acute coronary syndromes, especially acute myocardial infarction. CABG may be favored for: multi-vessel disease with LVEF<40% not amenable to complete revascularization by PCI; Left main coronary artery disease and / or proximal LAD disease with multi-vessel involvement; Interventional devices may be unable to access certain lesions, such as those with severe tortuosity, calcification, or chronic total occlusions; Patients with diabetes mellitus and diffuse multi-vessel disease precluding stent implantation; Alternating stenoses and aneurysmal dilatations; Or chronic total occlusion of the left anterior descending artery after anterior wall myocardial infarction where PCI is unlikely to be successful.

Furthermore, in addition to the above considerations, patient preferences should be incorporated into the choice of revascularization strategy for coronary artery disease. Individuals have diverse lifestyles, and when both PCI and CABG are viable options based on angiographic findings, eliciting the patient's perspective often plays a decisive role. For instance, patients desiring less discomfort, earlier recovery, and prompt return to work, while accepting a higher restenosis rate compared to CABG, may opt for PCI.

V Consultation Process

1. Assess appropriateness of revascularization: Based on the patient's survival or health status (symptoms, functional status and / or quality of life), revascularization is appropriate if the anticipated benefit outweighs the expected negative impacts of the procedure. In general, myocardial revascularization is appropriate for acute coronary syndromes and patients with severe symptoms and / or ischemia. Conversely, revascularization may be less appropriate for asymptomatic patients or those deemed low risk on non-invasive testing receiving optimal medical therapy.

2. Perform risk-benefit assessment: Using the SYNTAX Ⅱ score.

3. Myocardial revascularization strategy for coronary artery disease:

(1) For stable coronary disease: Refer to the 2016 Chinese Guidelines on Percutaneous Coronary Intervention.

(2) For non-ST-elevation acute coronary syndromes: First calculate the GRACE risk score to risk-stratify and guide timing of PCI.

(3) Patient preferences should also be considered when selecting the revascularization strategy. With equipoise between PCI and CABG for a given angiographic pattern, the patient's lifestyle perspectives often play a decisive role. For instance, patients desiring less discomfort, faster recovery and earlier return to work, while accepting a higher restenosis rate compared to CABG, may opt for PCI.

Section 9 Non-Invasive Assessment of Myocardial Ischemia

Current non-invasive methods for evaluating myocardial ischemia can be broadly classified into two categories: those that directly detect myocardial ischemia, primarily including characteristic clinical symptoms coupled with electrocardiographic changes, ambulatory ECG monitoring revealing characteristic patterns, exercise ECG testing, stress echocardiography, and myocardial perfusion scintigraphy, in addition to stress cardiac magnetic resonance imaging; and those that directly visualize coronary artery stenoses, mainly coronary CT angiography and coronary MR angiography which is still under investigation. These modalities employ different technical principles, resulting in varying diagnostic accuracy, specificity and sensitivity for myocardial ischemia, and consequently differing clinical utilities, necessitating optimal test selection.

I Non-Invasive Tests for Myocardial Ischemia

1. Resting ECG is the most direct and commonly used clinical method to detect myocardial ischemia. Characteristic ECG changes occur during an ischemic episode: ST-segment shifts (depression, elevation or pseudo-normalization), with rapid ST-segment resolution upon relief of chest pain, i.e. transient ST-T changes, support a diagnosis of ischemic angina; if typical evolutionary ECG patterns of myocardial infarction manifest, the diagnosis can be established.

Limitation: Non-specific ST-T changes (i.e. persistent rather than transient with ischemia) can be misdiagnosed clinically as coronary artery disease.

2. Ambulatory ECG Monitoring: If transient ST-T changes accompanied by significant heart rate increase or decrease are recorded, especially concurrent with typical angina symptoms, the diagnosis of myocardial ischemia is essentially established. Current ambulatory (Holter) ECG criteria for ischemia are: Horizontal or down-sloping ST-depression≥0.1 mV in≥2 contiguous leads, gradually developing, duration≥1 min, with post-episode ST resolution to baseline, and≥1 min between episodes, suggesting ischemic ST changes; concomitant ischemia-induced arrhythmias further support the diagnosis. Brief episodes of ST-elevation coinciding with angina symptoms are valuable for diagnosing variant angina due to coronary artery spasm. Furthermore, in established coronary artery disease with myocardial ischemia, 12-lead ambulatory ECG demonstrating characteristic transient ST-T changes can assist in diagnosing silent ischemia.

3. Exercise ECG Testing is primarily used clinically for routine screening of suspected or stable chronic coronary artery disease, with 60%-70% specificity and accuracy, but variable sensitivity depending on extent of disease. Exercise ECG testing includes treadmill or bicycle protocols, evaluating 12-lead ECG changes with exercise stress, with ST-segment shifts being the primary marker of ischemia. Abnormal blood pressure response and severe ventricular arrhythmias during exercise also suggest myocardial ischemia and severe coronary disease.

The advantages are simplicity, low cost, and widespread clinical use for CAD diagnosis, risk stratification and ischemia assessment. For women with normal resting ECGs able to exercise adequately, guidelines recommend exercise ECG as the initial ischemia detection method. However, exercise ECG has limited sensitivity for detecting non-obstructive (<70% stenosis) disease and is affected by age, sex, medications and comorbidities. Exercise testing is contraindicated in unstable clinical scenarios where increased cardiac demand may exacerbate unstable coronary lesions.

4. Stress Echocardiography principally detects ischemia by identifying wall motion abnormalities induced during exercise or pharmacologic stress. It has approximately 80% sensitivity and specificity for detecting ischemia, superior to exercise ECG alone. On dobutamine stress echocardiography, development of transient ischemic left ventricular dilation at peak stress highly suggests multi-vessel disease, with 85%-90% sensitivity and specificity.

5. Stress Myocardial Perfusion Imaging detects myocardial ischemia by identifying reversible perfusion defects during stress, with 70%-90% sensitivity, 75%-96% specificity and 85%-90% accuracy for diagnosing coronary artery disease. It is a relatively accurate non-invasive method for stable CAD diagnosis. Stress can be exercise or pharmacologic (adenosine, dipyridamole, dobutamine), useful in patients with resting ECG abnormalities unable to exercise adequately.

However, utility is limited by radioisotope supply issues, restricting routine use predominantly to tertiary centers. Additionally, perfusion imaging only detects advanced coronary stenoses but cannot identify early plaque or non-obstructive disease.

6. Coronary CT Angiography: Coronary CT Angiography is currently applied to coronary segments≥1.5 mm diameter, demonstrating 83%-93% sensitivity and 82%-97% specificity for detecting stenoses, with 71%-83% positive and 92%-98% negative predictive values. In patients with severe coronary calcification, sensitivity and negative predictive value are reduced. Clinical applications include symptomatic patients, ECG abnormalities, inability to exercise, or cases requiring evaluation for coronary disease. Multi-slice spiral CT (MDCT) can detect coronary artery plaques at an early stage and estimate their overall tissue composition and nature based on CT values. This includes calcified, fibrous, soft, and mixed plaques, allowing for a preliminary assessment of plaque vulnerability.

Coronary CT angiography can be affected by heart rate, rhythm, coronary calcification, stents, and pacemakers, making accurate quantification of luminal stenosis difficult, especially for mild to moderate stenosis. There are also radiation safety concerns, so indications must be strictly followed to avoid overuse. It should not be used for routine coronary artery disease screening in clinical practice. Patients with liver or kidney dysfunction or contrast allergies cannot undergo CTA.

7. MRI: Coronary MRI is still under investigation and not yet clinically applied.

Ⅱ Comparison of Methods

The specificity of coronary CT angiography can reach 97%, while other methods (ambulatory ECG, exercise ECG testing, dobutamine stress echocardiography, stress nuclear perfusion imaging) have 70%-75% specificity. Nuclear perfusion has the highest sensitivity, while ambulatory ECG monitoring has the lowest sensitivity. Although exercise ECG testing has relatively low specificity and sensitivity, it is simple, inexpensive and clinically useful as an initial screening test for myocardial ischemia. Exercise stress echocardiography provides better prognostic value than exercise ECG testing alone. The sensitivity, specificity and accuracy of adenosine stress echo in detecting myocardial perfusion abnormalities are comparable or even superior to nuclear perfusion imaging. Stress nuclear perfusion can detect myocardial ischemia and display coronary perfusion status. Coronary angiographic techniques can more directly and accurately reveal the degree and location of coronary stenoses. As imaging technology improves, image quality, specificity and sensitivity will continue to increase. Combining anatomic and functional ischemia testing aids in comprehensive diagnosis and risk stratification. Clinically, non-invasive ischemia detection should be applied reasonably for early diagnosis, risk stratification and selection of appropriate treatment to reduce costs and avoid wasted resources.

Ⅲ Consultation Process

1. Obtain a detailed medical history, including symptom onset, triggering / relieving factors, underlying cardiac or chronic systemic diseases, hypertension, diabetes, liver / kidney dysfunction, acute presentation, fever, cough, sputum, diaphoresis, cyanosis, hemoptysis, trauma, foreign body aspiration, or poisoning.

2. Rapidly assess vital signs based on level of consciousness, responses, heart rate, blood pressure and pulse oximetry.

3. Obtain a resting ECG promptly. Based on ECG and history, determine if the patient is in an unstable ischemic state, using non-exercise (e.g. ambulatory ECG, CT angiography) rather than exercise testing as the initial approach to avoid provoking severe ischemia.

4. Perform relevant physical exam (e.g. breath sounds, lip cyanosis, chest tenderness / percussion, asymmetric chest excursion, heart sounds / borders, jugular venous distension, neurological findings).

5. Rapid auxiliary examinations are necessary, such as bedside troponin tests, myocardial enzyme spectrum, blood gas analysis, renal function, electrolytes, chest X-rays, BNP or NT-proBNP, D-dimer, etc. If the preliminary test results rule out conditions such as acute myocardial infarction, acute pulmonary embolism, aortic dissection, and pneumothorax, further comprehensive examinations can be conducted to assess the presence of myocardial ischemia.

Section 10 Diagnosis and Treatment of Vulnerable Plaques

Coronary atherosclerotic heart disease (CHD) poses a severe threat to human health. Acute coronary syndromes (ACS) represent the acute manifestations of CHD. Pathologically, ACS results from progression of an atherosclerotic plaque to a vulnerable plaque that ruptures, causing complete or partial occlusive thrombosis.

Ⅰ Overview

A vulnerable plaque is one prone to thrombosis or rapid progression to culprit lesion, mainly including plaque rupture, erosive plaque, and partially calcified nodular plaque. Literature indicates patients with vulnerable plaque have a 4%-13% annual risk of cardiovascular events. Vulnerable plaques generally occur in the proximal coronary arteries and may not appear severely stenotic on angiography, potentially underestimating cardiovascular risk. Therefore, identifying vulnerable plaques is crucial. Plaque rupture accounts for 70%-75% of atherothrombosis, while erosive plaques are an important cause of coronary thrombosis / sudden death in premenopausal women. The vulnerability of partially calcified nodular plaques remains controversial. Plaque erosion exhibits distinct pathological and anatomical characteristics compared to plaque rupture.

Ⅱ Features

1. Large lipid core (>40% plaque volume);

2. Thin fibrous cap (<65 μm) with macrophage, activated T-lymphocyte, mast cell infiltration;

3. Decreased collagen, smooth muscle cells in fibrous cap;

4. Positive vascular remodeling;

5. Neovascularization;

6. Calcified nodules.

Ⅲ Biomarkers

1. C-Reactive Protein (CRP): Elevated high-sensitivity CRP reflects more vulnerable plaque in ACS patients and is the main serum marker. Plasma CRP independently predicts early and late mortality in intermediate / high-risk ACS, especially if troponin-positive.

2. Matrix Metalloproteinases (MMPs): MMPs are primarily activated and secreted by monocytes-macrophages and smooth muscle cells. The pathological mechanism of MMPs involves the degradation of the extracellular matrix, weakening the fibrous cap of plaques. Studies have indicated that the overexpression of MMPs is an independent risk factor for predicting the onset of Acute Coronary Syndrome (ACS), and their combined use with other inflammatory markers can enhance sensitivity.

3. Myeloperoxidase (MPO): A heme protein whose product HOCl can activate MMPs and inactivate MMP inhibitors.

4. Lipoprotein-associated Phospholipase A2: A zinc-binding protein from inflammatory bone marrow cells, secreted by macrophages / lymphocytes and upregulated by inflammatory mediators. Most binds LDL, hydrolyzing oxidized phospholipids to promote inflammation / atherosclerosis.

5. Adiponectin: An adipocyte-derived hormone that binds endothelial cells, inhibiting adhesion molecule expression and reducing inflammation. It also binds macrophage C1q, inhibiting phagocytic activity and foam cell formation. Research indicate that Low adiponectin levels strongly predict the presence of thin-capped fibroatheromas.

Ⅳ Imaging Examination

1. Angiography: Currently the "gold standard" for evaluating vascular stenosis. After contrast injection, vessels can be viewed from different angles to directly assess diameter and basic plaque morphology. The Ambrose angiographic classification divides plaques into 4 types: ① Concentric stenosis with smooth borders, relatively stable; ② Type Ⅰ eccentric stenosis with wide neck and smooth borders, relatively stable; ③ Type Ⅱ eccentric stenosis with irregular / overhanging / multiple borders forming a neck-like protrusion into the lumen, unstable and prone to rupture; ④ Multiple irregular stenoses, unstable and prone to rupture. Angiographically, vulnerable plaques often appear eccentric with irregular surfaces, filling defects, ulceration and thrombus.

2. Intravascular Ultrasound (IVUS): Widely used to detect plaque features like intraplaque hemorrhage, size, lipid pool, fibrous cap, vascular remodeling and calcification patterns. Sensitivity>90%, maximal resolution 100 μm (typically 100-250 μm). The limitation is modest resolution inadequate for precise vulnerable plaque characterization.

3. Virtual Histology IVUS (VH-IVUS): Based on IVUS, it identifies and color-codes plaque components by analyzing radio-frequency back-scatter signals, allowing visualization of necrotic core and fibrosis. Also limited by resolution.

4. Optical Coherence Tomography (OCT): Uses infrared light waves to image coronary artery wall structure, providing cross-sectional images of lumen dimensions, thrombus, plaque morphology / features like lipid burden, calcification, fibrous cap thickness. Can identify thrombus, dissection and stent positioning. Compared to angiography / IVUS, OCT more readily detects plaque rupture in ST-elevation ACS and thin-cap fibroatheroma, with 100% sensitivity for thrombus detection vs. 33% for IVUS. OCT also found plaque erosion in 23% of cases missed by IVUS / angiography.

5. Angioscopy: Plaque color (yellow, white) on angioscopy reflects composition and presence of intraluminal thrombus. Thin-cap fibroatheromas with lipid-rich cores appear yellow; thick-cap plaques rich in smooth muscle appear white. Platelet-rich thrombi at rupture sites are white granular deposits; fibrin / red cell-rich thrombi are irregular red intraluminal structures. Yellow lesions correspond to vulnerable plaques, with greater yellowness indicating higher rupture / thrombosis risk. However, in recent years, with the development of more advanced technologies such as Optical Coherence Tomography (OCT), the use of intravascular endoscopy has gradually decreased.

6. Multi-slice Coronary CT (MSCT): Can depict plaque composition based on differential CT attenuation values within the plaque. A disadvantage is that the examination has relatively high requirements for the patient.

7. MRI: Can differentiate lipid cores, calcification, fibrous caps and thrombus formation in unstable plaques. Sensitivity and specificity are 75% and 90% respectively for lipid necrotic core detection. T1-weighted hyper-intense signal suggests intraplaque hemorrhage, a marker of vulnerability.

8. Near-Infrared Spectroscopy (NIRS): Evaluates lipid and protein content of atherosclerotic plaques. Lipid core probability is displayed by color scale from red (low) to yellow (high). NIRS rapidly acquires data without obstructing coronary flow but is an invasive procedure.

V Treatment

1. Statins significantly lower LDL-C and have anti-inflammatory, anti-angiogenic effects. They reduce plaque volume, increase fibrous tissue, decrease lipid / inflammation within plaques and increase fibrous cap thickness, enhancing stability.

2. RAS inhibitors (ACEIs, ARBs) may stabilize vulnerable plaques in ACS and improve cardiac function. Beta-blockers are used empirically for vulnerable plaque, lacking robust evidence.

3. Antiplatelet therapy: Aspirin's role in secondary prevention of vulnerable plaque is well-

established. Clopidogrel or ticagrelor can be used if aspirin-intolerant. Other agents lack sufficient clinical evidence.

Ⅵ Consultation Process

1. ACS is often linked to vulnerable plaque, so clinically unstable angina (prone to evolve to AMI) should prompt consideration of vulnerable plaque.

2. In pre-procedural assessment, check for biomarkers like CRP, MMPs, MPO, Lp-PLA2, adiponectin suggesting vulnerable plaque.

3. If vulnerable plaque suspected pre-procedurally, perform relevant imaging and intensify plaque treatment peri-procedurally.

Section 11 Antiplatelet Therapy Strategies After PCI

Atherosclerosis and thrombosis are systemic, progressive diseases that commonly affect the heart, brain and peripheral arteries. Under the influence of cardiovascular risk factors, atherosclerotic plaques develop and their rupture triggers thrombus formation, leading to severe ischemic events. Patients with SCAD can progress to acute coronary syndromes (ACS) or even cardiac death.

The development of PCI has spanned plain old balloon angioplasty (POBA), bare metal stents (BMS), and drug-eluting stents (DES).

PCI effectively relieves angina, improves cardiac function / quality of life, and may extend survival—an indispensable therapy for coronary disease, especially as primary PCI has become one of the most effective treatments for ST-elevation myocardial infarction (STEMI). While reducing restenosis rates, first-generation non-degradable polymer DES had significantly higher late stent thrombosis risk than BMS. Current guidelines thus recommend at least 1 year of dual antiplatelet therapy (DAPT) after DES to reduce late stent thrombosis. However, prolonged DAPT is a double-edged sword—in addition to increased costs, it markedly elevates bleeding risk. Despite advances like new DES, technical improvements, intravascular imaging guidance and optimized periprocedural secondary prevention, optimal DAPT duration / dosing and management of clopidogrel resistance remain debated to balance ischemic and bleeding risks.

Ⅰ Antiplatelet Therapy Progress

Antiplatelet agents with different mechanisms act synergistically. Aspirin remains first-line for primary / secondary prevention of ischemic events; clopidogrel is "standard" after PCI; routine GPIIb / Ⅲa inhibitors are not recommended except for angiographically-proven thrombus burden or inadequate P2Y12 inhibitor loading. Recent PCI advances involve P2Y12 inhibitors and phosphodiesterase- Ⅲ inhibitors.

Prasugrel is a newer thienopyridine that metabolizes in the liver to an active P2Y12 inhibitor, with faster onset and 10-100x greater platelet inhibition than clopidogrel, less metabolic variation and no resistance. Loading 60 mg, maintenance 10 mg / day. Mainly used for defined lesions, clopidogrel resistance or diabetes. In TRITON-TIMI38, net clinical benefit favored prasugrel over clopidogrel in moderate / high-risk ACS undergoing PCI.

Ticagrelor is a newer cyclopentyltriazolopyrimidine that reversibly binds the P2Y12 receptor with faster, more potent platelet inhibition independent of metabolism. Loading 180 mg, maintenance 90 mg bid for≥1 year. It can be used in STEMI / NSTE-ACS regardless of initial treatment strategy. In the PLATO trial of 18,624 ACS patients randomized to ticagrelor or clopidogrel, ticagrelor reduced the composite endpoint by 16%, cardiovascular death by 21%, MI by 16% and definite stent thrombosis by 31%, without increased major bleeding.

Cilostazol is a selective phosphodiesterase-Ⅲ inhibitor with antiplatelet, vasodilatory and antiproliferative effects used for intermittent claudication (maintenance 100 mg bid). It is primarily used for high-risk ACS, especially clopidogrel resistance. Recent studies like the Korean DECLARE-LONG and DECLARE-DIABETES trials have highlighted the potential of triple anti-thrombotic therapy with cilostazol added to DAPT to reduce thrombotic events and restenosis after higher-risk DES implantation.

Ⅱ Antiplatelet Pretreatment for PCI

1. SCAD

(1) Elective PCI: Preload with aspirin 100-300 mg before elective stenting, then 100 mg / day maintenance. For PCI>6 h out, give clopidogrel 300-600 mg; for 2-6 h, 600 mg. For long-term 75 mg / day clopidogrel, reload 300-600 mg if proceeding to PCI.

(2) Intraprocedural: If no clopidogrel / aspirin pretreatment, recommend oral loading with clopidogrel 300-600 mg and aspirin 100-300 mg; consider GPIIb / Ⅲa inhibitor for urgent cases.

2. Non-ST Elevation ACS (NSTE-ACS): All patients without aspirin contraindication: initial aspirin load 100-300 mg then 100 mg / day maintenance. For early PCI, prefer ticagrelor (180 mg load, 90 mg bid maintenance) over clopido-grel. For intermediate-high ischemic risk (e.g. elevated troponin, including on clopidogrel), prefer ticagrelor. Clopidogrel: 600 mg load, 75 mg / day maintenance. GPIIb / Ⅲa can be considered for urgency or thrombotic complications; not recom-mended for pretreatment if no known coronary lesion.

3. ST Elevation MI (STEMI): All patients without aspirin contraindication: initial aspirin load 100-300 mg then 100 mg / day maintenance. Add a P2Y12 inhibitor—ticagrelor 180 mg load then 90 mg bid if no contraindication; clopidogrel 600 mg load then 75 mg / day if no ticagrelor access / contraindication. Use GPIIb / Ⅲa for urgency, no reflow or thrombotic complications. High-risk transfer for primary PCI can receive GPIIb / Ⅲa pretreated.

Ⅲ DAPT Duration

1. SCAD: Minimum 4 weeks after BMS; 4-6 weeks if BMS / POBA for elective non-cardiac surgery; 4-6 weeks if high bleeding risk, intolerant to 12 months DAPT or likely interruption within 12 months after BMS / POBA; 6 months after DES; consider<6 months if high bleeding risk after DES; 1-3 months if high bleeding risk, urgent non-cardiac surgery or oral anti-coagulation after DES;>6 months if high ischemic / low bleeding risk after DES; lifelong aspirin recommended after stopping P2Y12 inhibitor.

2. NSTE-ACS: Add P2Y12 inhibitor to aspirin for≥12 months unless contraindicated (e.g. high bleeding risk); if high ischemic / low bleeding risk, consider>1 year of DAPT.

3. STEMI: Add P2Y12 inhibitor to aspirin for≥12 months unless contraindicated (e.g. high bleeding risk).

Ⅳ Bleeding Risk Assessment and Prevention

Preventive measures for bleeding include: Pre-procedural bleeding risk assessment for all patients undergoing PCI, using the CRUSADE (Can Rapid risk stratification of Unstable angina patients Suppress Adverse outcomes with Early implementation) score (Tables 1-4, 1-5); preferential use of the radial artery approach; for high bleeding risk patients (e.g. renal dysfunction, advanced age, bleeding history, low body weight), prioritize anti-thrombotic agents with lower bleeding risk like bivalirudin or fondaparinux in the periprocedural period; weight-based anti-thrombotic dosing during PCI; and ACT monitoring to avoid over-systemic anti-coagulation.

Table 1-4 CRUSADE Scoring System

Variable Estimation	Range	Score
Baseline hematocrit (%)	<31	9
	31-33.9	7
	34-36.9	3
	37-39.9	2
	≥40	0
Creatinine clearance (mL / min)	≤15	39
	>15-30	35
	>30-60	28
	>60-90	17
	>90-120	7
	>120	0
Heart rate (bpm)	≤70	0
	71-80	1
	81-90	3
	91-100	6
	101-110	8
	111-120	10
	≥121	11
Sex	Male	0
	Female	8
Signs of heart failure	Yes	7
	No	0

(Continued)

Variable Estimation	Range	Score
Prior vascular disease (PAD or stroke)	No	0
	Yes	6
Diabetes mellitus	Yes	6
	No	0
Systolic blood pressure (mmHg)	≤90	10
	91-100	8
	101-120	5
	121-180	1
	181-200	3
	≥201	5

Table 1-5 Risk Stratification

Risk Level	Lowest Score	Highest Score	Bleeding Rate
Very Low	1	20	3.1%
Low	21	30	5.5%
Moderate	31	40	8.6%
High	41	50	11.9%
Very High	51	91	19.5%

Whether to stop or adjust antiplatelet / anticoagulant therapy after bleeding requires individualized assessment weighing bleeding vs recurrent ischemic event risk. Initial post-bleed management is usually non-pharmacologic, e.g. mechanical compression; recording timing / dosing of last anticoagulant or thrombolytic, liver / kidney function; estimating drug half-lives; identifying the bleeding source; checking CBC, coagulation tests, fibrinogen, creatinine; antiplatelet / anticoagulant activity assays if available; Ⅳ fluids and PRBC for hemodynamic instability; endoscopic, interventional or surgical local hemostasis if needed. If bleeding risk outweighs ischemic risk, anti-thrombotic agents should be stopped promptly. If inadequate response, pharmacologic measures can be tried: protamine to reverse unfractionated heparin at 1 mg / (80-100 U) heparin, maximum 50 mg; protamine can reverse 60% of low-molecular weight heparin (LMWH) at 1 mg / 100 U anti-Xa if given<8 h after LMWH, with an additional 0.5 mg / 100 U anti-Xa if ineffective. After withholding aspirin for 3 d, clopidogrel 5 d or ticagrelor 3 d, risks of bleeding vs recurrent ischemia should be re-evaluated to guide resumption of anti-thrombotic therapy.

V Summary

The optimal DAPT regimen (agents, doses, duration) after PCI requires further study due to conflicting evidence, lack of large-randomized trials, heterogeneous study populations, and variability in stent types / dosing / timing. Clinical practice should comprehensively consider ischemic risk, bleeding risk, medication adherence and cost to optimize individualized DAPT. High-risk features such as left main / bifurcation / bypass graft disease, ACS, diabetes, renal dysfunction or antiplatelet resistance should prompt treatment intensification via increased dosing, prolonged duration or agent adjustment. For lower risk, standard DAPT≥6 months is reasonable.

Ⅵ Consultation Process

Antiplatelet therapy is integral throughout coronary disease management, especially for patients undergoing PCI. Maximizing platelet inhibition while minimizing bleeding is challenging for the cardiovascular clinician and requires individualized risk assessment based on disease characteristics.

For established disease types / bleeding risks, follow the above principles strictly. If the clinical situation is unclear initially: First, assess urgency, prioritizing life-threatening conditions; second, clarify disease type and bleeding risk before initiating therapy; third, adjust strategy as the clinical course evolves; fourth, regardless of the ultimate regimen, thoroughly discuss the risks / benefits with the patient / family, inform about potential adverse events and management approaches.

Section 12 Anti-thrombotic Therapy After PCI in Atrial Fibrillation

Atrial fibrillation (AF) is the most common sustained cardiac arrhythmia, affecting around 1% of the population, with increasing prevalence by age nearly 70% of cases occur between 65-85 years old, and around 10% in those over 70. As two prevalent cardiovascular diseases, AF and coronary artery disease (CAD) share certain risk factors like diabetes and hypertension. Conversely, some clinical CAD scenarios like heart failure are also risk factors for AF. Therefore, CAD is one of the most common comorbidities in AF, with 20%-30% of AF patients having concomitant CAD.

AF treatment often requires oral anti-coagulation (OAC) to reduce stroke risk, while CAD necessitates long-term antiplatelet therapy to mitigate coronary events, especially after PCI where stent restenosis and thrombosis risks increase the complexity of anti-thrombotic management. Clinicians are thus faced with a dilemma in addressing both conditions concurrently, requiring a balanced approach to stroke versus bleeding risks.

Ⅰ Assessment of Stroke Risk in Patients with Atrial Fibrillation (AF)—The CHA2DS2-VASc Scoring System

In the past, the commonly used risk stratification method for atrial fibrillation was the CHADS2 scoring system. This method is simple, rapid, and easy to remember, but its shortcoming lies in its failure to recognize that risk is a continuous, unified entity. The CHADS2 score mainly focuses on selecting high-risk patients for anti-coagulation therapy. The 2010 ESC

Guidelines for Atrial Fibrillation introduced a new assessment method, CHA2DS2-VASc, also known as the "nine-point" evaluation method. This approach clarifies the low-risk factors for atrial fibrillation patients and scores based on major and minor risk factors. The guidelines tend to enhance the status of anti-coagulation therapy, emphasizing that 90% of patients require anti-coagulation treatment. The 2010 ESC Guidelines for Atrial Fibrillation recommend directly selecting anti-thrombotic therapy strategies based on risk factors. Patients with one major risk factor or two or more clinically relevant non-major risk factors, i.e., a CHA2DS2-VASc score≥2, should receive oral anticoagulants (OACs). For patients with one clinically relevant non-major risk factor, i.e., a CHA2DS2-VASc score of 1, either OACs or aspirin can be used, but OACs are preferentially recommended. For patients without risk factors, i.e., a CHA2DS2-VASc score of 0, aspirin or no anti-thrombotic therapy can be used, with no anti-thrombotic therapy being the preferred option. The 2016 ESC Guidelines continue to recommend the use of the CHA2DS2-VASc score as a stroke assessment tool. The guidelines indicate that for males with a CHA2DS2-VASc score≥2 and females with a score≥3, OACs are recommended. For patients with a CHA2DS2-VASc score of 1 or 2, the use of OACs can be considered. For patients suitable for new oral anticoagulants (NOACs), NOACs are preferentially recommended. For patients without other risk factors, neither anti-coagulation nor antiplatelet therapy is recommended.

Ⅱ Bleeding Risk Assessment in AF—HAS-BLED Score

For AF patients with multiple stroke risk factors, especially the elderly, the safety of OAC (major bleeding risk) remains clinically challenging. Based on the Euro Heart Survey on AF and SPORTIF Ⅲ / Ⅳ trials, the 2010 ESC AF guidelines recommend using the HAS-BLED score to assess bleeding risk, with a score≥3 indicating "high risk" requiring caution with OAC or aspirin. However, factors increasing stroke risk like advanced age, hypertension, prior stroke also elevate bleeding risk, making anti-thrombotic selection difficult in many high-risk patients despite the guideline's broader recommendations and enhanced practicality.

Ⅲ Anti-thrombotic Strategies After PCI in AF

1. Triple Therapy—Weighing Risks and Benefits: For post-PCI anti-thrombotic management in AF, the ACTIVE-W and ACTIVE-A trials showed warfarin was superior to combined aspirin / clopidogrel for thromboprophylaxis but with similar bleeding risks. Since dual antiplatelet therapy (DAPT) is the cornerstone of PCI and evidence-based for acute coronary syndromes, it cannot be omitted for CAD treatment. However, DAPT alone is insufficient for stroke prevention in AF. Consequently, in 2007, the American College of Cardiology (ACC) / American Heart Association (AHA) / Society for Cardiovascular Angiography and Interventions (SCAI) guidelines were modified and new recommendations regarding triple anti-thrombotic therapy with aspirin, clopidogrel, and warfarin were added.

For patients who underwent percutaneous coronary intervention (PCI) and had indications for anti-coagulation (such as atrial fibrillation or left ventricular thrombus), the addition of an anticoagulant was recommended. However, the guidelines simultaneously highlighted that triple anti-thrombotic therapy increases the risk of bleeding and advised that patients receiving triple therapy should be prescribed low-dose aspirin (75-81 mg / day) and clopidogrel (75 mg / day), while maintaining a strict international normalized ratio (INR) control between 2.0 and 2.5. Robust evidence supports DAPT for reducing coronary events and warfarin for stroke risk reduction in AF. So, the main concern with triple therapy is not its efficacy but the potential for increased bleeding. Clinicians often hesitate prescribing it despite meeting indications, due to the perceived elevated bleeding hazard. For example, in AF patients after PCI requiring triple therapy yet at high bleeding risk, antiplatelet therapy may be prioritized if the stent was placed in a critical location (e.g. left main, proximal LAD) where stent complications could be catastrophic, whereas anti-coagulation may take precedence for more distal or non-critical lesions simply aimed at improving quality of life.

2. Anti-thrombotic Treatment Plan After PCI in AF: The 2014 AHA / ACC / Heart Rhythm Society (HRS) AF Management Guideline recommends oral anticoagulants plus clopidogrel (without aspirin) for post-coronary revascularization AF patients with a CHA2DS2-VASc score≥2. On August 25, 2014, the ESC Thrombosis Working Group, European Heart Rhythm Association (EHRA), European Association of Percutaneous Cardiovascular Interventions (EAPCI), and Acute Cardiovascular Care Association (ACCA) jointly formulated and published the "Management of anti-thrombotic Therapy in Atrial Fibrillation Patients Presenting with Acute Coronary Syndrome and / or Undergoing Percutaneous Coronary or Valve Interventions: A Joint Consensus Document of the ESC / EHRA / EAPCI / ACCA." This consensus was also supported by the Heart Rhythm Society (HRS) and the Asia Pacific Heart Rhythm Society (APHRS). The interventional procedures covered by the consensus include percutaneous coronary intervention (PCI) and trans-catheter aortic valve implantation (TAVI). For atrial fibrillation patients with moderate-to-high thromboembolic risk (with an indication for oral anticoagulants) undergoing PCI, the recommended anti-thrombotic therapy strategies are presented in Table 1-6.

On August 27, 2016, the European Society of Cardiology (ESC) and European Association for Cardio-Thoracic Surgery (EACTS) jointly released the *2016 ESC Guidelines for the Management of Atrial Fibrillation*. The guidelines state that for stable coronary artery disease with atrial fibrillation, vitamin K antagonists can be used alone, while for ACS and / or PCI, antiplatelet therapy is needed in combination. The recommendations are: ① For atrial fibrillation with stable coronary disease and stroke risk, triple therapy (aspirin + clopidogrel + OAC) for 1 month after stenting to prevent coronary and cerebral ischemic events. ② For ACS, atrial fibrillation and stroke risk, triple therapy for 1-6 months after stenting to prevent coronary and cerebral ischemic events. ③ For ACS, atrial fibrillation and stroke risk without stenting, dual therapy (OAC + aspirin or clopidogrel) for 12 months to prevent coronary and cerebral ischemic events. ④ For patients on dual (especially triple) anti-thrombotic therapy, the ischemic and bleeding risks should be evaluated to achieve a balance between the two. ⑤ Dual therapy (OAC and clopidogrel 75 mg / d) may be used as an alternative to prior triple anti-thrombotic therapy in selected patients.

In summary, selecting an anti-thrombotic strategy after PCI in atrial fibrillation patients is highly challenging, as we are concerned about bleeding risk on one hand, but also worried

Table 1-6 Post-PCI Anti-thrombotic Regimens for Moderate-High Thromboembolism Risk AF Patients (OAC Indicated)

Bleeding Risk	Stroke Risk	Clinical Scenario	Recommendation
Low or Moderate (HAS-BLED 0-2)	Moderate Reproduced with permission from 365 Medical Network (CHA2DS2-VASC=1 for males)	Reproduced with permission from 365 Medical Network Stable Coronary Artery Disease	At least 4 weeks (up to 6 months): Triple anti-thrombotic therapy (OAC + aspirin 75-100 mg / d + clopidogrel 75 mg / d)[a] Treatment up to 12 months: OAC + clopidogrel 75 mg / d (or aspirin 75-100 mg / d)[b] Lifelong OAC[c]
	High Reproduced with permission from 365 Medical Network (CHA2DS2-VASC≥2)	Reproduced with permission from 365 Medical Network Stable Coronary Artery Disease	At least 4 weeks (up to 6 months): Triple anti-thrombotic therapy (OAC + aspirin 75-100 mg / d + clopidogrel 75 mg / d)[d] Treatment up to 12 months: OAC + clopidogrel 75 mg / d (or aspirin 75-100 mg / d) Lifelong OAC[c]
	Moderate Reproduced with permission from 365 Medical Network Reproduced with permission from 365 Medical Network (CHA2DS2-VASC=1 for males)	Reproduced with permission from 365 Medical Network Acute Coronary Syndrome	6 months: Triple anti-thrombotic therapy (OAC + aspirin 75-100 mg / d + clopidogrel 75 mg / d) Treatment up to 12 months: OAC + clopidogrel 75 mg / d (or aspirin 75-100 mg / d) Lifelong OAC[c]
	High Reproduced with permission from 365 Medical Network (CHA2DS2-VASC≥2)	Reproduced with permission from 365 Medical Network Acute Coronary Syndrome	6 months: Triple anti-thrombotic therapy (OAC + aspirin 75-100 mg / d + clopidogrel 75 mg / d) Treatment up to 12 months: OAC + clopidogrel 75 mg / d (or aspirin 75-100 mg / d) Lifelong OAC[c]
High Reproduced with permission from 365 Medical Network (HAS-BLED≥3)	Moderate Reproduced with permission from 365 Medical Network (CHA2DS2-VASC=1 for males)	Reproduced with permission from 365 Medical Network Stable Coronary Artery Disease	12 months: OAC + clopidogrel 75 mg / d Lifelong OAC[c]

(Continued)

Bleeding Risk	Stroke Risk	Clinical Scenario	Recommendation
	High Reproduced with permission from 365 Medical Network (CHA2DS2-VASC≥2)	Reproduced with permission from 365 Medical Network Stable Coronary Artery Disease	4 weeks: Triple anti-thrombotic therapy (OAC + aspirin 75-100 mg / d + clopidogrel 75 mg / d)[a] Treatment up to 12 months: OAC + clopidogrel 75 mg / d (or aspirin 75-100 mg / d) Lifelong OAC[c]
High Reproduced with permission from 365 Medical Network (HAS-BLED≥3)	Moderate Reproduced with permission from 365 Medical Network (CHA2DS2-VASC=1 for males)	Reproduced with permission from 365 Medical Network Acute Coronary Syndrome	4 weeks: Triple anti-thrombotic therapy (OAC + aspirin 75-100 mg / d + clopidogrel 75 mg / d)[d] Treatment up to 12 months: OAC + clopidogrel 75 mg / d (or aspirin 75-100 mg / d) Lifelong OAC[c]
	High Reproduced with permission from 365 Medical Network (CHA2DS2-VASC≥2)	Reproduced with permission from 365 Medical Network Acute Coronary Syndrome	4 weeks: Triple anti-thrombotic therapy (OAC + aspirin 75-100 mg / d + clopidogrel 75 mg / d)[d] Treatment up to 12 months: OAC + clopidogrel 75 mg / d (or aspirin 75-100 mg / d) Lifelong OAC[c]

Note: All patients should consider using a proton pump inhibitor (PPI), especially those on aspirin. For patients with lower bleeding risk, drug-eluting stents are preferred over bare metal stents; newer-generation drug-eluting stents are superior to bare metal stents, especially in patients with low bleeding risk (HAS-BLED 0-2). OAC: oral anticoagulant, including warfarin (INR: 2.0-2.5) or non-vitamin K antagonist oral anticoagulants (NOACs) at tested low doses, including: dabigatran 110 mg twice daily, rivaroxaban 15 mg once daily, or apixaban 2.5 mg twice daily.

a. Alternative options: OAC + clopidogrel 75 mg / d, or aspirin 75 mg / d + clopidogrel 75 mg / d.

b. Alternative option: aspirin 75 mg / d + clopidogrel 75 mg / d.

c. In special cases (e.g. left main, proximal bifurcation stenting, recurrent MI), single or dual antiplatelet therapy may be used alone or in combination. d. Alternative option: OAC + clopidogrel 75 mg / d.

about increased ischemic events when deescalating anti-thrombotic therapy. Theoretically, triple therapy should continue until stent endothelialization is complete. Therefore, to shorten the duration of triple therapy and reduce bleeding events, the most minimalistic stenting technique and rapidly endothelializing stents should be chosen. To reduce bleeding risk, NOACs can be used in combination with antiplatelet therapy. Additionally, for warfarin, close monitoring of the INR and maintaining it between 2.0-2.5 is crucial. For each patient, a comprehensive evaluation of thromboembolic, stent thrombosis, and bleeding risks should be performed, while respecting patient preferences, to individualize the anti-thrombotic regimen.

3. *2016 Chinese Guidelines on Anti-thrombotic Therapy After PCI in CAD with Atrial Fibrillation. The 2016 Chinese Guidelines for Percutaneous Coronary Intervention* provide the following recommendations on anti-thrombotic therapy after PCI in patients with CAD and atrial fibrillation: For SCAD with atrial fibrillation, CHA2DS2-VASc score≥2, and HAS-BLED≤2, OAC plus aspirin 100 mg / d and clopidogrel 75 mg / d for at least 1 month after BMS or new-generation DES implantation is recommended, followed by OAC plus aspirin 100 mg / d or clopidogrel 75 mg / d up to 1 year. For ACS with atrial fibrillation, if HAS-BLED≤2, regardless of stent type, OAC plus aspirin 100 mg / d and clopidogrel 75 mg / d for 6 months is recommended, followed by OAC plus aspirin 100 mg / d or clopidogrel 75 mg / d up to 1 year. For CAD patients (including SCAD and ACS) with HAS-BLED≥3 requiring OAC, regardless of stent type, OAC plus aspirin 100 mg / d and clopidogrel 75 mg / d for at least 1 month is recommended, followed by OAC plus aspirin 100 mg / d or clopidogrel 75 mg / d (duration based on clinical circumstances).

Ⅳ Consultation Process

Currently, there is a lack of large-scale clinical trial data on anti-thrombotic strategies after PCI in atrial fibrillation patients at high stroke risk. What clinicians need to do is: follow the guidelines, balance anti-coagulation and bleeding risks, individualize anti-thrombotic therapy based on risk stratification, in order to maximize benefit for atrial fibrillation patients undergoing PCI.

Section 13 Management of Periprocedural Bleeding in PCI Patients

Bleeding is a common complication during the periprocedural period of PCI and can be life-threatening in severe cases. Adequate pre-procedural evaluation, standardized intra-procedural techniques, and stringent post-procedural monitoring are key to reducing its occurrence. The management of periprocedural bleeding in PCI and common questions encountered during consultation are summarized below.

Ⅰ Bleeding Risk Assessment

The CRUSADE score (Table 1-7) is recommended for pre-procedural assess-ment of bleeding risk and risk stratification (Table 1-8) in PCI patients.

Table 1-7 CRUSADE Scoring System

Risk Factors	Baseline Hematocrit (%)							Gender	
Score	<31	31-33.9		34-36.9	37-39.9		≥40	Male	Female
	9	7		3	2		0	0	8
Risk Factors	Creatinine Clearance (mL / min)							Signs of Congestive Heart Failure	
Score	≤15	16-30	31-60	61-90	91-120		>120	No	Yes
	39	35	28	17	7		0	0	7
Risk Factors	Heart Rate (beats / min)							Diabetes	
Score	≤70	71-80	81-90	91-100	101-110	111-120	≥121	No	Yes
	0	1	3	6	8	10	11	0	6
Risk Factors	Systolic Blood Pressure (mmHg)							History of Peripheral Disease or Stroke	
Score	≤90	91-100	101-120	121-180	181-200		≥201	No	Yes
	10	8	5	1	3		5	0	6

Table 1-8 CRUSADE Scoring Risk Stratification

Score	≤20	21-30	31-40	41-50	>50
Risk Level	Very Low	Low	Moderate	High	Very High
Bleeding Risk (%)	3.1	4.5	8.6	11.9	19.5

Ⅱ Early Prevention

1. Improvement of Procedural Techniques and Equipment: To reduce bleeding related to arterial access, radial artery access should be utilized whenever possible; ultrasound or fluoroscopic guidance can be used for difficult access; if femoral artery access is unavoidable, relatively smaller sheaths should be used and removed early post-procedure.

2. Pharmacological Prevention: For patients at high risk of gastrointestinal bleeding, concomitant proton pump inhibitor (PPI) use is considered appropriate. anti-coagulation regimens should be selected rationally based on bleeding risk stratification: currently, the most effective anticoagulant combination for preventing ischemic events is low molecular weight heparin plus glycoprotein Ⅱb / Ⅲa inhibitor (GPI) or unfractionated heparin plus GPI, but with a significantly increased bleeding risk; regarding bleeding events, bivalirudin can significantly reduce major bleeding events, although foreign studies have reported an increased rate of stent thrombosis. However, the BRIGHT trial in a Chinese population did not show an increase in clinical ischemic adverse events.

Ⅲ Definitions and Classifications

The definitions and classifications of bleeding adopt the standards of the Bleeding Academic Research Consortium (BARC) as outlined in Table 1-9.

Table 1-9 Bleeding Academic Research Consortium (BARC) Bleeding Classification

Bleeding Type		Clinical Signs
0		No bleeding
1		Bleeding that does not necessitate immediate intervention; does not require medical attention or hospitalization, includes discontinuation of medication without consulting a physician
2		Any overt bleeding episodes with immediate intervention indications (e.g., bleeding volume greater than the estimated bleeding volume based on clinical conditions, including bleeding found only on imaging examinations), not meeting the criteria for types 3-5 but satisfying at least one of the following: ① Requiring medical, non-surgical intervention; ② Requiring hospitalization or escalation of care; ③ Requiring evaluation
3	3a	Overt bleeding with a decrease in hemoglobin of 30-50 g / L, requiring transfusion
	3b	Overt bleeding with a decrease in hemoglobin of≥50 g / L, cardiac tamponade, bleeding requiring surgical intervention or control (excluding dental, nasal, skin, and hemorrhoidal bleeding), or bleeding requiring intravenous administration of vasoactive drugs
	3c	Intracranial hemorrhage (excluding microhemorrhage and hemorrhagic transformation after cerebral infarction, including intraspinal hemorrhage); sub-types confirmed by autopsy, imaging examination, or lumbar puncture; bleeding causing visual impairment
4		Bleeding related to coronary artery bypass grafting (CABG), including: ① Intra-cranial bleeding within 48 hours perioperatively; ② Re-operation to control bleeding after closure of sternotomy; ③ Transfusion of≥5 units of whole blood or packed red blood cells within 48 hours postoperatively; ④ Chest tube output≥2 L within 24 hours
5 fatal hemorrhages	5a	Clinically suspected fatal bleeding without confirmation by autopsy or imaging examination
	5b	Definite fatal bleeding without confirmation by autopsy or imaging examination

Ⅳ Management of Bleeding

1. General Principles. Rapidly conduct a comprehensive assessment of bleeding and ischemia, strive for multidisciplinary collaboration, and make the best clinical decision. In hemodynamically stable patients, excessive blood transfusions are not recommended. Transfusion can be considered if hemoglobin is＜70 g / L, with a target of raising hemoglobin to 70-90 g / L.

2. Access Site Bleeding

(1) Local bleeding and hematoma: Confirm compression site and pressure, monitor closely. For active radial artery bleeding, watch for compartment syndrome. Stop anticoagulants and GPIs, but do not discontinue antiplatelet agents. Immobilize the affected limb, administer 20% mannitol intravenous infusion and apply local 50% magnesium sulfate cold compresses. If medical management fails or compartment pressure exceeds 30 mmHg, emergent surgical intervention should be considered.

(2) Arteriovenous fistula or pseudo-aneurysm: Attempt ultrasound-guided re-compression with 24-48 hours' compression dressing. Success is defined as resolution of bruit. Consider surgery if unsuccessful. Discontinuation of anticoagulants and GPIs is recommended, but not antiplatelet agents.

(3) Retro-peritoneal hematoma: First obtain abdominal CTA to localize bleeding source

and exclude active extravasation and manage shock aggressively. Discontinue anticoagulants and GPIs. Stop or taper antiplatelet agents based on risk stratification for recurrent ischemia after bleeding. Consider surgical intervention for progressive bleeding, hemodynamic instability, ipsilateral neurological deficits or severe pain.

3. Gastrointestinal Bleeding. For minor bleeding (e.g. BARC type$<$3), anti-thrombotic therapy can be continued with adequate hemostasis and close monitoring. For major bleeding (BARC$\geqslant$3), anti-thrombotic agents should be reduced or discontinued. If bleeding is uncontrolled or life-threatening, immediately discontinue all agents and provide fresh platelet transfusion. For high thrombotic risk patients (BMS$\leqslant$1 month or DES$\leqslant$3 months), pursue endoscopic hemostasis aggressively while maintaining dual antiplatelet therapy if possible, prioritizing resumption of P2Y12 inhibitor. For patients at high risk of recurrent ulcer bleeding, PPI plus aspirin is preferred over substituting clopidogrel for aspirin. Anti-platelets can be resumed 5 days after achieving hemostasis.

4. Intracranial Hemorrhage. Obtain non-contrast brain CT to assess bleed size. Anticoagulants and Anti-platelets should be held. For minor bleeds with minimal clinical impact in high thrombotic risk patients, antiplatelet therapy can be resumed after 7-10 days off medications, potentially reducing agents / doses based on clinical status. Concomitant GI bleeding warrants aspirin discontinuation.

Medical management includes blood pressure control and measures to reduce intracranial pressure. Neurosurgical intervention is indicated for: supratentorial bleed$\geqslant$30 mL, infratentorial bleed$\geqslant$10 mL with midline shift$\geqslant$1 cm, ventricular effacement, asymmetric / dilated pupil(s) or deteriorating mental status. Decompressive surgery may be pursued emergently for herniation, while other cases can be scheduled after 1 week off anti-coagulation.

5. Respiratory Bleeding. Minor hemoptysis does not necessitate antiplatelet discontinuation. Apart from STEMI patients within 48 hours who can continue anti-coagulation with monitoring, others may discontinue anticoagulants and GPIs.

Massive hemoptysis is defined as$\geqslant$100 mL per episode or$\geqslant$600 mL over 24 hours, constituting a high bleeding risk. Stop anticoagulants, GPIs and oral Anti-platelets. Position patient in lateral decubitus and obtain portable chest X-ray or CT to localize bleeding source and assess lung pathology. Avoid systemic hemostatic agents. Consider bronchoscopy and endobronchial therapy, surgical intervention if refractory.

6. Genitourinary Bleeding

(1) For microscopic hematuria, continue anti-thrombotic therapy. For gross hematuria, stop anticoagulants and GPIs (apart from STEMI within 48 hours who can continue with monitoring). Do not discontinue oral Anti-platelets.

(2) For uterine bleeding, use anticoagulant and antiplatelet strategies based on risk stratification. Consult gynecology to identify and treat underlying condition; emergent dilation and curettage or hysterectomy may be required.

7. Skin, Mucosal, Oral, Nasal and Ocular Bleeding. Do not discontinue antiplatelet therapy for skin, oral, nasal or non-vision threatening ocular bleeding. Apart from STEMI within 48 hours who can continue anti-coagulation with monitoring, stop anticoagulants and GPIs in other cases.

For vision-threatening ocular bleeding, stop anticoagulants and GPIs, and consider stopping or tapering oral Anti-platelets based on risk stratification.

V Bleeding Nursing Care

Provide patient education to ensure cooperation in prevention and early detection of bleeding. Closely monitor vital signs and access sites post-procedure, with enhanced care during immobilization. Ensure accurate administration of anticoagulant infusion rates and doses.

VI Consultation Process

Periprocedural bleeding in PCI can be challenging to manage. Close monitoring is required, with treatment adjustments based on the above principles. Revisit the antiplatelet strategy discussed in Section 11—pre-procedure bleeding risk assessment and discussion of bleeding risks with patients / families is crucial. Beyond pharmacotherapy, focus should be on modifiable factors contributing to bleeding, such as periprocedural blood pressure management (avoiding hypotension risking stent thrombosis, or hypertension increasing bleeding risk), dietary recommendations of bland, easily digested foods with adequate fiber, vitamins and micro-nutrients to avoid constipation and reduce bleeding risk.

Section 14 Common Questions in Consultation for Dyslipidemia

Lipids refer to cholesterol (TC), triglycerides and other lipid components such as phospholipids. TC and triglycerides are most clinically relevant, with TC comprising low-density lipoprotein cholesterol (LDL-C) and high-density lipoprotein cholesterol (HDL-C). The main clinical classifications of dyslipidemia include hypercholesterolemia, hypertriglyceridemia, mixed hyperlipidemia and low HDL-C.

Common lipid-lowering drugs: ① Statins, including atorvastatin, rosuvastatin, simvastatin, pravastatin, fluvastatin, etc. ② Fibrates, including fenofibrate, gemfibrozil, bezafibrate, ciprofibrate. ③ Cholesterol absorption inhibitors such as ezetimibe. ④ Newer lipid-lowering agents approved overseas include microsomal triglyceride transfer protein inhibitors, ApoB100 synthesis inhibitors, PCSK9 inhibitors.

I Rationale for Lipid-Lowering Therapy

Dyslipidemia, especially elevated LDL-C, is a key driver of atherosclerotic cardiovascular disease (ASCVD). Evidence shows that lowering LDL-C can stabilize, retard or regress atherosclerotic lesions, and significantly reduce the incidence, morbidity and mortality of ASCVD. As LDL-C plays a central role in ASCVD, lowering the LDL-C level is targeted for ASCVD risk reduction.

II Definition of ASCVD and Ten-year ASCVD Risk Assessment

ASCVD includes acute coronary syndromes, history of myocardial infarction, stable or unstable angina, coronary revascularization, atherosclerotic stroke or transient ischemic attack (TIA), peripheral arterial disease or revascularization—these patients are considered at extremely high risk. For those not meeting high or extreme ASCVD risk criteria, ten-year ASCVD risk should be estimated (Table 1-10).

ASCVD Overall Incidence Risk Assessment Flowchart

Individuals meeting any of the following criteria should be considered at high or very high risk:
Very High Risk: Patients with ASCVD.
High Risk: (1) LDL-C≥4.9 mmol / L or TC≥7.2 mmol / L. (2) Diabetic patients with LDL-C between 1.8 and 4.9 mmol / L, or TC between 3.1 and 7.2 mmol / L, and age≥40 years.

↓

Table 1-10 Ten-Year Risk Assessment for ASCVD

Risk Factors (Number) (Smoking, low HDL-C, men≥45 years or women≥55 years)		Serum Cholesterol Levels (mmol / L)		
		3.1≤TC<4.1 or 1.8≤LDL-C<2.6	4.1≤TC<5.2 or 2.6≤LDL-C<3.4	5.2≤TC<7.2 or 3.4≤LDL-C<4.9
Without Hypertension	0~1	Low Risk (5%)	Low Risk (5%)	Low Risk (5%)
	2	Low Risk (5%)	Low Risk (5%)	Medium Risk (5%-9%)
	3	Low Risk (5%)	Medium Risk (5%-9%)	Medium Risk (5%-9%)
With Hypertension	0	Low Risk (5%)	Low Risk (5%)	Low Risk (5%)
	1	Low Risk (5%)	Medium Risk (5%-9%)	Medium Risk (5%-9%)
	2	Medium Risk (5%-9%)	High Risk (≥10%)	High Risk (≥10%)
	3	High Risk (≥10%)	High Risk (≥10%)	High Risk (≥10%)

↓

Individuals with any two or more of the following risk factors are defined as high-risk for ASCVD:

- Systolic BP≥160 mmHg or diastolic BP≥100 mmHg.
- Non-HDL-C≥5.2 mmol / L (200 mg / dL).
- HDL-C<1.0 mmol / L (40 mg / dL).
- BMI≥28 kg / m^2.
- Smoking.

Ⅲ Key Populations Requiring Lipid Evaluation

1. Patients with a history of ASCVD.

2. Those with multiple ASCVD risk factors (e.g. hypertension, diabetes, obesity, smoking).

3. Those with a family history of premature cardiovascular disease (first-degree male relatives<55 years old or female relatives<65 years old with ischemic cardiovascular disease), or familial hyperlipidemia.

4. Those with presence of xanthomas or tendon thickening.

Ⅳ Procedures and Targets for Lipid-Lowering Therapy

1. Decide whether to initiate pharmacological lipid-lowering therapy based on individual ASCVD risk.

2. Lowering LDL-C is the primary intervention target for ASCVD prevention, with non-HDL-C as a secondary target.

3. Set lipid targets: LDL-C$<$1.8 mmol / L for very high risk,$<$2.6 mmol / L for high risk, $<$3.4 mmol / L for moderate and low risk.

4. If baseline LDL-C is elevated and target unachievable, aim for at least 50% LDL-C reduction. For very high risk with baseline LDL-C at goal, still pursue around 30% further reduction.

5. Statins are first-line for achieving lipid targets. Start with moderate-intensity statin and adjust dose based on individual LDL-C lowering and tolerability. If targets remain unmet, consider combination with other lipid-lowering agents.

V Long-Term Lipid-Lowering for Key Populations and Regimens

Long-term lipid-lowering therapy is primarily indicated for four statin-benefitting populations:

1. Established ASCVD: These patients have significantly increased future adverse cardiovascular event risk and require intensive secondary prevention including statins. Recommendations: High-intensity statin for ages 21-75 years; moderate-intensity for intolerance of high-intensity or age$>$75 years.

2. Baseline LDL-C$\geqslant$4.9 mmol / L, often seen in familial hypercholesterolemia. Even with combination lipid therapy, LDL-C$<$2.6 mmol / L may be difficult, but studies show$>$50% LDL-C lowering significantly reduces ASCVD risk. Recom-mendations: High-intensity statin; moderate-intensity if high-intensity not tolerated.

3. Diabetes without clinical ASCVD, age 40-75 years, LDL-C 1.8-4.9 mmol / L. Recommendations: Moderate-intensity statin; high-intensity if ten-year ASCVD risk$>$7.5%.

4. No clinical ASCVD or diabetes, LDL-C 1.8-4.9 mmol / L, ten-year ASCVD risk$\geqslant$7.5%. Recommendations: High or moderate-intensity statin.

VI Statin Intensities

1. High-intensity: Lowers LDL-C by$\geqslant$50%, e.g. atorvastatin 40-80 mg / d, rosuvastatin 20-40 mg / d.

2. Moderate-intensity: Lowers LDL-C by 30-$<$50%, e.g. atorvastatin 10 mg / d, rosuvastatin 10 mg / d, simvastatin 20-40 mg / d, pravastatin 40-80 mg / d, lovastatin 40 mg / d, fluvastatin 40 mg bid, pitavastatin 2-4 mg / d.

3. Low-intensity: Lowers LDL-C$<$30%, e.g. simvastatin 10 mg / d, pravastatin 10-20 mg / d, lovastatin 20 mg / d, fluvastatin 20-40 mg / d, pitavastatin 1 mg / d.

VII Statin Safety Assessment and Adverse Effect Management

1. Statins and Liver Function Abnormalities. Statin use is associated with elevated serum alanine aminotransferase (ALT) and aspartate aminotransferase (AST) levels. Liver function tests (LFTs) are recommended 4-8 weeks after statin initiation, and if normal, can be extended to every 6-12 months.

Clinical Management: If AST or ALT exceeds 3x upper limit of normal (ULN), the statin should be temporarily discontinued and LFTs checked weekly until normalization. Mild LFT elevations<3x ULN are not a contraindication; the statin can be continued as levels may decrease spontaneously in some patients.

Statins are contraindicated in active liver disease, persistently unexplained transaminase elevations>3x ULN, decompensated cirrhosis, and acute liver failure. They can be used safely in non-alcoholic fatty liver disease / steatohepatitis. Chronic liver disease or compensated cirrhosis are not contraindications.

2. Statins and Myopathy. Closely monitor for muscle pain or weakness. Recommend baseline creatine kinase (CK) before statin initiation and periodic monitoring. Promptly check CK if muscle symptoms, weakness or brown urine develop, as normal CK does not exclude statin-induced muscle injury if symptoms are present.

Clinical Management: Discontinue statin immediately if myopathy is suspected or confirmed. Other scenarios: ① Check thyroid function for hypothyroidism, a risk factor for myopathy, if muscle symptoms present. ② If muscle tenderness, pain or weakness (with or without CK elevation), rule out common causes like exercise / physical exertion and recommend moderate activity. ③ For muscle symptoms with normal or moderately elevated CK (3-10x ULN), follow CK levels weekly, and consider statin dose reduction or discontinuation if progressive CK elevation. ④ For rhabdomyolysis, immediately stop statin and provide intravenous hydration if needed.

For statin-associated myopathy, options include: ① Switch statins, preferring those with lower myopathy risk. ② Reduce statin dose during high-intensity therapy if myopathy develops, while monitoring symptoms / labs. ③ Intermittent dosing may be possible with longer acting rosuvastatin or atorvastatin. ④ Combination therapy by adding non-statin agents like ezetimibe can reduce statın dose requirements and myopathy risk.

3. Statins and Kidney Injury

(1) Statins do not cause acute kidney injury or chronic kidney disease independent of myopathy.

(2) Current data suggest statins do not cause chronic kidney disease; they may even retard renal function decline.

(3) No definitive evidence links statins to proteinuria.

(4) Statins appear safe in chronic kidney disease, with no differential impact on renal function across statin types.

4. Statins and New-Onset Diabetes. Long-term statin therapy is associated with increased risk of new-onset diabetes, a class effect seen in clinical trials of atorvastatin, simvastatin, rosuvastatin, pravastatin and lovastatin, with no difference between hydrophilic and lipophilic statins. However, the overall cardiovascular benefit-risk ratio of statins is 9:1, far outweighing the diabetes risk.

Clinical Management: At statin initiation for patients without diagnosed diabetes: ① Assess diabetes and cardiovascular risk, screening fasting glucose or HbA1c in high-risk individuals before starting statin. ② Emphasize diet and physical activity for weight management to reduce diabetes / CVD risk. Assess weight (without shoes / outerwear) and measure waist circumference at each visit. ③ Use guideline-recommended statin therapy to lower CVD risk unless contraindicated. ④ If diabetes develops during statin therapy, emphasize weight loss, antihyperglycemic medications if indicated to control glucose / HbA1c, and provide dietary / behavioral counseling.

5. Statins and Changes in Cognitive Function and Neurological Damage. Statin drugs have been associated with adverse effects of amnesia and confusion, although these events are generally not persistent in large clinical trials. When they do occur, they are usually not severe and typically resolve after discontinuation of the statin. The onset can vary greatly, from 1 day to many years after initiating statin therapy.

Clinical Management: The benefits of statins in reducing cardiovascular risk far outweigh the potential risk of cognitive impairment for most patients. Currently, there is insufficient or no medical evidence to establish a causal relationship between statin use and cognitive impairment. Given the severity of cognitive impairment, the widespread use of statins, and the high prevalence of cognitive impairment (due to many causes, especially aging), patient reports of cognitive issues should be taken seriously and properly evaluated, including appropriate neuropsychological testing in those who continue to experience symptoms after statin discontinuation. If cognitive impairment is determined to have no other cause, statin therapy should be discontinued after carefully considering the risk-benefit ratio.

If symptoms of peripheral neuropathy develop during treatment, secondary causes (e.g. diabetes, renal impairment, alcoholism, vitamin B12 deficiency, cancer, hypothyroidism, acquired immunodeficiency syndrome, heavy metal toxicity) should be ruled out. If no other cause is found, statin therapy may be discontinued for 3-6 months to determine if the peripheral neuropathy symptoms are related to statin use. If neurological symptoms do not improve after an appropriate period of statin discontinuation, whether to re-initiate statin therapy should be decided based on a risk-benefit analysis.

Ⅷ Patient Populations for Combined Lipid-Lowering Therapy and Common Combination Regimens

Combined lipid-lowering therapy is often used in patients who are statin-intolerant, do not achieve target cholesterol levels, or have severe mixed hyperlipidemia. The advantage is improved dyslipidemia control rates while reducing adverse event rates. Combination therapy typically consists of a statin plus another lipid-lowering drug with a different mechanism of action.

1. Statin plus Ezetimibe: These drugs affect cholesterol synthesis and absorption respectively, producing a beneficial synergistic effect. Combination therapy can lower LDL-C by around 18% beyond statin monotherapy without increasing adverse effects.

For patients whose cholesterol levels remain uncontrolled on moderate-intensity statin therapy or who are statin-intolerant, a low / moderate-intensity statin plus ezetimibe may be considered.

2. Statin plus Fibrate: Co-administration can more effectively reduce LDL-C, triglycerides, and increase HDL-C levels. However, as statins and fibrates share similar metabolic pathways with potential hepatotoxicity and myopathy risks, adverse events may be more likely with

combination use, necessitating careful safety monitoring. Start with low doses, administer the fibrate in the morning and statin in the evening to avoid significant increases in drug levels, and closely monitor liver and muscle enzymes. If no adverse effects occur, the statin dose can be gradually increased.

Indicated for high triglycerides with low HDL-C; severe hypertriglyceridemia with or without low HDL-C in mixed dyslipidemia, especially with diabetes and / or metabolic syndrome; high-risk ASCVD patients with sub-optimal triglyceride or HDL-C control despite statin therapy.

3. Statin plus PCSK9 Inhibitor: Though not yet marketed in China, statins plus PCSK9 inhibitors have become a combination therapy in Western countries for severe dyslipidemia, particularly familial hypercholesterolemia, providing greater LDL-C reductions and higher target attainment than any single agent.

For ASCVD patients whose LDL-C remains>2.6 mmol / L despite maximal lifestyle and drug therapy (e.g. statin + ezetimibe), a PCSK9 inhibitor can be added as a triple combination with different mechanisms of action.

4. Statin plus n-3 Fatty Acids: Often used for mixed dyslipidemia. However, high-dose n-3 polyunsaturated fatty acids may increase bleeding risk and caloric intake in diabetics and obese patients, so long-term use is not recommended. Whether this combination reduces cardiovascular events is still being explored.

Ⅸ Monitoring and Target Levels for Dyslipidemia Treatment in the Elderly

Lifestyle modification is the fundamental treatment for dyslipidemia in the elderly, including smoking cessation, salt restriction, alcohol limitation, reducing saturated fat and cholesterol intake, increasing vegetables, fruits, fish, nuts, whole grains / high-fiber foods rich in plant sterols, appropriate weight loss, and regular aerobic exercise. Lipid levels should be re-checked at 6-8 weeks; if at target or significantly improved, lifestyle changes should continue with follow-up at 3-6 months. If still at target, re-evaluate every 6-12 months.

In elderly patients on statin therapy, monitor for muscle pain, tenderness, weakness, fatigue, and gastrointestinal symptoms. Check lipids, liver and muscle enzymes, and renal function before and 4 weeks after initiation. If not at target by 3-6 months, adjust statin type or dose. Once at target, follow up every 6-12 months (Table 1-11).

Table 1-11 Lipid Target Levels for Dyslipidemia Treatment in the Elderly (mmol / L)

Clinical Condition and / or Risk Factors	LDL-C Target	Non-HDL-C Target	Clinical Condition and / or Risk Factors	LDL-C Target	Non-HDL-C Target
Atherosclerotic Cardiovascular Disease	<1.8	<2.6	Chronic Kidney Disease	<2.6	<3.4
Diabetes + Hypertension or Other Risk Factor	<1.8	<2.6	Hypertension + 1 Other Risk Factor	<2.6	<3.4
Diabetes	<2.6	<3.4	Hypertension or 3 Other Risk Factors	<3.4	<4.1

Note: Non-HDL-C=TC - HDL-C; Other risk factors include age (≥45 for men, ≥55 for women), smoking, HDL-C<1.04 mmol / L, BMI≥28 kg / m^2, premature familial CVD history.

X How to Manage Dyslipidemia in Organ Transplant Recipients?

Dyslipidemia is a common complication in solid organ transplant recipients and a major risk factor for coronary heart disease and stroke. The prevalence of hyperlipidemia is 40%-80%, manifesting as elevated total cholesterol, LDL-C, and triglycerides. In addition to standard risk factors, immunosuppressive drugs have a clear association with post-transplant dyslipidemia (Tables 1-12, 1-13).

Table 1-12 Effects of Commonly Used Immunosuppressants on Lipid Levels

Drug	Effect on Lipids	Mechanism
Glucocorticoids	Increased VLDL, Total Cholesterol (TC), Trigly-cerides (TG); De-creased HDL	Accelerate lipolysis, inhibit lipogenesis, increase blood glucose levels, promote shift from glucose to lipid metabolism, induce insulin resistance and metabolic syndrome. Cumulative effect with long-term use
Cyclosporine	Increased LDL, TC	Reduce bile acid synthesis, down-regulate LDL receptor function, inhibit cholesterol clearance, induce cholesterol synthesis, promote VLDL→LDL conversion. Additional lipid-raising effect when combined with glucocorticoids
Tacrolimus	Mildly Increased LDL, Total Chol-esterol (TC)	Similar class as cyclosporine but weaker lipid-raising effect
Sirolimus, Everolimus	Increased Total Chole-sterol (TC), Trigly-cerides (TG)	Increase hepatic lipogenesis, decrease lipid clearance, inhibit insulin and insulin-like growth factor pathways

Table 1-13 Lipid Metabolism Reference Ranges and Risk Stratification for Transplant Recipients (mmol / L)

Classification	TC	LDL-C	HDL-C	TG
Optimal Value		<2.59(100)		
Desirable Range	<5.18(200)	<3.37(130)	≥1.04(40)	<1.70(150)
Marginally Elevated	5.18-6.21 (200-239)	3.37-4.13 (130-159)		1.7-2.25 (150-199)
Elevated	≥6.22(240)	≥4.14(160)	≥1.55(60)	≥2.26(200)
Extremely High		>4.93(190)		>5.67(500)
Decreased			<1.04(40)	

For transplant recipients, LDL-C is the primary target for lipid-lowering therapy, with TG, TC and HDL-C as secondary targets.

1. Lipid Management in Kidney Transplant Recipients. Drug selection must consider interactions with immunosuppressants and other medications, as well as effects on transplanted kidney function. If hepatic or renal impairment exists, drugs with minimal or no hepatorenal effects should be preferred. Dosage adjustments may be required based on the recipient's glomerular filtration rate (GFR) (Table 1-14).

Table 1-14 Recommended Statin Dosages for Kidney Transplant Recipients (mg / day)

Statin	GFR Level (mL / min / 1.73 m^2)		Combined with Cyclosporine
	≥30	<30 or Dialysis	
Atorvastatin	10-80	10-80	10-80
Fluvastatin	20-80	10-40	10-40
Lovastatin	20-80	10-40	10-40
Pravastatin	20-40	20-40	20-40
Simvastatin	20-80	10-40	10-40

2. Lipid Management in Heart Transplant Recipients. Regardless of baseline lipid levels, statin therapy should be initiated 1-2 weeks post-transplant. Considering drug interactions between statins and calcineurin inhibitors and the associated risk of myopathy, starting statin doses in heart transplant recipients should be lower than general lipid-lowering recommendations (Table 1-15).

Table 1-15 Recommended Statin Dosages for Heart Transplant Recipients (mg / day)

Drug	Recommended Dose	Drug	Recommended Dose
Pravastatin	20-40	Lovastatin	20
Simvastatin	5-20	Atorvastatin	10-20
Fluvastatin	40-80	Rosuvastatin	5-20

3. Lipid Management in Liver Transplant Recipients. Statins are the first-line pharmacotherapy for hypercholesterolemia after liver transplantation, but 7%-10% of statin-induced liver injury has been reported. Therefore, statins should be initiated at low doses with gradual titration and close liver function monitoring. Discontinuation may be required. All statins except pravastatin undergo CYP450 metabolism, necessitating immunosuppressant level monitoring and dose adjustments during statin therapy. The safety of ezetimibe post-liver transplant remains to be confirmed so it is not currently recommended. For isolated hypertriglyceridemia, fish oils are first-line, with fenofibrate or gemfibrozil as alternatives if response is sub-optimal (Table 1-16).

Table 1-16 Recommended Post-Transplant Statin Dosages for Liver Recipients (mg / day)

Drug	Standard Dose	Post-Liver Transplant Dose	Drug	Standard Dose	Post-Liver Transplant Dose
Atorvastatin	10-80	10-40	Simvastatin	20-40	20-40
Rosuvastatin	5-40	5-20	Pravastatin	40-80	20-40
Lovastatin	40-80	20-40	Fluvastatin	80	40

4. Lipid Management in Lung Transplant Recipients. Post-transplant immunosuppressant use can induce hyperlipidemia, occurring in approximately 20.5% of 1-year and 52.2% of 5-year survivors. Glucocorticoid and calcineurin inhibitor-induced hyperlipidemia is recognized to promote atherosclerosis and requires aggressive management.

Primary hyperlipidemia prevention usually starts 3 months post-transplant, including dietary control, exercise, and management of other cardiovascular risk factors to reduce risks of cardiovascular disease and renal impairment. For patients with established ASCVD, secondary hypercholesterolemia prevention begins once vitals are stable post-transplant, with an initial LDL-C target<2.0 mmol / L and concomitant aspirin 100 mg / day. Drug options and starting doses (max recommended) are shown in Table 1-17.

Table 1-17 Recommended Statin Dosages (mg / day) for Lung Transplant Recipients

Drug	Recommended Dose		Remarks
	Starting Dose	Maximum Dose	
Atorvastatin	10	80	Preferred
Fluvastatin	20	80	
Pravastatin	10	40	

XI Consultation Process

1. Achieving lipid targets is crucial for preventing and treating cardiovascular and cerebrovascular diseases, and can often be accomplished through interventions like dietary control, exercise, and medication.

2. Pay close attention to populations that require lipid monitoring. Based on the patient's specific circumstances, such as risk factors, presence of atherosclerotic cardiovascular disease, hypertension, diabetes, etc., establish corresponding lipid goals, with low-density lipoprotein cholesterol being particularly important.

3. Understand the lipid-lowering effects of different drugs and inform patients about potential adverse effects like liver dysfunction, myopathy, renal impairment, dysglycemia, etc. Educate on early detection through monitoring for muscle pain, regular liver / kidney function tests, etc.

4. If lipid targets are not met despite dietary, exercise, and single drug interventions, combination drug therapy can be considered (e.g. statin plus ezetimibe, statin plus fibrate).

5. For organ transplant recipients like liver, heart, kidney, lung, etc., manage lipid levels according to the above principles.

Section 15 Thrombolytic Therapy for Acute Myocardial Infarction

I Definition of Acute ST-Segment Elevation Myocardial Infarction (STEMI)

STEMI refers to the clinical syndrome of acute myocardial ischemic necrosis, often caused by rupture or erosion of an unstable coronary plaque, endothelial injury and subsequent thrombus formation leading to acute, persistent, complete coronary occlusion. This results in sudden reduction or cessation of blood supply, causing myocardial ischemia, injury and necrosis.

Ⅱ Diagnostic Criteria for STEMI

1. Infarction-type angina: Severe, crushing, constrictive, suffocating chest pain / tightness lasting>20 min, unrelieved by nitroglycerin, isosorbide dinitrate or fast-acting angina medications.

2. Dynamic ECG ST-T changes (T wave widening & peaking → ST-T segment merging & elevation → uniphasic ST elevation → pathological Q wave formation).

3. Elevated myocardial necrosis biomarkers: CK-MB, cTnI / T>2x upper reference limit.

Note: Early STEMI may only show T wave widening / peaking and reciprocal changes! Biomarkers may not be elevated within the first 2 hours of STEMI onset! Hence, early STEMI diagnosis and treatment should not wait for: biomarker elevation, typical uniphasic ST elevation, or pathological Q waves. Early STEMI diagnosis is based on: ① Infarction-type angina; ② ECG showing T wave widening / peaking and ST-T segment merging / elevation.

Ⅲ Differential Diagnosis of STEMI (Table 1-18)

Ⅳ Thrombolytic Therapy for STEMI

The extent of myocardial infarction in STEMI is closely related to the total ischemic time, so the core concept in STEMI management is minimizing total ischemic time as much as possible.

Reperfusion therapy is the key to successful STEMI treatment. Ample evidence-based medicine and clinical practice have shown that thrombolytic therapy within 3 hours of STEMI onset has similar efficacy to primary PCI, and is more rapid, convenient and accessible. Hence it remains extremely valuable for primary care hospitals and patients presenting>3 hours from PCI-capable centers. If PCI cannot be performed within 120 minutes, thrombolysis should be initiated within 30 minutes. However, it must be emphasized that thrombolysis is only the start, not the end, of STEMI reperfusion therapy. Patients should be promptly transferred 3-24 hours post-thrombolysis to a higher-level facility for coronary angiography or PCI to further confirm, remedy, optimize and consolidate reperfusion therapy efficacy.

While reperfusion is key to STEMI treatment success, standardized management of all aspects is closely linked to final outcomes. The following operations need to be coordinately implemented in an integrated diagnostic-therapeutic approach.

Immediate Blood Tests: Complete blood count (CBC), coagulation function, electrolytes, myocardial necrosis markers	+	Basic Treatment: Appropriate positioning / psychological counseling / ECG monitoring / defibrillation preparation / oxygen therapy / sedation and analgesia / nitroglycerin	+	Core Treatment: Heparinization anti-coagulation, dual antiplatelet aggregation (aspirin 300 mg + clopidogrel 300-600 mg or ticagrelor 180 mg loading dose), prevention and treatment of malignant ventricular arrhythmias: β-receptor blockers + potassium supplementation

Table 1-18 Differential Diagnosis of STEMI

Clinical Manifestations	Differential Diagnosis	Etiology or Inducing Factors	Disease Characteristics	Accompanying Symptoms and Signs	Auxiliary Examinations
Retrosternal or precordial pain	Angina pectoris	Onset after fatigue, emotional agitation, cold exposure, or overeating	Pain location and nature are similar, but myocardial infarction is more severe. Dura-tion is shorter, generally not exceeding 15 min	Rarely fever or asthma, no pericardial friction rub; blood pressure elevated or unchanged. Can be significantly relieved after taking nitroglycerin	ECG shows no change or temporary ST-segment and T-wave changes
Precordial pain, fever	Acute pericarditis	Caused by infection	Severe, persistent precordial pain; pain and fever often occur simultaneously, aggravated by breathing and coughing, relieved by sitting and leaning forward; pericardial fric-tion rub may be present in early stage	Systemic symptoms are not as severe as myocardial infarction	ECG shows ST-segment arcuate elevation in all leads except aVR, T-wave inversion, and no abnormal Q-waves
Chest pain, dyspnea, shock	Acute pulmonary embolism	Embolus blocking pulmonary artery	Sudden chest pain, hemo-ptysis, dyspnea, shock; cyanosis	Accentuated second heart sound in pulmonary valve area, jugular venous disten-tion, hepatomegaly, lower extremity edema	ECG shows deepened S-wave in lead Ⅰ, significant Q-wave and T-wave inversion in lead Ⅲ, leftward shift of transition zone in chest leads, and T-wave inversion in right chest leads; pulmonary vascular CTA
Severe chest pain, shock	Aortic dissection	Vascular tear, blood seeping into aortic wall	Chest pain peaks imme-diately, often radiating to back, ribs, abdomen, waist, and lower limbs	There may be a significant difference in blood pressure and pulse between the two upper limbs, and temporary paralysis, hemiplegia, and aortic valve insufficiency manifesta-tions in the lower limbs	Echocardiography, X-ray, or MRI can help diagnose
Chest pain, shock	Acute abdomen	Often has a corresponding disease history	Corresponding characteri-stics of various factors causing acute abdomen	Board-like abdomen, abdo-minal tenderness, and rebound pain	Careful history taking, physical examination, ECG, and myocardial enzyme spectrum can help differentiate

1. Indications for Thrombolysis. ① Age$<$75 years, symptom onset$<$12 hours - proceed with immediate thrombolysis once STEMI diagnosed, if no contraindications. ② Age$>$75 years—consider reduced or half-dose thrombolysis after carefully weighing ischemic vs. bleeding risks. ③ Symptom onset 12-24 hours—thrombolysis may be considered if ongoing ischemic chest pain or hemodynamic instability with persistent ST elevation.

2. Absolute Contraindications to Thrombolysis. ① Any prior intra-cranial hemorrhage. ② Structural cerebrovascular lesions (e.g. arteriovenous malformations). ③ Intracranial malignancy (primary or metastatic). ④ Acute ischemic stroke or transient ischemic attack within 3 months. ⑤ Suspected or confirmed aortic dissection. ⑥ Active bleeding or bleeding diathesis (excluding menses). ⑦ Significant closed head / facial trauma within 3 months.

3. Relative Contraindications to Thrombolysis. ① Uncontrolled severe hypertension (SBP$\geqslant$180 mmHg or DBP$\geqslant$110 mmHg) —thrombolysis may begin after BP control (SBP$<$160 mmHg). ② Prolonged ($>$10 min) or traumatic CPR (rib fractures, pericardial effusion). ③ Dementia or known intracranial pathology. ④ Major surgery or trauma within 3 weeks, internal bleeding within 4 weeks. ⑤ Major non-compressible vascular puncture within 2 weeks. ⑥ Infective endocarditis. ⑦ Pregnancy. ⑧ Active peptic ulcer disease. ⑨ Terminal cancer or severe hepatic / renal disease. ⑩ Anticoagulant use—bleeding risk increases with higher INR.

4. Thrombolytic Agent Selection. Fibrin-specific agents (e.g. tenecteplase) are preferred. Non-fibrin-specific agents (e.g. streptokinase) should only be used if fibrin-specific agents are unavailable (see Table 1-19).

5. Assessing Thrombolytic Efficacy

(1) $\geqslant$50% ST segment resolution within 60-90 minutes post-thrombolysis.

(2) Earlier cTn peak within 12 hours and CK-MB peak within 14 hours of symptom onset.

(3) Significant chest pain relief within 2 hours post-thrombolysis.

(4) Reperfusion arrhythmias 2-3 hours post-thrombolysis e.g. accelerated idioventricular rhythm, transient AV / bundle branch blocks.

6. Management of Thrombolytic Complications. The main risk of thrombolytic therapy is bleeding, especially intracranial hemorrhage (0.9%-1%) and bleeding from visceral organs (e.g. gastrointestinal bleeding), which can significantly increase mortality if occurred. For intracranial hemorrhage, immediately stop thrombolysis, anti-thrombotic and anticoagulant treatment, and use mannitol to reduce intracranial pressure; if unfractionated heparin was used within 4 hours, protamine sulfate is recommended to reverse heparin (1 mg protamine can neutralize 100 U unfractionated heparin); immediately transfer to a higher-level hospital capable of PCI. For bleeding from other organs, reduce or stop anticoagulant and anti-thrombotic drugs, provide symptomatic treatment such as blood transfusion, and transfer to a higher-level hospital as soon as possible.

7. Post-Thrombolytic Management for STEMI

(1) anti-coagulation and anti-thrombotic therapy: After using unfractionated heparin for 48 hours, gradually reduce the dose and switch to subcutaneous low molecular weight heparin. Currently, evidence-based medicine recommends enoxaparin: for age$<$75 years, 1 mg / kg subcutaneously every 12 hours for 8 days; for age$>$75 years, 0.75 mg / kg subcutaneously

Table 1-19 Methods of Using Various Thrombolytics

Heparin Treatment			Intravenous injection of unfractionated heparin 5000U (60-80U / kg) Followed by continuous intravenous infusion of 12U / (kg•h) Monitor aPTT or ACT to 1.5-2.0 times control value (aPTT: 50-70s) during and after thrombolysis	
Thrombolytic Agents - Plasminogen Activators	Specificity	Alteplase (rt-PA) Prourokinase (Pro-UK)	Full-dose Administration (100 mg):	On the basis of heparin therapy, inject 15 mg rt-PA intravenously → 0.75 mg / kg intravenous infusion for 30 min (usually not exceeding 50 mg) → 0.5 mg / kg intravenous infusion for 60 min (usually not exceeding 35 mg) → Continue heparin maintenance for 48 h
			Half-dose Administration (50 mg):	On the basis of heparin therapy, dissolve 50 mg rt-PA in 50 mL dedicated solvent → Inject 8 mg intravenously → 42 mg intravenous infusion for 90 min → Continue heparin maintenance for 48 h
		Reteplase (r-PA)	On the basis of heparin therapy, dissolve 20 mg Pro-UK in 10 mL normal saline and intravenously push for 3 min → Dissolve 30 mg Pro-UK in 90 mL normal saline and intravenously infuse for 30 min → Continue heparin maintenance for 48 h	
		Tenecteplase (TNK-tPA)	On the basis of heparin therapy, dissolve 10 mU r-PA in 5-10 mL water for injection and intravenously push for more than 2 min → Repeat the above dose after 3 min → Continue heparin maintenance for 48 h	
		Urokinase (UK)	On the basis of heparin therapy, dissolve 30-50 mg TNK-tPA in 10 mL normal saline and intravenously push (dose is 30 mg for body weight<60 kg, increase dose by 5 mg for every 10 kg increase in body weight) → Continue heparin maintenance for 48 h	
	Non-specificity	Alteplase (rt-PA)	On the basis of heparin therapy, add 1.5 million U UK to 100 mL normal saline and intravenously infuse for 30 min or intravenously infuse 22,000 U / kg for 30 min → Continue heparin maintenance for 48 h	

every 12 hours for 8 days; for creatinine clearance$<$30 mL / min regardless of age, 1 mg / kg subcutaneously once daily. Dual antiplatelet therapy is recommended after thrombolysis.

(2) For STEMI patients without contraindications, beta-blockers should be routinely administered within 24 hours, starting with a low dose and gradually increasing. After 24 hours of onset, all STEMI patients without contraindications are recommended for long-term ACE inhibitor treatment; if not tolerated, consider ARBs. Statins have lipid-lowering, anti-inflammatory, endothelial function improvement, and antiplatelet effects. In the absence of contraindications, statin therapy is recommended early during hospitalization, regardless of cholesterol levels.

Thrombolytic therapy for STEMI patients in primary care hospitals or non-PCI hospitals is the initiation, not the end, of reperfusion therapy. STEMI patients should be transferred to a PCI hospital for coronary angiography within 3-24 hours after thrombolysis.

V Consultation Procedures

1. For patients suspected of having acute myocardial infarction, attention should be paid to taking a medical history, presenting symptoms, determining time of onset and time of exacerbation, and closely monitoring changes in electrocardiogram, enzymes, and cardiac biomarkers.

2. For early-onset STEMI, the diagnosis is mainly based on characteristics of acute myocardial infarction chest pain, widened and elevated T waves on ECG, and ST-T segment elevation. Early diagnosis of STEMI allows timely coronary revascularization.

3. With the widespread establishment of chest pain centers, patients with confirmed STEMI are recommended to undergo coronary angiography and percutaneous coronary intervention as soon as possible to limit further myocardial necrosis.

4. Pre-procedure, maintain the patient's vital signs (strict bed rest, oxygen, ECG monitoring, analgesia, prevention and monitoring of arrhythmias, electrolyte management, etc.).

5. Pay attention to the use of antiplatelet drugs pre-procedure.

6. If the patient refuses percutaneous coronary intervention, thrombolytic therapy can be considered. Note the indications and contraindications for thrombolysis, and inform the patient and family of potential complications. Rescue percutaneous coronary intervention should be performed within 3-24 hours.

7. Inform the patient of the severity of STEMI and the need for long-term medication.

Section 16 Mechanical Complications of Acute Myocardial Infarction

I Definition

Mechanical complications are serious sequelae of acute myocardial infarction (AMI), including papillary muscle dysfunction and rupture, ventricular aneurysm formation, and cardiac rupture. Cardiac rupture includes free wall rupture, ventricular septal defect, and papillary muscle rupture—life-threatening complications.

In recent years, treatment of AMI has significantly improved, but mortality from mechanical complications remains high at 2.8%-3.5% in AMI patients. New cardiac murmurs and acute hemodynamic changes are important indirect clinical indicators of mechanical complications post-AMI. Direct diagnosis relies on echocardiography, cardiac catheterization, and left ventriculography. Once mechanical complications occur in AMI, the prognosis is grave with extremely high mortality. Therefore, in AMI treatment, it is crucial to enhance awareness of mechanical complications for early diagnosis and timely intervention to reduce AMI mortality.

Ⅱ Classification

1. Left ventricular free wall rupture is the most common form of cardiac rupture. Becker and van Mantgem classify it into 3 types:

(1) Type Ⅰ rupture: Characterized by acute disruption of the left ventricular free wall. In most cases, wall thickness is not significantly thinned, suggesting type I rupture occurs early after infarction as an acute process. More common in single-vessel disease.

(2) Type Ⅱ rupture: Characterized by well-demarcated myocardial infarction in progression, with the rupture site surrounded by necrotic tissue and thrombus, suggesting type Ⅱ is a subacute process occurring after myocardial erosion. More common in multi-vessel disease.

(3) Type Ⅲ rupture: Occurs in areas with extensive myocardial thinning and concomitant aneurysm formation, representing a subacute or chronic process.

Rupture is most often localized to the central portion of the ventricular aneurysm. Extent of coronary disease varies.

In general, around 50% of type Ⅰ ruptures occur early after infarction, mostly within 24 hours, while types Ⅱ and Ⅲ have a wider window, occurring around day 8 and 21 post-infarction.

2. Ventricular septal rupture can be simple or complex:

(1) Simple: Direct rupture from left to right ventricle with relatively straight tract and minimal intra-myocardial hemorrhage. Rupture site commonly involves the mid to apical ventricular septum, often related to acute anterior wall MI.

(2) Complex: Rupture frequently involves the basal septum with serpingous tracts and intra-myocardial hemorrhage. Mostly due to acute inferior wall MI, difficult to treat with high mortality.

3. Complete papillary muscle rupture causing acute severe mitral regurgitation is relatively rare but often fatal. Incidence is＜1%, with 80% mortality in complete papillary muscle rupture. As the posterior papillary muscle has a single blood supply, its rupture rate is 5-10 times that of the anterior muscle. Partial papillary muscle rupture is more common than complete rupture and amenable to surgery. Similar to left ventricular free wall and septal rupture, papillary muscle rupture mostly occurs within 1 week post-AMI.

Ⅲ Clinical Features and Diagnosis

1. Clinical Features. The most serious complication of AMI is rupture of myocardial tissue. Clinical manifestations of cardiac rupture can vary significantly depending on the rupture site,

which may involve the papillary muscles, ventricular septum, or left ventricular free wall.

(1) Left Ventricular Free Wall Rupture: Clinically more common in elderly and female patients, those with hypertension compared to normotensive individuals, and first-time MI sufferers. Free wall rupture typically leads to hemopericardium and cardiac tamponade causing death. The clinical course can be acute or subacute. Acute rupture (within 24 hours) presents with sudden confusion, electromechanical dissociation on ECG monitoring, undetectable blood pressure, absent arterial pulsations, and immediate death from acute cardiac tamponade. Subacute rupture (24-48 hours) results from initially contained myocardial hemorrhage due to endocardial tear, which subsequently extends to the epicardial surface.

(2) Ventricular Septal Rupture: More likely in patients without collateral circulation, transmural MI, elderly, females, and those with hypertension. Rarely occurs with prior old MI, diabetes, or severe coronary artery disease. Typically presents within 7 days post-MI, most often after anterior wall MI. The rupture site correlates with MI location—apical septal rupture in anterior MI and basal septal rupture in inferior MI. Clinical presentation and prognosis depend on the degree of shunting and hemodynamic impairment. May manifest as acute respiratory distress and pulmonary edema, with a characteristic new harsh pansystolic murmur at the left sternal border and thrill.

(3) Papillary Muscle Rupture: Complete papillary muscle rupture causing acute severe mitral regurgitation is relatively rare but often fatal, with 80% mortality mainly from massive mitral regurgitation leading to acute pulmonary edema. Partial papillary muscle rupture, usually of the head or tip, is more common and results in severe mitral regurgitation. A new late systolic murmur or marked accentuation of a pre-existing murmur is heard at the mitral area.

2. Diagnosis. The diagnosis of left ventricular free wall rupture is not difficult based on clinical features, but confirmatory tests include echocardiography and pericardiocentesis. In AMI patients at risk for cardiac rupture who develop acute decompensation, especially new murmurs and pulmonary edema, ventricular septal rupture and papillary muscle rupture should be considered first. Definitive diagnosis is made by physical examination and echocardiography.

Ⅳ Treatment Principles

1. Medical Management

(1) General measures as for AMI—oxygen, sedation, activity restriction.

(2) Invasive hemodynamic monitoring to assess vital signs and cardiac function.

(3) Maintain respiratory stability with supplemental oxygen, invasive or non-invasive ventilation to increase PaO_2 and oxygen saturation.

(4) Intravenous inotropes (e.g. dopamine and / or dobutamine), vasodilators (e.g. nitroprusside or nitrates), and diuretics (furosemide and hydrochlorothiazide) to reduce preload and after-load while maintaining systolic BP$>$90 mmHg, pulmonary capillary wedge pressure 12-15 mmHg, and cardiac index$>$2 L / m^2.

(5) In hemodynamically unstable AMI with mechanical complications, intra-aortic balloon counter-pulsation (IABP) is crucial for stabilization, improving ischemia, and maintaining hemodynamics. IABP enhances coronary diastolic flow and organ perfusion, reduces left

ventricular after-load and systemic vascular resistance, decreases myocardial work and oxygen demand, and corrects low cardiac output. It provides circulatory support as a bridge to surgery.

2. Surgical Treatment

(1) Left Ventricular Free Wall Rupture: Medical management of free wall rupture post-AMI has very high mortality. Clinically, except for subacute free wall rupture and pseudo-aneurysms amenable to emergency surgery, most patients die within minutes and surgical survival is also very low. Surgery aims to relieve cardiac tamponade, repair the ventricular rupture, and achieve complete coronary revascularization.

(2) Ventricular Septal Rupture: Besides medical management, treatment options include surgical repair or percutaneous septal occluder device closure. Medical therapy alone is ineffective with poor prognosis. Surgical repair remains the most effective treatment currently. The optimal timing for surgery is controversial—the traditional view favored delaying surgery for 2-4 weeks until scar formation due to edema, tissue friability, and necrosis in the acute phase. However, these patients deteriorate rapidly with 65% mortality within 2 weeks. With advances in surgical techniques, anesthesia, and perioperative care, many experts now recommend emergency surgery once diagnosed, especially for larger defects, regardless of cardiogenic shock status. Surgical timing: ①Large defects with pulmonary-to-systemic flow ratio＞2：1 without shock—urgent post-cath surgery within 24 hours. ②With severe cardiogenic shock—initial medical stabilization followed by surgery within 48 hours of hemodynamic stability. ③Small defects with flow ratio＜1.5：1 without hemodynamic compromise—elective surgery at 3-6 weeks is safer.

(3) Papillary Muscle Rupture: Acute moderate-to-severe ischemic mitral regurgitation from papillary muscle rupture post-AMI causes rapid decompensation and cardiogenic shock with dismal prognosis. Over-all in-hospital mortality is 55%-71% with medical therapy and 40% with surgery. Early mitral valve repair / replacement and emergency CABG is recommended. Isolated emergency CABG without addressing mitral regurgitation adversely impacts outcomes. Regarding timing, earlier consensus favored delaying surgery due to friable myocardium post-AMI, but increasing evidence shows no benefit in waiting, supporting early surgical intervention within 24 hours.

V Common Questions in Consultation

1. How to assess risk of mechanical complications post-AMI? Mechanical complications are rare but well-recognized as typically fatal sequelae of AMI, the third leading cause of death after malignant arrhythmias and cardiogenic shock.

2. What are the risk factors for mechanical complications post-AMI? More common in elderly, females, post-thrombolysis, low BMI, and delayed reperfusion therapy. Emergency PCI reduces mechanical complication rates while thrombolysis decreases AMI mortality but increases mechanical complication rates. Persistent post-infarct angina, excessive physical activity, and pericarditis also increase risk.

3. How to determine optimal timing of surgery for mechanical complica-tions post-AMI?

(1) Left ventricular free wall rupture—emergency surgery, despite high risks and mortality, as medical management alone is universally fatal. Surgery offers a chance of survival.

(2) Ventricular septal rupture: ①Large defects with pulmonary-to-systemic flow ratio>2:1 without shock—urgent post-cath surgery within 24 hours. ②With severe cardiogenic shock—initial medical stabilization followed by surgery within 48 hours once stable. ③Small defects with flow ratio<1.5 : 1 without hemodynamic compromise—elective surgery at 3-6 weeks is safer.

(3) Papillary muscle rupture: Despite temporary stabilization with medical therapy, rapid decompensation is possible with poor outcomes. Therefore, early surgery should be undertaken after comprehensive evaluation.

4. Is concomitant CABG recommended with repair / replacement surgery? There is debate around performing concomitant CABG with mitral valve repair or replacement surgery, but most experts believe that revascularization of significant multi-vessel coronary disease can improve long-term survival, left ventricular function, and prognosis.

Ⅵ Consultation Process

1. Mechanical complications of acute myocardial infarction often occur within 1 week after onset. The risk of complications should be fully communicated to the patient and their family, and they should be informed on how to cooperate with treatment, such as absolute bed rest, maintaining regular bowel movements, eating a light diet, maintaining a peaceful state of mind, and ensuring adequate sleep.

2. Closely observe the patient's vital signs, clinical symptoms, cardiopulmonary physical examination, relevant biochemical indicators, internal environment balance, etc. Promptly identify and solve problems to minimize the occurrence of mechanical complications of acute myocardial infarction.

3. If mechanical complications of acute myocardial infarction occur, fully explain the condition to the patient's family and actively treat the patient based on the above treatment principles.

Chapter 2

Heart Failure

Section 1 Differential Diagnosis Approach for Dyspnea

Dyspnea is caused by various systems, including respiratory, cardiovascular, digestive, neurological, hematological, and psychiatric. During consultation, a systematic clinical thinking approach is required, sometimes involving multidisciplinary consultation.

I Definition

Dyspnea refers to the patient's subjective experience of varying degrees and types of air insufficiency, breathing discomfort, labored breathing, and suffocation, with or without signs of respiratory effort such as mouth breathing, nasal flaring, and accessory respiratory muscle involvement. It may also be accompanied by changes in respiratory rate, depth, and rhythm. The patient's mental state, living environment, education level, psychological factors, and the nature of the disease can influence their description of dyspnea.

II Classification

1. Based on duration, dyspnea can be classified as acute (course$<$3 weeks) or chronic (course$\geqslant$3 weeks).

2. Based on etiology, dyspnea can be classified as: ① Cardiac dyspnea: seen in heart failure caused by various heart diseases and large pericardial effusions; ② Pulmonary dyspnea: mainly caused by ventilation and gas exchange dysfunction due to various diseases of the airways, pulmonary circulation, chest wall, and respiratory muscles; ③ Toxic dyspnea: caused by respiratory center stimulation or drug suppression; ④ Hematologic dyspnea: caused by reduced oxygen-carrying capacity of red blood cells or stimulation of the respiratory center by massive hemorrhagic shock, seen in severe anemia, shock, etc.; ⑤ Neuropsychiatric and muscular dyspnea: often caused by increased intracranial pressure and decreased cerebral blood supply, suppressing the respiratory center, or respiratory muscle weakness due to neuromuscular paralysis, resulting in ventilation insufficiency; ⑥ Dyspnea caused by other diseases: such as massive ascites, giant abdominal tumors, late pregnancy, acute infectious diseases with high fever, etc. Pulmonary dyspnea can be further divided into expiratory, inspiratory, and mixed dyspnea.

Ⅲ Etiology

Based on pathophysiology, common causes of dyspnea include:

1. Ventilatory mechanical dysfunction: Massive abdominal or thoracic masses; bronchial asthma, emphysema, bronchitis; endotracheal tumors; pulmonary interstitial fibrosis; kyphoscoliosis; lymphangioleiomyomatosis, obesity; central and peripheral airflow limitation; pleural thickening; restriction of chest wall and diaphragm expansion or diaphragmatic paralysis; pulmonary expansion restriction; and tracheal or laryngeal edema or stenosis.

2. Respiratory pump dysfunction: Severe hyperinflation; neuromuscular diseases; obesity; pleural effusion; pneumothorax; and poliomyelitis.

3. Increased respiratory drive: Decreased cardiac output; decreased effective hemoglobin, such as poisoning; hypoxemia; renal diseases; and increased excitation of pulmonary receptors.

4. Ineffective ventilation: Pulmonary capillary destruction; and pulmonary vascular obstruction.

5. Psychological abnormalities: Anxiety; somatization disorder; depression; and malingering.

Ⅳ Description of Dyspnea Characteristics

The nature of dyspnea is mainly determined by the patient's self-description, which may provide diagnostic clues to the cause. The specific expressions of dyspnea vary among patients, and common terms include "chest tightness," "wheezing" "shortness of breath" "rapid breathing" "gasping" "suffocation""air hunger" "difficulty breathing" "chest constriction" "labored breathing" "pressure sensation" "choking sensation", etc. The description of dyspnea symptoms should have specific content. For example, if the patient describes dyspnea as exertional, it often suggests cardiopulmonary diseases, most commonly seen in heart failure, bronchial asthma, chronic obstructive pulmonary disease, and diseases affecting respiratory muscles. Dyspnea with a sensation of chest tightness is often a feeling during bronchial constriction. Studies have shown that chest tightness is a major symptom of early asthma, originating from the sensation of stimuli from the lungs, rather than an exertion-related feeling. Air hunger / unsatisfied inspiration is a sensation of air insufficiency, indicating a mismatch between the patient's ventilation and respiratory drive, triggered by increased respiratory drive.

Ⅴ Assessment Methods for Dyspnea

Currently, there is no universal assessment method for dyspnea. It generally includes three aspects: clinical sensation assessment, severity assessment of dyspnea sensation, and the impact and burden of dyspnea symptoms. It should be noted that the severity of dyspnea sensation is often inconsistent with the severity of the underlying disease-causing dyspnea, so they cannot be used interchangeably. For acute dyspnea, clinical sensation assessment and severity assessment should be the focus; for chronic dyspnea, the impact and burden of dyspnea symptoms should be emphasized. When conducting a clinical assessment, a detailed history, the patient's symptom experience, and diagnostic tests are important foundations for diagnosing dyspnea.

For dyspnea of unknown cause, multidisciplinary expert consultation is often required.

First, it is necessary to assess whether the patient has emergency symptoms and whether vital signs are stable, and a rapid judgment and evaluation should be made, especially to identify hidden and atypical potentially life-threatening emergency symptoms. The following are urgent situations that require immediate appropriate treatment: dyspnea at rest or with minimal activity in patients with heart failure; acute chest pain, sweating, tachycardia or bradycardia, hypertension or hypotension, and syncope in patients with coronary heart disease; dyspnea at rest, fever, hypoxemia, tachycardia, and hypertension in patients with pulmonary embolism; decreased oxygen saturation, feeling of weakness and shortness of breath, rapid respiratory rate (>30 breaths / min), tachycardia, decreased blood pressure, and high / moderate pneumonia severity scores in patients with pneumonia; restlessness in patients with pneumothorax; peak expiratory flow (PEF)<80% of predicted value, tripod position, paradoxical pulse, and silent lung in patients with chronic obstructive pulmonary disease and bronchial asthma; respiratory rate>20 breaths / min, progressive cyanosis, restlessness in patients with dyspnea due to acute pancreatitis, severe trauma such as chest and abdominal trauma, amputation, massive wounds, and fractures.

Ⅵ Auxiliary Examinations

Among the causes of dyspnea, cardiac and pulmonary origins account for about 75%, while other causes account for about 25%. Appropriate examinations should be selected and evaluated for differential diagnosis.

1. Electrocardiogram (ECG) is important for dyspnea caused by heart failure triggered by myocardial ischemia, myocardial infarction, arrhythmias, etc.

2. Chest X-ray is convenient and quick, clearly showing the size and shape of the heart, lungs, and chest lesions, especially suitable for rapid diagnosis of pulmonary congestion, pulmonary edema, pneumonia, pneumothorax, pleural effusion, etc.

3. Elevated serum brain natriuretic peptide (BNP) and N-terminal pro-B-type natriuretic peptide (NT-proBNP) levels can be used as rapid diagnostic markers of cardiac dyspnea and determine the severity of heart failure (evidence level IA).

4. Cardiac troponin (T or I) is important for diagnosing acute myocardial infarction. Recent studies have found that cardiac troponin T or I may increase in heart failure, especially in acute decompensated heart failure, and its level may decrease after treatment, indicating myocardial injury during acute heart failure. The *2013 AHA / ACC Heart Failure Guidelines* state that cardiac troponin measurement is recommended to clarify the prognosis or severity of acute decompensated heart failure (evidence level IA).

5. Other biomarkers such as myocardial fibrosis markers, soluble ST2, and galectin-3 play important roles in the differential diagnosis of heart failure and predicting heart failure prognosis and mortality.

6. D-dimer is a monitoring indicator of thrombotic diseases, with higher sensitivity than specificity. It is mainly used to differentiate pulmonary embolism in the differential diagnosis of dyspnea. When D-dimer is<0.5 mg / L, pulmonary embolism can be basically excluded, while when D-dimer is>0.5 mg / L, it should be highly suspected and comprehensively judged in

combination with the patient's history and other examination results.

7. Cardiac Doppler ultrasound can accurately evaluate the size, structure, valvular morphology, activity, myocardial contraction, diastolic function, and cardiac function of the heart, thus playing an important role in the differential diagnosis of heart diseases and being simple and easy to perform.

8. Pulmonary function tests can help clarify the nature and extent of respiratory dysfunction; bronchodilation and airway provocation tests can be performed to assist in the diagnosis of suspected asthma. At the same time, pulmonary function tests are important for determining the severity and prognosis of pulmonary diseases.

9. Lung CT and CTA: High-resolution CT has incomparable advantages in diagnosing lung tumors, pulmonary interstitial fibrosis, and other diseases. Therefore, it has special diagnostic value in clarifying dyspnea caused by the above diseases. Pulmonary artery CTA is relatively inexpensive, non-invasive, safe, simple to operate, and highly reproducible, with a diagnostic agreement rate comparable to pulmonary angiography, gradually replacing pulmonary angiography.

10. Other examinations: When deep breathing and expiration have a rotten apple smell, check blood ketones and perform blood gas analysis; if hematological diseases are suspected, complete blood count, coagulation function, and bone marrow aspiration should be performed; if dyspnea caused by uremia or chemical toxins is suspected, renal function and related toxin tests are needed; if dyspnea is suspected to be related to brain diseases, neurological examinations are required.

Ⅶ Differential Diagnosis of Dyspnea

Many diseases can cause dyspnea. A comprehensive and systematic understanding of the patient's condition should be obtained, and the principles of "systematic, orderly, fast, and accurate" should be followed for the differential diagnosis of dyspnea, emphasizing the physician's comprehensive judgment ability.

The "systematic" principle means that dyspnea involves not only respiratory diseases but also extrapulmonary diseases, such as cardiovascular system (heart failure), nervous system (neuropathy), motor system (muscle diseases), and hematological diseases, avoiding preconceived notions. The "orderly" principle means that attention should be paid to the severity and urgency of diseases in the differential diagnosis of dyspnea, following a certain order, such as first excluding life-threatening acute and severe conditions, such as cardiac diseases (acute heart failure, myocardial infarction, and cardiac tamponade), airway foreign bodies, spontaneous pneumothorax, pulmonary embolism, etc., and then differentiating other chronic diseases. The "fast" principle means that it should be quickly determined whether it is a life-threatening acute or severe condition to reduce the risk in the differential diagnosis process of dyspnea. The "accurate" principle means that based on systematic examinations, efforts should be made to accurately judge the nature and degree of dyspnea and initiate effective treatment targeting the cause as early as possible.

Differential diagnosis can proceed based on the characteristics of dyspnea, including the mode of onset, precipitating factors, associated symptoms, physical findings, and suspected etiologies. Targeted investigations can then confirm or exclude specific diseases based on these initial assessments. Associated symptoms and physical findings can also aid in differential diagnosis. Although no unified diagnostic algorithm exists, patient history and physical examination are crucial, along with proper interpretation of ancillary test results.

Ⅷ Management of Dyspnea

The management of dyspnea is usually divided into general treatment, emergency treatment and symptomatic treatment, causal treatment or special treatment, etc. Due to the different causes of dyspnea, it is difficult to have a common treatment model applicable to all dyspnea. For dyspnea caused by any reason, the most fundamental treatment measure is the treatment of the primary disease, i.e., causal treatment.

The effect of oxygen therapy on relieving dyspnea is still controversial, and it may be beneficial for those with dyspnea at rest or with mild activity. For patients with acute dyspnea of unknown cause, their airway, breathing, and circulation status should be rapidly assessed and judged, while collecting relevant medical history and conducting focused physical examinations. Based on the results of preliminary examinations and vital signs, it is determined whether the patient needs to be hospitalized. When acute dyspnea symptoms are urgent and vital signs are unstable, vital signs should be immediately monitored, intravenous access established, and oxygen administered, while initiating preliminary treatment targeting the possible causes and then admitting the patient for further diagnosis and treatment; for those with urgent symptoms but stable vital signs, vital sign monitoring should be immediately provided, while initiating preliminary treatment targeting the possible causes. If the patient's symptoms or vital signs worsen after preliminary treatment, intravenous access should be established, oxygen administered, and the patient admitted for treatment, while those with milder symptoms can be further diagnosed and treated in the outpatient clinic; for those with mild symptoms and stable vital signs, they can be diagnosed and treated in the outpatient clinic, with detailed history taking and physical examination, and medication treatment and adjustment. If the patient's symptoms or vital signs worsen, they should be admitted for diagnosis and treatment.

Ⅸ Consultation Considerations

1. First, assess the urgency of symptoms, identify respiratory distress, stabilize vital signs, quickly treat fatal causes, and stabilize the patient for stepwise evaluation.

2. The significance of comorbid symptoms for cause differentiation: dyspnea with fever suggests infectious diseases (pneumonia, pulmonary tuberculosis, lung abscess); with chest pain suggests pulmonary infarction, pneumothorax, acute myocardial infarction, pleurisy; with wheezing suggests bronchial asthma, cardiac asthma; with frothy sputum—acute left heart failure, organophosphate poisoning; with coma suggests intracranial lesions, uremia, severe pneumonia, or poisoning.

3. Significance of physical findings in differential diagnosis: Jugular venous distension suggests increased right atrial pressure, as seen in right heart failure and pericardial effusion;

tracheal tugging suggests upper airway obstruction; barrel chest suggests chronic obstructive pulmonary disease; bilateral diffuse crackles that vary with position suggest left heart failure; diffuse wheezing suggests asthma; clubbing suggests bronchiectasis, lung abscess, or interstitial fibrosis; unilateral absent breath sounds suggest pneumothorax, massive pleural effusion, or large space-occupying lesion.

4. Distinguish functional from organic dyspnea:

(1) Organic dyspnea: Objectively, in addition to changes in respiratory rate and pattern, patients experience a sense of respiratory impairment, inspiratory or expiratory effort, use of accessory muscles, audible wheezing or rhonchi, and worsening of dyspnea in supine position or with exertion. Physical examination may reveal abnormal cardiorespiratory or systemic findings. If organic dyspnea is confirmed, life-threatening conditions like myocardial infarction, pulmonary embolism, heart failure, airway foreign body, or pneumothorax should be considered first.

(2) Functional dyspnea: Patients subjectively experience a sense of respiratory effort, but objectively appear to breathe smoothly apart from rapid rate, without wheezing, rhonchi, or a sense of airway obstruction. No tracheal tugging is present, and dyspnea is unchanged between sitting and supine positions. Blood pressure may be elevated, and heart rate slightly increased, but without cyanosis. Cardiopulmonary examination is normal, with normal oxygen saturation. Psychological factors are often involved, with emotional changes like crying during presentation.

5. Simple, valuable ancillary tests: Arterial blood gas analysis, serum biochemistry, electrocardiogram, chest radiography, B-type natriuretic peptide (BNP), and D-dimer measurement can help diagnose most common causes of dyspnea.

X Consultation Process

1. Assess vital signs; if instability like hypoxemia, tachypnea, hypotension, or malignant arrhythmias is present, initiate emergency measures like mechanical ventilation, cardioversion, temporary pacing, anti-arrhythmic drugs, and vasopressors.

2. Supplement critical history, including underlying heart or lung disease, diabetes or renal impairment, acute onset, associated chest discomfort or diaphoresis, cyanosis or hemoptysis, trauma or foreign body aspiration, fever, cough, or sputum production, or potential poisoning.

3. Perform focused physical examination, assessing postural effects on dyspnea, asymmetry of breath sounds, barrel chest, cyanosis, cardiac dullness, crackles or wheezes, jugular venous distension, peripheral edema (unilateral or bilateral), and mental status or neurological deficits.

4. Rapidly obtain ancillary tests like arterial blood gases, renal function, electrolytes, electrocardiogram, chest radiography, BNP or NT-proBNP, and D-dimer. If pulmonary embolism is suspected, pursue computed tomographic pulmonary angiography. If heart failure is considered, promptly obtain echocardiography.

5. After diagnosis, initiate treatment: for acute myocardial infarction, pursue urgent revascularization; for pneumothorax or massive effusion, perform drainage; for pulmonary embolism, consider thrombolysis or anti-coagulation; for heart failure, provide diuretics, vasodilators, inotropic support, or device therapy as needed, followed by comprehensive

evaluation with echocardiography and coronary angiography; for severe pneumonia, provide antimicrobials and supportive care; for acute exacerbations of chronic lung disease, provide bronchodilators or mechanical ventilation; for diabetic ketoacidosis, uremia, intracranial pathology, poisoning, or airway compression / obstruction, provide condition-specific and supportive treatment.

6. After excluding the above urgent and life-threatening causes and common causes, investigate respiratory difficulties or functional respiratory difficulties caused by diseases of the nervous system, muscular system, blood system, etc.

Section 2 Advances in the Diagnosis and Treatment of Acute Left Heart Failure

Acute heart failure is a syndrome characterized by a significant, abrupt decrease in cardiac output due to an acute cardiac condition, resulting in inadequate tissue and organ perfusion and acute pulmonary edema. Common etiologies include acute myocardial infarction, hypertensive emergencies, valvular heart disease, and cardiomyopathies. Clinically, acute left heart failure is more prevalent, manifesting primarily as acute pulmonary edema or cardiogenic shock, with occasional presentations of cardiogenic syncope or cardiac arrest. Dyspnea is the most common and prominent symptom of left heart failure. Acute left heart failure is a cardiac emergency requiring prompt resuscitative treatment, and the short-term prognosis is influenced by the underlying cause, the degree of cardiac decompensation, and the timeliness and appropriateness of resuscitation.

I Epidemiology

Despite decreasing incidence and mortality rates for major cardiovascular diseases like coronary artery disease and hypertension, the incidence of heart failure continues to rise. In the Framingham cohort of 5,192 men and women followed for 20 years, the incidence of heart failure was 3.7% in men and 2.5% in women. In the United States, over 2 million individuals have heart failure diagnosed by the National Heart, Lung, and Blood Institute, with approximately 400,000 new cases of acute heart failure diagnosed annually.

II Causes of Acute Left Heart Failure

1. Myocardial infarction related to coronary artery disease, particularly extensive anterior wall myocardial infarction, papillary muscle or chordae tendineae rupture, and ventricular septal defects.

2. Acute valvular regurgitation due to infective endocarditis causing valve perforation or chordae tendineae rupture.

3. Others: Abrupt hypertensive emergencies in patients with hypertension, rapid arrhythmias or severe bradyarrhythmias in the setting of underlying heart disease, excessive or rapid blood transfusion or fluid administration.

Ⅲ Pathophysiology of Acute Left Heart Failure

The pathophysiological basis of acute left heart failure is a sudden severe reduction in myocardial contractility, leading to an abrupt decrease in cardiac output, or acute valvular regurgitation into the left ventricle, resulting in a rapid rise in end-diastolic pressure, impaired pulmonary venous drainage, and an accompanying increase in pulmonary capillary wedge pressure. As pulmonary capillary pressure rapidly increases, fluid extravasates into the pulmonary interstitium and alveoli, causing acute pulmonary edema.

The pulmonary circulation is a low-pressure system compared to the systemic circulation, with a mean pulmonary capillary pressure of 7.5-10 mmHg and a colloid osmotic pressure of approximately 27 mmHg, favoring the retention of fluid within the vascular space under normal conditions. In left ventricular dysfunction, elevated left ventricular end-diastolic pressure leads to corresponding increases in left atrial and pulmonary capillary pressures. When the mean pulmonary capillary pressure exceeds 25 mmHg, the critical level is surpassed, and fluid begins to accumulate in the pulmonary interstitium as lymphatic drainage becomes overwhelmed, ultimately extravasating into the alveoli and causing pulmonary edema.

Ⅳ Clinical Manifestations of Acute Left Heart Failure

1. Dyspnea is the most common and prominent symptom of left heart failure, with patients experiencing a sense of breathlessness requiring forceful and rapid respirations, often reaching 20-30 breaths per minute.

(1) Orthopnea: A distinctive sign of acute left heart failure, manifesting as severe dyspnea in the supine position with relief upon sitting upright. In severe cases, patients are forced to assume a semi-upright or seated position, hence the term "orthopnea". In the most severe instances, patients may sit upright at the bedside or in a chair, with their legs dangling and their torso leaning forward to enhance the action of the respiratory muscles. This mechanism compensates for pulmonary congestion. In healthy individuals, lung volumes decrease by an average of 5% in the supine position, whereas in orthopnea, lung volumes decrease by an average of 25%, indicating more severe pulmonary congestion and lung stiffening. The mechanisms underlying dyspnea include: ① Increased pulmonary capillary pressure stimulates vagal afferents adjacent to the pulmonary vascular bed, reflexively exciting the respiratory center and triggering the Churchill-Cope reflex, leading to tachypnea; ② Increased pulmonary blood volume and enlarged pulmonary capillary bed reduce alveolar volume, decreasing lung compliance and requiring greater negative inspiratory pressures for lung expansion and greater positive expiratory pressures for lung deflation, necessitating increased respiratory muscle effort; ③ The enlarged pulmonary capillary bed compresses small airways, increasing airway resistance. Patients assume an upright posture to redistribute blood away from the pulmonary circulation, alleviating symptoms.

(2) Paroxysmal Nocturnal Dyspnea: A clinical manifestation of acute left heart failure with pulmonary edema or acute exacerbation of chronic pulmonary edema. Paroxysmal dyspnea can be classified into two types: ① Caused by acute left heart failure, with predominant left

ventricular failure, more common; ② Caused by mitral stenosis, with predominant left atrial failure. However, the clinical presentations are similar. Typically, patients experience sudden awakening from sleep, often after several hours in the recumbent position, with severe dyspnea necessitating an upright position and accompanied by cough. Mild cases resolve within minutes of sitting upright, while severe cases are accompanied by cough, frothy sputum, and wheezing, termed "cardiac asthma". The mechanism involves fluid mobilization from peripheral edema 1-2 hours after falling asleep, increasing venous return and cardiac preload. Respiratory center insensitivity during sleep delays the perception of dyspnea until pulmonary congestion and hypoxia reach a critical threshold. During cardiac asthma episodes, elevated arterial pressure leads to increased pulmonary artery and capillary pressures, with sudden decreases in arterial pressure being an ominous sign.

2. Acute Pulmonary Edema results from a rapid and sustained increase in pulmonary capillary pressure, representing a qualitative change from the preceding forms of dyspnea, as capillary fluid extravasates in quantities exceeding lymphatic clearance capacity. Fluid initially accumulates in the pulmonary interstitium, compressing alveoli and reducing the effective gas exchange surface area while decreasing lung compliance, leading to severe dyspnea. Interstitial fluid can also compress small airways, further exacerbating dyspnea and producing wheezing, termed "cardiac asthma". Acute pulmonary edema occurs when left ventricular end-diastolic pressure, left atrial pressure, and pulmonary capillary pressure exceed 30 mmHg. Based on the progression and clinical manifestations, pulmonary edema can be categorized into five stages:

(1) Prodromal Stage: Atypical symptoms, with shortness of breath and occasional anxiety. Physical examination may reveal pale, clammy skin and tachycardia. Chest radiography may show characteristic perihilar haziness or a "butterfly" pattern.

(2) Interstitial Pulmonary Edema Stage: Dyspnea without frothy sputum. Orthopnea, pallor, and occasional cyanosis may be present. Some patients may exhibit jugular venous distension, wheezing on lung auscultation, and occasional fine crackles.

(3) Alveolar Pulmonary Edema Stage: Frequent cough, severe dyspnea, and pink, frothy sputum. Diffuse rhonchi and crackles are audible throughout both lung fields.

(4) Shock Stage: Hypotension, thready pulse, pallor, worsening cyanosis, diaphoresis, and altered mental status.

(5) Agonal Stage: Severe respiratory and cardiac dysrhythmias, imminent death.

3. Cardiac Syncope. Cardiac syncope refers to a temporary loss of cons-ciousness caused by reduced cardiac output and subsequent cerebral hypo-perfusion due to impaired cardiac pumping function itself. During an attack that lasts for a few seconds, symptoms such as limb convulsions, respiratory arrest, and cyanosis may manifest, known as Stokes-Adams syndrome. Attacks are typically brief, with consciousness promptly regaining afterward. This condition mainly occurs in cases of acute cardiac outflow obstruction or severe arrhythmias.

4. Cardiogenic Shock. Cardiogenic shock is shock induced by insufficient cardiac output resulting from depressed cardiac pumping capability. When the reduction in cardiac output is sudden and significant, compensatory mechanisms like increasing circulating blood volume cannot be initiated promptly, though neurogenic reflexes may cause marked peripheral and

visceral vasoconstriction to maintain blood pressure and preserve cerebral and coronary perfusion. Clinically, in addition to general signs of shock, cardiogenic shock often presents with evidence of cardiac decompensation, elevated pulmonary capillary wedge pressure, and jugular venous distension.

V Common Signs of Left Heart Failure

1. Pulsus alternans: Regular rhythm but alternating strong and weak pulse volumes. As left ventricular failure worsens, pulsus alternans can be detected by palpating peripheral arteries. Mechanisms include: ① Different numbers of contracting myocardial fibers between beats. During a weak pulse, some fibers are in a relative refractory period and fail to contribute to ventricular contraction, whereas all fibers are excitable during a strong pulse. ② Varying degrees of myocardial relaxation preceding each contraction.

2. Gallop rhythm is a common sign of left heart failure, best audible at the apex or para-apical area in the left lateral decubitus position and accentuated by expiration.

3. Initially lungs may be clear or just wheezy, but moist rales rapidly develop in bilateral lung bases and progress upwards to involve the entire lung fields. In severe cases, coarse rales resembling boiling water can be auscultated throughout all lung zones.

Ⅵ Complications of Acute Left Heart Failure

1. Cardiogenic shock: In 50% of acute left ventricular failure cases with markedly and abruptly reduced cardiac output, severe right ventricular dysfunction unresponsive to preload occurs, leading to hypotension, poor end-organ perfusion, and cardiogenic shock.

2. Multiple organ dysfunction: Acute cardiac decompensation, especially cardiogenic shock, can cause acute hypoxia and dysfunction of vital organs like the kidneys, brain and liver before compensatory mechanisms take effect, resulting in multiple organ failure that further exacerbates cardiac dysfunction.

3. Electrolyte and acid-base disturbances: Use of diuretics, salt restriction, poor intake, as well as nausea, vomiting and diaphoresis can lead to hypokalemia, hyponatremia, hypochloremic metabolic alkalosis and metabolic acidosis.

Ⅶ Laboratory and Auxiliary Tests

1. Arterial blood gas may show significantly reduced oxygen saturation, normal or low carbon dioxide levels, and low pH level.

2. Chest X-ray may reveal bat-wing pulmonary edema extending from the hilar regions, cardiomegaly, and diminished cardiac pulsations.

3. ECG may show sinus tachycardia or various arrhythmias, myocardial injury, left atrial and ventricular hypertrophy.

4. Echocardiography may demonstrate chamber dilation and reduced left ventricular ejection fraction (LVEF < 40%).

5. Natriuretic peptides are useful for diagnosing and differentiating acute heart failure (Class Ⅰ, Level A): BNP < 100 ng / L or NT-proBNP < 300 ng / L can reasonably exclude acute heart

failure.

6. Cardiac troponin T or I levels may rise>3-5 folds in acute myocardial infarction, but can remain elevated in decompensated heart failure, providing risk stratification and severity assessment (Class I, Level A).

Ⅷ Diagnosis of Acute Left Heart Failure

The diagnosis can usually be made without difficulty based on clinical history, typical symptoms / signs, and auxiliary test results.

Ⅸ Differential Diagnosis of Acute Left Heart Failure

1. Bronchial asthma: Both cardiac asthma and bronchial asthma present with acute onset of cough, dyspnea and wheezing, but require very different management principles. Bronchial asthma is a reversible obstructive pulmonary disease with increased airway hyperreactivity. Patients often have a longstanding history of recurrent wheezing or atopy. It is more common in young adults, with a cough productive of scanty, tenacious sputum or none unless infected. Physical exam may show hyperinflation but is often clear without crackles unless pneumonia or atelectasis coexists. Cardiac findings are typically normal. Pulmonary function tests show increased airway resistance and blood eosinophilia (eosinophil count often>250-400 / μL).

2. Acute respiratory distress syndrome (ARDS): Also known as shock lung, wet lung, pump lung or adult respiratory distress syndrome, ARDS can be confused with acute left heart failure due to shared features like dyspnea, cyanosis, crackles and wheezing. However, ARDS often lacks a preceding pulmonary history and can follow any acute insult causing direct or indirect lung injury like trauma, drowning, shock, cardiopulmonary bypass, bacterial / viral pneumonia, or pancreatitis. Onset is typically after the initial illness or within 24-48 hours of the insult. Dyspnea is severe but rarely requires sitting upright. Hypoxemia progressively worsens despite supplemental oxygen. Wheezing and crackles may be present, but no gallop, cardiomegaly or organic murmurs. Treatment measures for cardiac asthma often have no obvious effect; the floating catheter shows pulmonary capillary wedge pressure<15 mmHg (1.99 kPa). Positive end-expiratory pressure ventilation is effective in assisting treatment, and ARDS often involves multiple organ failure.

X Treatment of Acute Left Heart Failure

1. Principles: Remove precipitating factors, treat underlying causes, reduce left ventricular filling pressures, augment cardiac output, and reduce circulating blood volume.

(1) Immediately have the patient assume an upright or semi-upright position with legs dependent, or apply sequential tourniquets to the extremities, releasing one limb every 15 minutes rotationally. This reduces venous return and alleviates pulmonary edema.

(2) Oxygen Therapy: Promptly initiate high-flow oxygen via nasal cannula at 10-20 L / min. For critically ill patients, apply face mask or non-invasive positive pressure ventilation. If arterial PO_2 cannot be maintained above 60 mmHg, initiate positive pressure ventilation. Immediately initiate oxygen therapy and defrothing measures. Pre-bubbling oxygen through 40%-70% ethanol

humidification can reduce alveolar surface tension, promoting froth clearance and improving ventilation.

(3) Establish Intravenous Access Quickly: Rapidly secure intravenous access to enable drug administration and sampling for electrolytes, renal function, etc. Send blood gas samples for urgent analysis.

(4) ECG, blood pressure, and other monitoring: To deal with various potentially serious arrhythmias at any time.

2. Sedation: Immediately intravenously inject 3-5 mg of morphine, which can be repeated if necessary, with a total amount not exceeding 15 mg. Morphine not only has sedative effects, relieves the patient's anxiety, and slows breathing but also dilates veins and arteries, thereby reducing cardiac preload and afterload and improving pulmonary edema. Note that it is contraindicated in patients with respiratory failure and should be used with caution or contraindicated in the elderly, asthma, coma, severe lung disease, respiratory depression, and bradycardia or atrioventricular block.

3. Rapid diuresis: Fast-acting and potent diuretics should be immediately selected, commonly loop diuretics, among which furosemide is frequently used. First, intravenously inject 20-40 mg, followed by an intravenous infusion of 5-40 mg / h, with a total dose not exceeding 80 mg in the initial 6 h and 160 mg in the initial 24 h. Torasemide 10-20 mg can also be administered intravenously. If loop diuretics are used for routine treatment, the initial intravenous dose should be equal to or greater than the long-term daily dose. Note: When using diuretics, do not overdose, especially avoid causing hypokalemia. Furosemide 20-40 mg intravenous injection should be completed within 2 minutes, taking effect within 10 minutes, and lasting for 3-4 h; it can be repeated after 4 h. In addition to its diuretic effect, this drug also has a venodilating effect, which is beneficial for the relief of pulmonary edema.

4. Vasodilators: For simple emergency treatment, first sublingually administer 0.5 mg of nitroglycerin every 5-10 minutes. If the effect is not significant, intravenous infusion of vasodilators can be used instead, with common preparations including nitroglycerin, sodium nitroprusside, and phentolamine. If blood pressure is $<$90 / 40 mmHg (12 / 5.3 kPa) during the use of vasodilators, dopamine can be added to maintain blood pressure, and the dosage or infusion rate of vasodilators can be adjusted accordingly. Note: When using vasodilators, prevent blood pressure from dropping too quickly.

(1) Nitroglycerin: Patients' tolerance to this drug varies greatly among individuals. It can be started at 5-10 μg / min and then adjusted every 10 minutes, with each increase of 5-10 μg / min. Adverse reactions include headache, tachycardia, nausea, vomiting, flushing, and methemoglobinemia.

Nitrate drugs such as nitroglycerin, when continuously intravenously infused for more than 72 h, can easily develop drug resistance. Attention should be paid to switching to other vasodilators or using them intermittently.

(2) Sodium nitroprusside: Start with an intravenous infusion at a concentration of 50 mg / 500 mL and a rate of 0.5 μg / (min·kg), and gradually adjust the dose according to the therapeutic response, increasing by 0.5 μg / kg per minute. The commonly used dose is 3 μg / kg per minute,

with a maximum of 10 μg / kg per minute. Adverse reactions of sodium nitroprusside include: ① When the blood drug concentration is high and the drug is suddenly discontinued, rebound hypertension may occur; ② Excessively rapid and severe blood pressure reduction, resulting in dizziness, sweating, headache, muscle tremors, nervousness or anxiety, restlessness, stomach pain, reflex tachycardia or arrhythmia, with the occurrence of symptoms related to the intravenous administration rate rather than the total amount. Dose reduction or discontinuation can lead to improvement; ③ Thiocyanate toxicity, which may cause ataxia, blurred vision, delirium, dizziness, headache, unconsciousness, nausea, vomiting, tinnitus, and shortness of breath. The drug should be discontinued, and symptomatic treatment should be provided.

Precautions for the use of sodium nitroprusside: ① Light-sensitive, the infusion solution should be freshly prepared, and the infusion bottle should be quickly wrapped with black paper to avoid light; ② Other drugs should not be added to the solution. The prepared solution can only be administered by slow intravenous drip, preferably using a microinfusion pump, which can accurately control the administration rate; ③ During the use of this drug, blood pressure should be frequently measured, preferably in the monitoring room; ④ For patients with renal insufficiency and using this drug for more than 48-72 h, plasma cyanide or thiocyanate should be measured daily, maintaining thiocyanate not exceeding 100 μg / mL and cyanide not exceeding 3 μmol / mL.

5. Positive inotropic drugs: Positive inotropic drugs are suitable for patients with acute left heart failure accompanied by hypotension and can be used alone or in combination. Generally, they should be started at medium or small doses and gradually increased as needed. For patients with significantly reduced blood pressure, hydroxylamine (aramine) can be briefly combined to rapidly increase blood pressure and ensure blood perfusion to the heart and brain.

(1) Dopamine: Low-dose dopamine (<2 μg / kg per minute) can reduce peripheral resistance and dilate renal and coronary small veins.

Higher-dose dopamine (>2 μg / kg per minute) can increase myocardial contractility and cardiac output. It can be used in patients with pulmonary edema accompanied by hypotension.

(2) Dobutamine: The starting dose is 2-3 μg / kg per minute, and the maximum dose can be up to 20 μg / kg per minute.

(3) Phosphodiesterase inhibitors: Mainly milrinone is used, with an initial dose of 25-75 μg / kg intravenous injection (>10 min), followed by an intravenous infusion of 0.375-0.750 μg / (kg·min). Levosimendan (Class Ⅱa, Level B): Its positive inotropic effect is independent of β-adrenergic stimulation and can be used in patients currently receiving β-blocker therapy. The initial dose is 12 μg / kg intravenous injection (>10 min), followed by an intravenous infusion of 0.1 μg / (kg·min), which can be halved or doubled as appropriate. For patients with a systolic blood pressure<100 mmHg, no loading dose is required.

6. Cardiotonic drugs: Digitalis drugs are most suitable for patients with atrial fibrillation accompanied by a rapid ventricular rate and known ventricular enlargement with left ventricular systolic dysfunction. Digitalis has a good therapeutic effect on cardiac pulmonary edema with pressure overload, such as aortic stenosis and hypertension. It has a more life-saving benefit for acute pulmonary edema with severe mitral stenosis accompanied by rapid atrial fibrillation.

Digitalis drugs are not recommended for use within 24 h of the acute phase in patients with acute myocardial infarction and are contraindicated in patients with severe mitral stenosis accompanied by sinus rhythm. The first choice is often proscillaridin A (lanatoside C). For those without a recent medication history, the initial dose can be 0.4-0.8 mg intravenous injection, and 0.2-0.4 mg can be given again after 2 h if necessary.

7. Treatment of bronchospasm: Based on typical symptoms and signs, attention should be paid to the differentiation between acute dyspnea and bronchial asthma. Coughing up pink frothy sputum and a gallop rhythm at the apex of the heart help diagnose pulmonary edema and differentiate cardiogenic shock coexisting with pulmonary edema from shock caused by other reasons. Aminophylline 0.25 g can be slowly injected intravenously in 20 mL of 5% glucose solution, or 500 mg can be added to 250 mL of 5% glucose solution for intravenous drip, which is especially suitable for patients with obvious wheezing, as it can alleviate bronchospasm and enhance the diuretic effect.

8. Treatment of inducing factors and causes: After the acute symptoms are alleviated, treatment of the inducing factors and underlying causes should be initiated. For example, antihypertensive measures should be taken for hypertensive patients, and rapid ectopic arrhythmias should be corrected.

9. Adrenocortical hormones have anti-allergic, anti-shock, anti-exudative, and stress-reducing effects. Generally, dexamethasone 10-20 mg is selected for intravenous injection or intravenous drip. It should be used with caution or contraindicated in patients with active bleeding. In the case of acute myocardial infarction, it is generally not routinely used unless accompanied by heart block or shock.

10. Application indications for mechanical ventilators: Cardiac and respiratory arrest requiring cardiopulmonary resuscitation and combined with type I or type Ⅱ respiratory failure. There are two methods: ① Non-invasive ventilator-assisted ventilation (Class Ⅱa, Level B): It is divided into continuous positive airway pressure ventilation and biphasic positive airway pressure ventilation. It is recommended for pulmonary edema combined with respiratory failure that cannot be corrected by routine oxygen therapy and medication, with a respiratory rate$>$20 breaths / min, and for patients who can cooperate with ventilator ventilation, but it is not recommended for patients with a systolic blood pressure$<$85 mmHg; ② Endotracheal intubation and mechanical ventilation: The application indications are during cardiopulmonary resuscitation, severe respiratory failure that cannot be improved by routine treatment, especially for patients with obvious respiratory and metabolic acidosis affecting the state of consciousness.

11. Precautions: During the treatment process, electrocardiographic and hemodynamic monitoring should be performed.

XI Consultation Considerations

1. Quickly perform clinical assessment and monitoring after examining the patient: The assessment should quickly clarify the volume status; whether there is insufficient circulatory perfusion; whether there are inducing factors and (or) complications of acute heart failure. Non-

invasive monitoring (Class Ⅰ, Level B) continuously measures heart rate, respiratory rate, blood pressure, oxygen saturation, arterial blood gas, electrocardiogram, etc. For patients with unstable hemodynamic status, severe condition, and unsatisfactory treatment effect, such as those with pulmonary edema (or) cardiogenic shock, hemodynamic monitoring should be provided, with the main methods being right heart catheterization and peripheral arterial catheterization.

2. Valuable and easy-to-perform examinations: Arterial blood gas analysis, chest X-ray, electrocardiogram, BNP or NT-proBNP, and troponin levels can be instructed to be performed when receiving the consultation call. Echocardiography is of great significance for determining the cause and cardiac function status, so larger centers should be equipped with bedside machines.

3. The most meaningful treatment measures are firstly maintaining vital signs, and the fastest ways to relieve symptoms are, in order, morphine, diuretics, and vasodilators, paying attention to the improvement and stabilization of the internal environment.

Ⅻ Consultation Process

1. Assess the patient's vital signs. If unstable, such as decreased oxygen saturation, shallow rapid breathing, hypotension, or malignant arrhythmias, immediately provide emergency treatment like mechanical ventilation, defibrillation, temporary pacemaker, antiarrhythmic drugs, and vasopressors.

2. Supplement key medical history, such as underlying heart disease, chest discomfort or pain, diaphoresis, alcohol abuse, peripartum period, or family history of cardiomyopathy. Recent infections, fluid overload, or increased water intake that may exacerbate heart failure should also be noted.

3. Pay attention to important physical examination findings, such as blood pressure (noting sudden after-load increase causing heart failure or cardiogenic shock), arrhythmias, pulmonary rales, jugular venous distension, peripheral edema, cardiomegaly, heart murmurs, or gallop rhythm.

4. Rapidly perform auxiliary tests like arterial blood gas, renal function, electrolytes, electrocardiogram, chest X-ray, BNP or NT-proBNP, and echocar-diography once stable. Pursue urgent revascularization if electrocardiogram suggests acute myocardial infarction.

5. Promptly relieve symptoms. The fastest-acting drugs are morphine (contraindicated in altered mental status, significant hypoxia, hypotension, or chronic obstructive pulmonary disease), diuretics, and vasodilators to reduce preload and after-load. Avoid vasodilators in hypertrophic obstructive cardiomyopathy or severe valvular stenosis; if symptoms persist, use positive inotropes. For severe cases unresponsive to medical therapy or unstable vitals, promptly initiate non-pharmacological treatments like non-invasive or invasive ventilation, ultrafiltration, continuous renal replacement therapy, intra-aortic balloon pump (for ischemic cardiomyopathy), or extracorporeal membrane oxygenation, while maintaining internal environment stability.

6. Once symptoms improve, complete relevant examinations to determine the underlying cause of heart failure.

Section 3 Heart Failure with Preserved Ejection Fraction

I Definition and Classification

Based on left ventricular ejection fraction (LVEF), heart failure can be classified into heart failure with reduced ejection fraction (HFrEF), heart failure with mid-range ejection fraction (HFmrEF), and heart failure with preserved ejection fraction (HFpEF).

Generally, HFrEF refers to the traditional concept of systolic heart failure, while HFpEF refers to diastolic heart failure. With preserved or normal LVEF, systolic function may still be abnormal, and some heart failure patients may have co-existing systolic and diastolic dysfunction. LVEF is an important indicator for classifying heart failure patients and is also associated with prognosis and treatment response (Table 2-1).

Table 2-1 Classification of HFrEF, HFmrEF, and HFpEF

Heart Failure Type		HF-REF	HF-mrEF	HF-PEF
	1	Symptoms ± signs	Symptoms ± signs	Symptoms ± signs
	2	LVEF<40%	41%<LVEF-49%	LVEF>50%
	3	—	1. Elevated natriuretic peptide levels	1. Elevated natriuretic peptide levels
			2. At least one of the following additional criteria:	2. At least one of the following additional criteria:
			a. Relevant structural heart disease (LVH) and / or LAE	a. Relevant structural heart disease (LVH) and / or LAE
			b. Diastolic dysfunction	b. Diastolic dysfunction

LAE=left atrial enlargement; LVH=left ventricular hypertrophy

a. In early heart failure (especially HFpEF) and with diuretic treatment, signs may be absent.

b. BNP>35 pg / mL, and / or NT-proBNP>125 pg / mL

II Diagnosis

1. The diagnosis of HFpEF should fully consider the following two aspects:

(1) Main clinical manifestations: ① Typical symptoms and signs of heart failure; ② Normal or mildly reduced LVEF (≥45%) with non-dilated left ventricle; ③ Evidence of relevant structural heart disease (such as left ventricular hypertrophy, left atrial enlargement) and / or diastolic dysfunction; ④ Echocardiography excludes valvular heart disease, pericardial discasc, hypertrophic cardiomyopathy, restrictive (infiltrative) cardiomyopathy, etc.

(2) Other factors to consider: ① Should conform to the epidemiological characteristics of the disease: mostly elderly female patients with hypertension or long-standing hypertension history as the underlying cause of heart failure, some with comorbidities like diabetes, obesity, atrial fibrillation; ② BNP and / or NT-proBNP measurements are valuable references, albeit controversial. Mildly to moderately elevated levels, or at least in the "gray zone", support the diagnosis.

2. Auxiliary Examinations: Echocardiographic parameters for diagnosing left ventricular diastolic dysfunction lack accuracy and reproducibility, therefore, a comprehensive evaluation of cardiac structure and function should integrate all relevant 2D and Doppler parameters. Early diastolic mitral annular velocity (e') can assess myocardial relaxation, while E / e' relates to left ventricular filling pressures. Evidence of diastolic dysfunction on echocardiography may include reduced e' (average<9 cm / s), increased E / e' (>15), abnormal E / A ratio (>2 or<1), or a combination. At least two abnormal indices and / or presence of atrial fibrillation increase the likelihood of diastolic dysfunction.

Ⅲ Treatment

1. Clinical trials in HFpEF (PEP-CHF, CHARM-Preserved, I-Preserve, J-DHF, etc.) have failed to demonstrate that medications effective for HFrEF, such as ACEIs, ARBs, and beta-blockers, can improve outcomes or reduce mortality in HFpEF patients.

The VALIDD trial suggests blood pressure lowering is beneficial for heart failure patients with hypertension. A comprehensive treatment approach targeting HFpEF symptoms, comorbidities, and risk factors is recommended.

2. Aggressively control blood pressure: Target lower than standard for uncomplicated hypertension, i.e.<130 / 80 mmHg systolic (Class Ⅰ, Level A). All 5 major antihypertensive drug classes can be used, with preference for beta-blockers, ACEIs or ARBs.

3. Diuretic use: Relieving fluid retention and edema is crucial to alleviate pulmonary congestion and improve cardiac function. However, excessive diuresis should be avoided to prevent preload reduction and hypotension (Class Ⅰ, Level C).

4. Control and treat other underlying conditions and complications: Control ventricular rate in chronic atrial fibrillation (Class Ⅰ, Level C) with beta-blockers or non-dihydropyridine CCBs (diltiazem or verapamil). If possible, restore and maintain sinus rhythm for patient benefit (Class Ⅱb, Level C). Actively treat diabetes and control blood glucose. Weight loss for obese patients. For left ventricular hypertrophy, ACEIs, ARBs, beta-blockers, etc. may be used to promote regression and improve diastolic function (Class Ⅱb, Level C). Digoxin cannot increase myocardial relaxation and is not recommended.

5. Revascularization: Since myocardial ischemia can impair ventricular diastolic function, coronary revascularization should be performed in symptomatic coronary artery disease patients or those with proven myocardial ischemia (Class Ⅱa, Level C).

6. If concomitant HFrEF is present, prioritize its treatment.

Ⅳ Common Questions in Consultation

1. What is the pathophysiological mechanism of HFpEF? HFpEF, commonly referred to as diastolic heart failure, has an unclear pathophysiological mechanism. Current understanding suggests impaired left ventricular active relaxation during diastole and decreased myocardial compliance, i.e. increased stiffness (myocyte hypertrophy with interstitial fibrosis), leading to impaired left ventricular filling during diastole, reduced cardiac output, elevated end-diastolic pressure, and consequent heart failure.

2. What are the epidemiological characteristics of HFpEF? HFpEF can coexist with systolic dysfunction or occur in isolation. HFpEF accounts for approximately 50% of all heart failure cases (40%-71%), with a prognosis similar to or slightly better than HFrEF. Asymptomatic left ventricular diastolic dysfunction is associated with increased heart failure incidence and mortality rates. An epidemiological survey from the United States found that 21% of the community population had asymptomatic mild diastolic dysfunction, and 7% had moderate-to-severe diastolic dysfunction.

3. What methods are used to diagnose HFpEF? Symptoms ± signs; LVEF≥ 50%; elevated natriuretic peptide levels; at least one of the following: relevant structural heart disease (left ventricular hypertrophy and / or left atrial enlargement), diastolic dysfunction.

4. What are the treatment methods and precautions for HFpEF? First, treat the underlying disease and complications, such as hypertension, diabetes, coronary artery disease, atrial fibrillation, and left ventricular hypertrophy. Second, select appropriate medications, including ACEIs, ARBs, beta-blockers, CCBs, etc.

V Consultation Process

1. Assess the patient's vital signs. If unstable, such as decreased oxygen saturation, shallow rapid breathing, hypotension, or malignant arrhythmias, immediately provide emergency treatment like mechanical ventilation, defibrillation, temporary pacemaker, antiarrhythmic drugs, and vasopressors.

2. Supplement key medical history, such as recent infections, fluid overload, increased water intake, or new-onset arrhythmias that may exacerbate heart failure.

3. Pay attention to important physical examination findings, such as blood pressure (noting sudden after-load increase causing heart failure or cardiogenic shock), arrhythmias, pulmonary rales, jugular venous distension, peripheral edema, cardiomegaly, heart murmurs, or gallop rhythm.

4. Rapidly perform auxiliary tests like arterial blood gas, renal function, electrolytes, electrocardiogram, chest X-ray, BNP or NT-proBNP, and follow up with echocardiography once stable.

5. Promptly relieve symptoms. The fastest-acting drugs are morphine (contraindicated in altered mental status, significant hypoxia, hypotension, or chronic obstructive pulmonary disease), diuretics, and vasodilators to reduce preload and after-load. Avoid vasodilators in hypertrophic obstructive cardiomyopathy or severe valvular stenosis. If medical therapy cannot relieve severe symptoms or vital signs remain unstable, promptly initiate non-pharmacological treatments like non-invasive or invasive ventilation, ultrafiltration, continuous renal replacement therapy, intra-aortic balloon pump (for ischemic cardiomyopathy), or extracorporeal membrane oxygenation, while maintaining internal environment stability.

6. HFpEF patients are often elderly with multiple comorbidities. Control blood pressure, heart rate, and blood glucose, perform revascularization and / or secondary coronary artery disease prevention, and provide anti-coagulation for atrial fibrillation patients.

Section 4 Pharmacological Treatment of Chronic Heart Failure

I Drug Therapy

1. Diuretics

(1) Indications: All heart failure patients with evidence of fluid retention should receive diuretic therapy (Class Ⅰ, Level C).

(2) Administration: Start with low doses, gradually increasing until diuresis occurs, aiming for 0.5-1.0 kg of daily weight loss. Once symptoms improve and the condition is controlled, maintain the lowest effective dose long-term, adjusting as needed based on fluid status. Daily weight change is the most reliable indicator for monitoring diuretic effect and dose titration.

(3) Agent selection: Commonly used diuretics include loop diuretics and thiazides. Prefer loop diuretics such as furosemide or torsemide, especially for significant fluid overload or renal impairment. Furosemide dose has a linear relationship with effect and is not dose-limited, though very high doses are not clinically recommended. Thiazides are only suitable for heart failure patients with mild fluid retention, hypertension, and normal renal function. Hydrochlorothiazide 100 mg daily reaches maximum effect (dose-response curve plateaus), with no additional benefit from higher doses. The newer diuretic tolvaptan, a vasopressin V2 receptor antagonist with aquaretic but not natriuretic effects, demonstrates greater efficacy in refractory edema or hyponatremia.

(4) Adverse effects: Electrolyte disturbances are common, such as hypokalemia, hypomagnesemia, and hyponatremia. Distinguish between depleted-volume and dilutional hyponatremia, treating the latter as diuretic resistance. Diuretic use can activate endogenous neurohormonal systems, particularly the renin-angiotensin-aldosterone system (RAAS) and sympathetic nervous system, necessitating concomitant use with ACEIs or ARBs and Beta-blockers.

It is crucial to discern whether symptoms such as hypotension and worsening renal function are adverse reactions to diuretics, indicative of worsening heart failure, or a manifestation of hypovolemia.

2. ACE Inhibitor (ACEI)

(1) Indications: All patients with reduced left ventricular ejection fraction (LVEF) must use ACEIs for life unless contraindicated or not tolerated (Class Ⅰ, Level A). For populations at high risk of heart failure (Stage A), consider ACEI for prevention (Class Ⅱa, Level A).

(2) Contraindications: Fatal adverse reactions such as laryngeal edema, severe renal failure, and pregnancy. Use with caution in bilateral renal artery stenosis, serum creatinine $>$265.2 μmol / L (3 mg / dL), serum potassium $>$5.5 mmol / L, symptomatic hypotension (systolic blood pressure $<$ 90 mmHg), and left ventricular outflow tract obstruction.

(3) Administration: Begin with a low dose and gradually increase to the target dose, typically doubling the dose every 1-2 weeks. Dosage titration and maintenance should be personalized, with lifelong use once an appropriate dose is established. Avoid abrupt discontinuation. Monitor blood pressure, serum potassium, and renal function; decrease dose if creatinine rises $>$30%, and

discontinue if levels continue to increase.

(4) Adverse Effects: Commonly related to angiotensin Ⅱ (Ang Ⅱ) suppression, such as hypotension, renal impairment, and hyperkalemia; or related to accumulation of bradykinin, such as cough and angioedema.

3. Beta-Blockers

(1) Indications: For structural heart disease with reduced LVEF, asymptomatic heart failure regardless of myocardial infarction status, and symptomatic or previously symptomatic NYHA Class Ⅱ-Ⅲ stable chronic heart failure patients requiring lifelong use unless contraindicated or not tolerated. Also applicable under close monitoring and specialist guidance for NYHA Class Ⅳ a heart failure.

(2) Contraindications: Contraindicated in patients with second-degree or higher atrioventricular block, active asthma, and reactive respiratory diseases.

(3) Administration: Recommended agents include metoprolol succinate, bisoprolol, or carvedilol, which improve prognosis. Initiate beta-blockers as soon as diagnosed with heart failure with reduced LVEF if symptoms are mild or improved unless symptoms are recurrent or progressing. The majority of clinical studies utilize metoprolol succinate, with more substantial evidence than metoprolol tartrate; however, initial treatment may transition using metoprolol tartrate.

(4) Beta-blocker therapy for heart failure should aim to achieve the target dose or the maximum tolerable dose. The target dose is validated as effective in past clinical trials. Start with a small dose, typically 1 / 8 of the target dose, increasing every 2-4 weeks with individualized titration. This method is determined by the unique biological effects of beta-blockers, which often take 2-3 months of continuous medication to develop. Initial pharmacologic effects include inhibiting myocardial contractility, which may induce or worsen heart failure, thus starting doses should be low, and increments slow. Resting heart rate is an indicator of effective cardiac beta-blockade, typically aiming for 55-60 beats per minute as the target or maximum tolerable dose.

(5) Adverse Effects: Early non-severe side effects generally do not require discontinuation; instead, delay dose increases until they resolve. If initial treatment causes fluid retention, increase diuretic dosage until pre-treatment body weight is restored before continuing increments.

1) Hypotension: Typically occurs within the first 24-48 hours of the initial dose or upon increasing the dose, usually asymptomatic and self-resolving. Consider discontinuing medications that affect blood pressure, such as vasodilators, reduce the diuretic dose, or temporarily decrease the ACEI dose.

If low blood pressure accompanied by symptoms of low perfusion occurs, it may be necessary to reduce or discontinue beta-blockers and reassess the patient's clinical status.

2) Fluid Retention and Worsening Heart Failure: If heart failure mildly to moderately worsens during medication, diuretic dosages should be increased. If deterioration is related to the initiation or increase of beta-blockers, a temporary dose reduction or reversion to the previous dose may be appropriate. If deterioration is not associated with beta-blockers, discontinuation is not required; instead, identify and manage exacerbating factors and intensify treatment measures.

3) Bradycardia and Atrioventricular Block: If the heart rate falls below 55 beats per minute, or symptoms such as dizziness occur, or second or third-degree atrioventricular block develops, a dose reduction or discontinuation may be necessary.

4. Aldosterone Receptor Antagonists

(1) Indications: Patients with LVEF≤35% and NYHA Ⅱ-Ⅳ; symptomatic patients despite treatment with ACEIs (or ARBs) and beta-blockers (Class Ⅰ, Level A); post-AMI patients with LVEF≤40%, symptoms of heart failure, or a history of diabetes (Class Ⅰ, Level B).

(2) Administration: Start with a low dose and gradually increase, particularly with spironolactone recommended in smaller doses—eplerenone starting at 12.5 mg once daily, target dose 25-50 mg once daily; spironolactone starting at 10-20 mg once daily, target dose 20 mg once daily.

(3) Precautions: Not advisable for patients with serum potassium>5.0 mmol / L, impaired renal functiom [creatinine>221 μmol / L (2.5 mg / dL) or eGFR<30 mL / min / 1.73 m^2]. Regular monitoring of serum potassium and renal function is required; reduce or discontinue if serum potassium exceeds 5.5 mmol / L. Avoid NSAIDs and COX-2 inhibitors, particularly in the elderly. Spironolactone may cause reversible gynecomastia, disappearing after discontinuation. Eplerenone has fewer adverse reactions.

5. ARBs

(1) Indications: Similar to ACEIs, recommended for patients who cannot tolerate ACEIs (Class Ⅰ, Level A). Also for symptomatic heart failure patients dissatisfied with outcomes after diuretics, ACEIs, and beta-blockers, and who cannot tolerate aldosterone antagonists (Class Ⅱb, Level A).

(2) Administration: Start with a low dose, gradually increasing to the recommended target dose or maximum tolerable dose.

(3) Precautions: Similar to ACEIs, potential for inducing hypotension, renal impairment, and hyperkalemia; monitor blood pressure (including postural changes), renal function, and serum potassium within the first 1-2 weeks of initiation or dose change. ARBs generally have fewer adverse reactions such as dry cough and are less likely to cause angioedema compared to ACEIs.

6. Digoxin

(1) Indications: Suitable for chronic HF-REF patients who remain symptomatic despite therapy with diuretics, ACEIs (or ARBs), beta-blockers, and aldosterone antagonists, with LVEF≤45%, particularly appropriate for patients with atrial fibrillation and rapid ventricular rates (Class Ⅱa, Level B). Digoxin should not be discontinued lightly in patients already on it. Not recommended for patients with NYHA Class Ⅰ.

(2) Administration: Maintenance a dosage of 0.125-0.25 mg / day, dosage halved for elderly or those with renal impairment. For controlling rapid ventricular rates in atrial fibrillation, doses can be increased to 0.375-0.50 mg / day. Strict monitoring for digoxin toxicity and drug concentrations is necessary.

7. Ivabradine

(1) Indications: Suitable for HF-REF patients with sinus rhythm. Used when recommended doses or maximum tolerated doses of ACEIs or ARBs, beta-blockers, and aldosterone antagonists

have been reached, yet heart rate remains≥70 bpm with persistent symptoms (NYHA Ⅱ-Ⅳ), Ivabradine may be added (Class Ⅱa, Level B). Also, for symptomatic patients who cannot tolerate beta-blockers with heart rate≥70 bpm (Class Ⅱb, Level C).

(2) Administration: Starting dose of 2.5 mg twice daily, adjusted based on heart rate, with a maximum dose of 7.5 mg twice daily. The resting heart rate should ideally be controlled around 60 bpm, not falling below 55 bpm.

(3) Adverse Reactions: Rare incidences of bradycardia, phosphenes, blurred vision, palpitations, and gastrointestinal reactions.

8. Controversial, Investigational, or Uncertain Efficacy Medications

(1) Vasodilators: There is no supporting evidence for the use of direct-acting vasodilators or α-blockers in the treatment of chronic heart failure. Nitrates are commonly used to alleviate symptoms of angina or dyspnea but lack evidence for heart failure treatment.

(2) Traditional Chinese Medicine: Several studies in China have explored the use of traditional medicine for heart failure. A multicenter, randomized, placebo-controlled study using biomarkers as surrogate endpoints showed that the adjunctive use of specific traditional Chinese medicine on top of standard and optimized heart failure treatment significantly reduces NT-proBNP levels in patients with chronic heart failure. Future studies should aim for mortality as a primary endpoint to provide more convincing clinical evidence.

(3) n-3 Polyunsaturated Fatty Acids (n-3 PUFAs): While n-3 PUFAs can reduce cardiovascular mortality, they do not decrease hospitalization rates for heart failure. Their effects on post-AMI patients are unclear.

(4) Metabolic Modulators: Exploratory research on certain agents that improve myocardial energy metabolism, such as trimetazidine, coenzyme Q10, and L-carnitine, has been conducted, but overall evidence remains weak, lacking large-scale prospective studies. Trimetazidine is recommended in recent international guidelines for coronary artery disease, hence its application could be considered in heart failure with concurrent coronary artery disease.

(5) Renin Inhibitors—Aliskiren: Aliskiren shows no significant improvement in cardiovascular mortality or heart failure hospitalization rates and increases the risk of hyperkalemia, hypotension, and renal failure, particularly not recommended for use in patients with diabetes.

(6) Statins: Currently, statins are not recommended for the treatment of heart failure. However, if the etiology or underlying condition of the chronic heart failure patient involves coronary artery disease, or other conditions necessitate routine and long-term use of statins, their use is acceptable.

(7) Calcium Channel Blockers (CCBs): Most CCBs, especially short-acting dihydropyridines and those with negative inotropic effects (like verapamil and diltiazem), should be avoided in chronic HF-REF patients. However, if a heart failure patient suffers from severe hypertension or angina that other medications cannot control, amlodipine or felodipine may be used safely in the long term, although they do not improve survival rates but do not adversely affect prognosis.

(8) Anticoagulants and Antiplatelet Agents: Routine anticoagulation or antiplatelet therapy is generally unnecessary in chronic heart failure. Patients with dilated cardiomyopathy and heart

failure without other indications should not use aspirin. Antiplatelet and / or anticoagulant drugs should be considered based on individual risk factors for thromboembolism and other underlying conditions.

(9) Not Recommended Medications: Thiazolidinediones (glitazones) can exacerbate heart failure and increase the risk of heart failure hospitalization. NSAIDs and COX-2 inhibitors can cause sodium retention, worsen renal function, and exacerbate heart failure and should be avoided.

Ⅱ Common Questions in Consultations

1. Combining Neuroendocrine Inhibitors

(1) ACEIs and Beta-Blockers: The combination of these medications, termed the "golden pair", produces additive or synergistic benefits, further reducing mortality risk. After initiating both drugs, doses should be alternated and gradually increased to reach each drug's target dose or maximum tolerated dose. To avoid hypotension, beta-blockers and ACEIs can be administered at different times of the day.

(2) ACEIs and Aldosterone Antagonists: Clinical studies confirm that combining these reduces the mortality rate in chronic heart failure patients (Class Ⅰ, A-level), and is relatively safe, but strict monitoring of serum potassium is necessary, usually combined with potassium-sparing diuretics to prevent hyperkalemia. On top of the "golden pair" basis of ACEIs and beta-blockers, adding an aldosterone antagonist forms a "golden triangle", becoming a fundamental treatment scheme for chronic HF-REF.

2. Evaluating the Combination of ACEIs, ARBs, and Other Medica-tions: ACEIs are the first-class medications proven to reduce mortality in heart failure patients and are the cornerstone of heart failure treatment with the most accumulative evidence from evidence-based medicine. The combination of ACEIs and ARBs is still debated, with inconsistent findings from clinical trials regarding their co-use in treating heart failure. Such combinations, especially in post-AMI heart failure patients, are generally discouraged due to potential adverse effects like hypotension, hyperkalemia, elevated creatinine levels, and even increased incidence of renal impairment (ONTARGET trial). Following recent clinical trials, the use of aldosterone antagonists has been actively recommended after ACEIs and beta-blockers, making the addition of ARBs generally unnecessary, especially the concurrent use of ACEIs, ARBs, and aldosterone antagonists is contraindicated.

3. Mechanisms and Evidence-Based Medicine for Beta-Blockers in Treating Heart Failure: Chronic over-activation of the sympathetic nervous system in heart failure patients leads to downregulation and impairment of myocardial β_1 receptors. Beta-blocker therapy can restore the normal function of these receptors. Studies indicate that long-term use (over three months) can improve cardiac function and increase LVEF; treatments lasting 4-12 months also reduce ventricular mass and volume, improve ventricular shape, indicating a delay or reversal in myocardial remodeling. This is due to the "biological effect" of beta-blockers on enhancing intrinsic myocardial function, distinct from their acute pharmacological actions. Three classic large-scale clinical trials for chronic systolic heart failure—CIBIS-Ⅱ, MERIT-HF, and

COPERNICUS—using selective β_1 receptor blockers bisoprolol, metoprolol succinate, and non-selective β_1 / β_2, α_1 receptor blocker carvedilol, respectively showed a relative risk reduction in mortality by 34%, 34%, and 35%, while also reducing heart failure rehospitalization rates by 28%-36%. A unique feature of beta-blocker therapy in heart failure is its significant reduction in sudden death rates by 41%-44%.

Ⅲ Consultation Process

1. Complete Echocardiographic Examination: Determine the type of chronic heart failure (reduced EF, preserved EF, mid-range EF).

2. Comprehensive Diagnostic Assessment: Complete coronary angiography, ambulatory ECG, and echocardiography. If necessary, conduct cardiac MRI to clarify the underlying etiology of heart failure and target etiological treatment.

3. Important Medical History Review: Note any recent symptoms such as new onset of chest discomfort or pain, signs of infection like fever or cough, or signs of fluid retention such as edema, increased heart rate, and weight gain.

4. Physical Examination Emphasis: Check blood pressure, heart rate, rhythm, presence of dry or wet rales in the lungs, jugular vein distention, and lower limb edema.

5. Control and Avoidance of Heart Failure Precipitants: Avoid infections, excessive fluid intake, heavy physical labor, emotional stress, and over-tiredness.

6. Treatment: For heart failure with preserved or mid-range EF, provide symptomatic treatment such as diuresis and blood pressure control. For reduced EF heart failure, unless contraindicated, the "golden triangle" medications must be used to improve prognosis (ACEI / ARB / ARNI, beta-blockers, aldosterone antagonists), starting with low doses of ACEI / ARB / ARNI and beta-blockers and gradually increasing to maximum tolerable doses. Diuretics should be used as needed. If resting heart rate remains $\geqslant$70 bpm despite these medications, consider adding Ivabradine. Assess the need for ICD or CRT-D implantation. If symptoms persist despite these treatments, consider adding digoxin. For refractory end-stage heart failure, evaluate the need for heart transplantation or ventricular assist devices.

Section 5 Device Therapy for Heart Failure

Heart failure is a common issue in cardiovascular consultations, with most patients improving through pharmacotherapy. However, a small subset requires mechanical circulatory support (MCS), which has become a crucial strategy for treating end-stage heart failure, cardiogenic shock, and pump failure. Device therapy for heart failure encompasses a wide range of interventions, including implantable cardiac defibrillators (ICDs), cardiac resynchronization therapy (CRT-P / D), intra-aortic balloon pumps (IABP), extracorporeal membrane oxygenation (ECMO), ventricular assist devices (VADs), and total artificial hearts. Cardiovascular specialists primarily consult on these interventions in the ICU and thoracic and cardiovascular surgery settings. IABP and ECMO are the primary devices used during consultations, with IABP being more widely utilized in China, while ECMO is used by a few hospitals. This section focuses on IABP, while ICD and CRT-P / D implantations are performed within the cardiovascular department, and implantable left ventricular assist devices are managed by cardiac surgery.

I Intra-aortic Balloon Pump (IABP)

1. Overview: The IABP is one of the most widely used and effective adjunct devices in clinical cardiovascular medicine. The concept of aortic counter-pulsation was first proposed by Harken in 1958, with Nantrowitz successfully applying it clinically in 1967. Professor Bregman, a renowned expert on IABP, has conducted extensive research on the technology, leading to improvements in device quality, reduced complication rates, and enhanced rescue success rates. IABP has become recognized as a critical method for managing intractable heart failure.

The intra-aortic balloon pump (IABP) catheter is percutaneously inserted via the femoral artery and positioned approximately 1-2 cm distal to the subclavian artery opening in the descending thoracic aorta. During ventricular diastole, the balloon inflates, elevating diastolic pressure within the aorta, which enhances coronary blood flow and improves myocardial perfusion and oxygenation. Conversely, during ventricular systole, balloon deflation causes a sharp drop in aortic pressure, reducing left ventricular ejection resistance. This alleviates the left ventricular after-load, decreases cardiac workload, and thus improves ventricular function.

2. Pre-operative Preparation

(1) Equipment Preparation:

1) Balloon Catheter: Constructed from polyurethane, this catheter features a thin, transparent, yet resilient and sturdy balloon.

A slender catheter runs inside the balloon, equipped with multiple small holes to facilitate even gas exchange.

Balloon catheters vary in size from those suitable for children to adults, chosen based on the patient's age, weight, and height. Typically, adult males use a 40 mL balloon, whereas adult females often require a 30-35 mL balloon. The size for children is adjusted based on body weight.

2) Counter-pulsation Pump: Includes a power system, drive system, monitoring system, adjustment system, and triggering system. Ensure helium is adequately stocked, connect the power, and set the triggering mode (electrical or pressure trigger), frequency, and counter-pulsation timing. Adjustments may be made during operation based on the patient's condition, and some pumps can auto-adjust counter-pulsation timing by tracking the electrocardiogram.

(2) Patient Preparation:

1) Skin preparation.

2) Administration of sedatives, analgesics, and local anesthesia.

3) Monitoring hemodynamic and electrocardiographic changes.

3. Indications

(1) Poor cardiac function pre-cardiac surgery, hemodynamic instability, heart function class Ⅳ, LVEF＜30%.

(2) Post-open heart surgery complications such as difficulty weaning from cardiopulmonary bypass or severe low cardiac output syndrome, mean arterial pressure＜50 mmHg, left atrial

pressure>20 mmHg, cardiac index<2.0 L / (min·m²), central venous pressure>15 cm H_2O, urine output<0.5 mL / (kg·h), requiring multiple inotropic drugs with continued hypotension.

(3) Unstable angina, extensive myocardial infarction, ventricular septal rupture, cardiogenic shock, papillary muscle rupture, severe mitral regurgitation.

(4) Severe myocarditis with unstable hemodynamics.

(5) Pre-heart transplant IABP support while awaiting a donor heart.

4. Contraindications

(1) Aortic valve insufficiency.

(2) Aortic dissection or aneurysms, including those who have undergone aortic arch surgery and / or have aortic injury.

(3) Severe atherosclerotic or calcific narrowing of the aorta or femoral arteries.

(4) Irreversible brain damage.

(5) Severe coagulopathy.

5. Nursing Care. Post-IABP Insertion Post-IABP insertion care and clinical monitoring are crucial, encompassing several key aspects.

(1) Accurately monitor vital signs such as heart rate, temperature, respiratory rate, blood pressure, cardiac output, cardiac index (CI), and urine output to evaluate the effectiveness of the IABP.

(2) Obtain an immediate chest X-ray post-insertion to confirm the position of the balloon within the aorta; ideally, the balloon's tip should be located between the second and third ribs (1 cm below the descending aortic arch). Improper balloon positioning can either obstruct the subclavian artery if too high or renal arteries if too low, leading to renal ischemia and renal failure. Monitor the patient's left radial artery pulse and urine output. Check for abdominal pain and auscultate bowel sounds; severe abdominal pain or absent bowel sounds might indicate mesenteric artery occlusion by the catheter, necessitating immediate adjustment.

(3) Per medical orders, monitor the activated clotting time (ACT) every 4-6 hours, maintaining ACT values between 150-180 seconds, and adjust heparin dosage accordingly. Monitor platelet counts and be vigilant for signs of bleeding and thrombus formation.

(4) Observe the IABP counter-pulsation timing and counter-pulsation effect, and gradually adjust various IABP parameters to achieve optimal assisted effect [stable blood pressure, systolic pressure>90 mmHg, CI>2.5 L / (min·m²), urine output>1 mL / (kg·h), gradually reduced dosage of positive inotropic drugs, warm peripheral circulation].

(5) Continuously monitor for any blood outflow from the balloon catheter outer sheath, which may indicate balloon rupture. In the event of balloon rupture, immediately remove the IABP catheter, and if continued assisted support is required, re-insert a new catheter.

(6) Regularly monitor renal function parameters such as blood urea nitrogen (BUN) and creatinine (Cr) to promptly detect any signs of renal insufficiency.

(7) Observe the skin temperature and color of the limb on the catheter insertion side, palpate the dorsalis pedis and posterior tibial arteries, and if necessary, use Doppler to detect and record blood flow. Pay particular attention to potential compartment syndrome caused by compression or ischemia of major vessels, manifested as limb swelling. If present, measure limb circumference

regularly at 15 cm below the patella for the calf and 20 cm above the patella for the thigh.

(8) Patients requiring IABP are typically critically ill and bedridden, necessitating enhanced basic nursing care to prevent pressure sores and passive limb movements to reduce thrombus formation. For the catheterized limb, hip immobilization is advisable, but below-knee self-assisted movements can be allowed to a moderate extent. Maintain a semi-recumbent position $<30°$ to avoid hip flexion, which could kink the balloon catheter, and buttock bending, which could displace the balloon towards the aortic arch, risking aortic injury.

(9) IABP patients have restricted mobility and require assistance with daily activities, potentially causing agitation and anxiety. Therefore, timely explanations and reassurance should be provided to encourage better cooperation with treatment.

(10) IABP removal can be accomplished through different approaches, guided by the principle of gradually reducing assisted conditions and evaluating hemodynamic outcomes after each step.

To remove the IABP catheter, first taper vasoactive medication doses gradually. If the patient's condition stabilizes, reduce the counter-pulsation frequency to 1∶2 or 1∶3 intervals or lower the counter-pulsation pressure. Concurrently, monitor hemodynamic parameters; if stable, catheter removal can be considered. During removal, allow a small amount of blood to expel from the puncture site to flush out any potential thrombi, then apply pressure for 30 minutes, followed by elastic bandage compression for 6 hours and bed rest for 12-24 hours. Observe for local bleeding or oozing, monitor lower limb perfusion, and track hemodynamic changes.

Ⅱ Extracorporeal Membrane Oxygenation (ECMO)

ECMO is an extracorporeal circulation technique extended beyond the cardiac surgery suite. The principle involves draining venous blood from the patient, oxygenating it extra-corporeally through a specialized artificial heart-lung bypass circuit, and then returning it to the patient's arterial or venous system, partially substituting cardiopulmonary function to maintain tissue oxygenation.

The basic ECMO structure includes intravascular cannulae, connecting tubing, a driving pump (artificial heart), an oxygenator (artificial lung), oxygen supply lines, and monitoring systems.

ECMO is used to support patients with severe cardiopulmonary dysfunction. Common types include veno-arterial (VA) and veno-venous (VV) configurations. Only the former provides cardiac support by draining blood from the femoral vein, oxygenating it extra-corporeally, and returning it to the femoral artery. ECMO is often employed for long-term mechanical circulatory support or as a bridge to transplantation. Compared to other novel left ventricular assist devices, ECMO has a longer history and more robust evidence base from clinical studies, along with advantages of compact size and portability. The German-developed Cardio-help and LIFEBRIDGEB2T portable ECMO systems have successfully been deployed in pre-hospital emergency settings. However, due to the high cost of the complete ECMO system, few hospitals offer this capability, and it is not a typical consultation issue. Detailed information can be found in dedicated textbooks.

Ⅲ Consultation Process

1. Assess if heart failure patients have indications for device therapy, including cardiac resynchronization therapy (CRT), CRT with defibrillator (CRT-D) implantation, non-invasive ventilation, invasive mechanical ventilation, intra-aortic balloon pump (IABP), ultra-filtration, continuous renal replacement therapy (CRRT), extracorporeal membrane oxygenation (ECMO), or left ventricular assist devices.

2. For patients with implanted implantable cardioverter-defibrillators (ICDs), evaluate for any ventricular arrhythmia events or shocks and the need for anti-arrhythmic drug adjustment. For CRT recipients, assess heart failure symptom improvement, LVEF changes, and QRS width; if no response, optimize device programming with echocardiographic guidance.

3. For patients on non-invasive ventilation, monitor oxygen saturation, mental status, tolerance, and symptom improvement, considering transition to invasive mechanical ventilation if necessary.

4. For IABP recipients, evaluate therapeutic effect (invasive blood pressure, counter-pulsation pressure, heart rate, symptom relief) and adverse events (bleeding, renal dysfunction, mesenteric ischemia, arteriovenous fistula, local hematoma). Consider IABP removal when vasoactive medications can be tapered, and the patient stabilizes.

5. For heart failure patients undergoing ultra-filtration, monitor continuous anticoagulation (ACT or aPTT) and maintain fluid balance and electrolyte homeostasis.

Section 6 Differential Diagnosis of Edema

Edema is a common clinical symptom with complex etiologies. Other departments frequently consult cardiovascular physicians to establish or exclude cardiac causes of edema.

Ⅰ Overview

Edema refers to the pathological accumulation of excess fluid in interstitial spaces, manifesting clinically as swelling. Mild fluid retention may not cause visible edema, which typically occurs with over 4-5 kg of retained fluid. Edema can be generalized or localized. Generalized edema results from diffuse interstitial fluid distribution, presenting as swelling in multiple areas with pitting on prolonged pressure. Localized edema occurs when fluid accumulates in specific interstitial spaces. Pleural, pericardial, and peritoneal fluid accumulation are termed pleural effusion, pericardial effusion, and ascites, respectively—special forms of edema.

Ⅱ Brief Mechanisms of Edema

Edema arises from imbalances in fluid distribution between the vascular, lymphatic, and interstitial compartments, which leads to increased interstitial volume. Key causes include decreased plasma osmotic pressure, increased capillary permeability, elevated capillary hydrostatic pressure, and lymphatic obstruction. Fluid accumulation activates the renin-angiotensin-aldosterone system and anti-diuretic hormone, promoting sodium and water retention, perpetuating edema formation.

Ⅲ Diagnostic Approach

An accurate etiological diagnosis can be established through history taking, physical examination, laboratory tests, and diagnostic procedures, which guides clinical management. However, for edema, the priority is addressing any organ system dysfunction or life-threatening factors first.

1. History: ① Onset, duration, gradual or sudden; ② Localization, generalized or confined to specific areas, unilateral or bilateral; ③ Characteristics, pitting or non-pitting edema, pain, tenderness; ④ Associated symptoms like weight gain / loss, exertional dyspnea, paroxysmal nocturnal dyspnea, orthopnea; ⑤ Exacerbation with dependent positioning or prolonged standing / sitting, relief with elevation; excessive salt intake, new medications or dose changes; trauma, immobility; ⑥ Severity, ambulation ability, tightness of shoes or belts.

2. Physical Examination: Perform a comprehensive exam based on potential edema etiologies. Note important positive findings like jugular venous distension, cardiomegaly, abnormal heart sounds / murmurs, lung crackles, ascites, hepatojugular reflux. For unilateral leg edema, compare sides—a$>$1 cm ankle or$>$2 cm calf circumference difference warrants further evaluation.

3. Diagnostic Tests: Thorough history and examination are often sufficient for diagnosis, but tests can aid diagnosis in early / mild cases or intermittent edema. Electrocardiogram, chest X-ray, complete blood count, biochemistry, thyroid function, brain natriuretic peptide, urinalysis evaluate renal, hepatic, thyroid, and nutritional status and screen for cardiopulmonary disease. Echocardiography is crucial for cardiac edema. In unexplained leg edema, especially in older adults, echocardiography should assess pulmonary pressures regardless of symptoms.

Ⅳ Differentiating Cardiovascular Edema

1. Cardiac Edema: Prioritize cardiac etiologies as they can be life-threatening. Predictors include elevated jugular venous pressure, tachycardia, dyspnea, fatigue, weight gain, angina, orthopnea, crackles, electrocardiographic changes, elevated natriuretic peptides, and echocardiographic abnormalities. Features are bilateral pitting edema, with dependent edema in severe cases like bedridden decompensated heart failure.

2. Venous Edema: Deep vein thrombosis (DVT) is the most common cause of leg edema. Risk factors include venous stasis, vascular injury, and hypercoagulability. Signs like pain, tenderness, swelling, and erythema is often unilateral. Diagnosis utilizes Doppler ultrasound, D-dimer, and contrast venography.

3. Drug-induced Edema: Bilateral, gradually progressive edema can result from various medications like anti-hypertensives that cause vasodilation, activating renin-angiotensin-aldosterone and promoting sodium / water retention. Risk increases with calcium channel blockers (CCBs), β-blockers, central α-agonists, and peripheral α-antagonists. Women and the elderly on CCBs are prone to warm weather or dose increase-related edema, worsening during

the day and improving at night with recumbency. Non-dihydropyridine CCBs like verapamil / diltiazem reduce peripheral edema risk.

V Treatment

Cardiac edema is managed according to heart failure principles. For deep vein thrombosis (DVT), evaluate for concomitant pulmonary embolism and involve vascular surgery. For antihypertensive-induced edema, combine low-dose diuretics, switch to non-dihydropyridine calcium channel blockers (CCBs) with angiotensin-converting enzyme inhibitors / angiotensin Ⅱ receptor blockers, or change anti-hypertensive agents if edema is intolerable.

Ⅵ Consultation Process

1. Supplement key history: underlying heart disease, liver / renal dysfunction, dyspnea, palpitations, anorexia, jaundice, abdominal distension, oliguria, leg pain / discoloration / temperature changes, and skin changes.

2. Emphasize physical exam: arrhythmias, lung crackles / wheezes, jugular venous distension, cardiomegaly, murmurs, pulsus alternans; symmetric leg edema; temperature / color changes; and pitting edema.

3. Expedite testing: liver / renal function, urinalysis, chest X-ray, natriuretic peptides, thyroid studies, echocardiography, and leg Doppler ultrasound.

4. After excluding organic causes, consider drug-induced edema.

5. Treat the underlying etiology.

Section 7 Advances in Right Heart Failure

I Overview

Right heart failure (RHF) is a clinical syndrome of impaired right ventricular (RV) systolic and / or diastolic function from any cause, inadequate to meet metabolic demands, with at least two features: ① Symptoms / signs consistent with RHF; ② Objective evidence of RV structural / functional abnormalities or elevated intracardiac pressures.

In 1616, Harvey and William first proposed the RV's role in pumping blood to the lungs rather than nutritive support. RV research has lagged behind the left ventricle, with limited evidence and guidelines on RHF and RV function. However, RHF carries higher morbidity and mortality than left heart failure and independently impacts its prognosis.

RV characteristics: ① Thin-walled, compliant, peristaltic contraction (similar to gastrointestinal smooth muscle); ② Relatively insensitive to preload, with modest preload increases slightly augmenting stroke volume; ③ Sensitive to after-load, with acute RHF from abrupt pulmonary artery pressure elevations; ④ More susceptible than the left ventricle to oxidative stress and cell death pathway activation; ⑤ Poor response to inotropes, diuretics, and vasodilators.

Ⅱ Etiologies of RHF

1. Secondary to left heart failure: Hemodynamic features include elevated pulmonary venous and pulmonary capillary wedge pressures (PCWP > 15 mmHg) and pulmonary artery pressures.

2. Respiratory diseases / hypoxia: COPD, interstitial lung diseases, obstructive sleep apnea, chronic high-altitude diseases.

3. Chronic thromboembolic pulmonary hypertension.

4. Idiopathic pulmonary arterial hypertension: Elevated pulmonary artery pressure, and normal PCWP.

5. Pulmonary vascular disease from connective tissue disorders.

6. Congenital heart diseases like atrial septal defects, pulmonic stenosis, Ebstein's anomaly, residual pulmonary regurgitation after tetralogy of Fallot repair, ruptured sinus of Valsalva aneurysm into right atrium, and Eisenmenger syndrome (RHF from structural, contractile and conduction defects).

7. Tricuspid regurgitation: Organic or functional.

8. RV cardiomyopathies: Amyloidosis, restrictive cardiomyopathy, arrhythmo-genic RV cardiomyopathy, and RV infarction.

9. Hyperthyroid heart failure: RHF is more common, as hyperthyroidism increases cardiac output and venous return, potentially causing pulmonary endothelial damage over time, RV dilation, functional tricuspid regurgitation and eventual RHF.

Ⅲ Clinical Manifestations of RHF

1. The clinical manifestations of right heart failure include the following aspects.

(1) Early manifestations include abdominal bloating, anorexia, dyspnea, etc.

(2) Fluid retention leads to generalized edema, leg swelling, and ascites.

(3) Reduced cardiac output manifests as fatigue, weakness, and exercise intolerance.

(4) Impaired contractile reserve.

(5) ECG changes: Right axis deviation, right ventricular hypertrophy, atrial / ventricular arrhythmias, S waves in lead I, ST-T wave changes in precordial leads.

(6) Physical exam: Left sternal heave, jugular venous distension, and hepatomegaly.

2. RV Diastolic Dysfunction

(1) Often precedes systolic dysfunction, dilation or hypertrophy.

(2) May aid early detection of RV involvement.

(3) Echocardiography provides quantitative assessment. 3D echo allows RV volume / ejection fraction measurement in most patients.

3. Stages of RHF

Stage A: Risk factors but no RV structural changes or symptoms.

Stage B: RV structural / functional abnormalities but no symptoms.

Stage C: Structural changes and symptoms of RHF.

Stage D: Refractory RHF (requiring specialized interventions like maximal medical therapy or procedures / surgeries, yet with persistent severe symptoms at rest and refractory arrhythmias).

Ⅳ Treatment of RHF

1. Treatment Principles

(1) Implement appropriate preventive and therapeutic measures based on RHF stage.

(2) Primarily address the underlying etiology driving RHF.

(3) Optimize preload reduction, after-load reduction, and inotropy while maintaining sinus rhythm and atrioventricular / inter-ventricular synchrony.

2. Acute RHF Management

(1) Volume status: Adequate preload, mildly elevated venous pressures to maintain systemic perfusion.

(2) Augment RV performance with inotropes: ① Milrinone (preferred phosphodiesterase-Ⅲ inhibitor) increases RV output, reduces pulmonary vascular resistance; ② Dopamine or epinephrine if hypotensive to increase biventricular inotropy; ③ Control pulmonary inflammation, hypoxia, hypercapnia; sedate adequately; minimize ventilatory support.

3. Chronic RHF Management

(1) Vasoactive Drugs

1) Nitrates / nitroprusside: Venodilate and arteriodilate to reduce preload / after-load, suitable for RHF from left ventricular systolic / diastolic dysfunction; contraindicated in pulmonary hypertension as non-selective pulmonary vasodilation worsens hypoxia / acidosis.

2) Dobutamine / dopamine: First-line agents for severe RHF. Dobutamine is a synthetic catecholamine with dose-dependent β_1 / β_2 agonism increasing cardiac output without preload effects. Low-dose dopamine induces renal vasodilation; intermediate doses are inotropic; higher doses vasoconstrict and increase blood pressure. For hypotension, start dopamine 2 μg / (kg·min), titrating up to 8 μg / (kg·min).

3) ACE inhibitors and beta-blockers: In patients with global heart failure, ACE inhibitors can increase right ventricular ejection fraction, reduce right ventricular end-diastolic volume, and lower right ventricular filling pressures; beta-blockers such as carvedilol or bisoprolol can improve right ventricular function.

4) In patients with right heart failure caused by pulmonary hypertension, ACE inhibitors do not increase exercise tolerance or improve hemodynamics; instead, they may worsen the condition due to a drop in blood pressure. beta-blockers also tend to worsen exercise tolerance and hemodynamics.

(2) Selective Pulmonary Vasodilators

1) Calcium channel blockers (CCBs) are strongly contraindicated in patients who have not undergone acute vasoreactivity testing or had a negative vasoreactivity test. Patients already on CCBs with sub-optimal response should have the dose gradually weaned off, and vasoreactivity re-assessed before deciding on re-initiation.

2) CCB therapy should be limited to vasoreactive patients; however, a positive vasoreactive response does not necessarily guarantee efficacy with CCBs.

3) CCBs should be started at low doses and gradually uptitrated over weeks to the maximum tolerated dose, provided there are no significant changes in systemic blood pressure.

4) After one year of therapy, repeat acute vasoreactivity testing to re-evaluate sustained responsiveness, as only long-term responders should continue CCB treatment.

5) Monitor for adverse effects like ventilation / perfusion mismatch, right-to-left shunting, paradoxical pulmonary hypertension, decompensation, sudden death, and reduced RV filling.

(3) Diuretics: In RHF patients, diuretics can markedly reduce preload and alleviate the burden on the right ventricle, thereby improving symptoms. Clinical studies demonstrate that diuretics rapidly ameliorate symptoms in RHF and reduce fluid overload within hours to days. Diuretics are not only a principal therapeutic modality for RHF but also pivotal in determining treatment success. Research indicates that all heart failure patients presenting with overt symptoms have fluid overload, warranting diuretic administration. However, in cor pulmonale secondary to chronic obstructive pulmonary disease, potent diuretics should be avoided to prevent metabolic alkalosis. Concurrently, close monitoring of blood gases, blood pressure, and electrolytes is imperative during diuretic therapy to prevent hypotension or electrolyte disturbances.

4. Main Therapeutic Approaches for Pulmonary Arterial Hypertension (PAH)

(1) Endothelin Pathway: In 1985, endothelium-derived coronary vasocon-strictors were first reported. Endothelin-2 was discovered in 1988 and published in *Nature*. In 2001, bosentan became the first approved endothelin receptor antagonist for PAH. Endothelins cause endothelial, smooth muscle, and fibro-blast dysfunction, leading to proliferation, hypertrophy, and fibrosis. Bosentan dosing is weight-based; for ≥40 kg patients, the recommended initial dose is 62.5 mg twice daily, uptitrated to 125 mg twice daily after 4 weeks. Liver function should be monitored at least monthly during treatment. Ambrisentan is dosed at 2.5, 5, or 10 mg daily. Sitaxentan is dosed at 100 mg daily, with monthly liver function monitoring. Sitaxentan interacts with warfarin, necessitating dose reduction to avoid elevated INR.

(2) Nitric Oxide Pathway: Sildenafil, tadalafil, vardenafil.

(3) Prostacyclins: Epoprostenol, iloprost. Animal studies suggest iloprost plus sildenafil is superior to monotherapy for hemodynamics.

5. Arrhythmia Management

(1) QRS prolongation > 180 ms in RHF predisposes to ventricular tachycardia and sudden death.

(2) Primarily by treating the underlying RHF etiology.

(3) Catheter ablation for inducible monomorphic VT.

(4) ICD for high sudden death risk.

6. Refractory RHF

(1) Identify and address precipitants.

(2) Ⅳ dobutamine, milrinone, digoxin.

(3) Combination pulmonary vasodilators.

(4) Ⅳ iloprost 0.5-4 ng / (kg·min).

(5) CRT.

(6) Percutaneous tricuspid valve repair.

(7) Atrial septostomy.

(8) RV assist devices.

(9) Heart / lung transplantation.

V Future Outlook

Right heart failure is a common cardiovascular disorder with a progressive course and poor prognosis. Although research on RHF in China is still in its infancy, increasing attention has been devoted to this condition in recent years. Randomized controlled trials are being conducted to enhance our understanding of RHF etiologies and pathogenic mechanisms, providing a more evidence-based approach to clinical diagnosis and management, ultimately improving patients' quality of life and survival.

VI Common Questions in Consultation

1. Is leg edema synonymous with RHF? While generalized edema, leg swelling, and ascites are frequent manifestations of RHF due to fluid overload, they are non-specific findings requiring differentiation from hypoproteinemia, hypothyroidism, deep vein thrombosis, and constrictive pericarditis.

2. Can RHF exist independently? RHF can arise secondary to left heart failure as part of global heart failure, but it can also occur in isolation, such as in congenital heart diseases with elevated pulmonary pressures and right-to-left shunting, leading to right ventricular dysfunction.

VII Inpatient Attending Consultation Process

1. Assess the patient's vital signs and hemodynamic stability. If there are signs of instability such as decreased oxygen saturation, shallow and rapid breathing, hypotension, or malignant arrhythmias, immediately provide emergency treatment such as endotracheal intubation, mechanical ventilation, cardioversion, temporary pacemaker, antiarrhythmic drugs, and vasopressors to maintain blood pressure.

2. Obtain key medical history, including the presence of underlying heart diseases: congenital heart disease, tricuspid regurgitation, right ventricular cardiomyopathy, right ventricular myocardial infarction, hyperthyroid heart disease, etc.; respiratory diseases / hypoxia such as COPD, OSAS, etc.; chronic pulmonary embolism; idiopathic pulmonary arterial hypertension; connective tissue disease-related pulmonary vascular disease, etc. Also, note any triggering factors such as fever, fatigue, pregnancy, long-distance air travel, or high-altitude travel.

3. Pay attention to important physical examination findings, such as cyanosis of the lips, jugular venous distention, thyroid enlargement, barrel chest, decreased breath sounds, dry or moist rales in both lungs, palpable heave at the left sternal border, enlarged cardiac dullness on percussion, cardiac murmurs, associated hepatomegaly, ascites, joint redness and deformity, lower extremity edema (unilateral or bilateral), etc.

4. Rapidly perform auxiliary examinations such as blood gas analysis, renal function, electrolytes, electrocardiogram (preferably 18-lead), chest X-ray, BNP or NT-proBNP, D-dimer, troponin, etc. If acute pulmonary embolism is suspected, promptly perform pulmonary artery

CTA. Quickly complete echocardiography to further clarify the etiology. Also, perform pericardial echocardiography to exclude the possibility of pericardial effusion.

5. Identify acute or chronic right heart failure. If acute right heart failure is confirmed, rapidly differentiate the etiology and correct the cause as soon as possible. For example, if the electrocardiogram suggests acute right ventricular myocardial infarction, perform early revascularization treatment. For patients with pulmonary embolism, evaluate and select thrombolytic therapy, anticoagulation therapy, or pulmonary artery embolectomy. For sepsis, administer antibiotics and correct hypoxia, acidosis, etc. If chronic right heart failure is confirmed, complete right heart catheterization, cardiac MRI, and other examinations to further clarify the etiology. Use vasoactive drugs, pulmonary vasodilators, diuretics, etc., as appropriate.

Section 8 Cardiogenic Shock

I Overview

Cardiogenic shock results from a failure of the heart's pumping function, which is unable to maintain minimal cardiac output, leading to a drop in blood pressure and inadequate blood supply to vital organs and tissues. This induces a systemic micro-circulatory dysfunction, characterized by a series of pathophysiological processes such as ischemia, hypoxia, metabolic disorders, and significant organ damage.

The primary cause of cardiogenic shock is acute myocardial infarction, with 5%-10% of patients experiencing shock. In China, the incidence of cardiogenic shock complicating acute myocardial infarction is 6%-8%. Despite significant advances in percutaneous interventions and myocardial revascularization in treating acute myocardial infarction, the mortality rate for cardiogenic shock remains high, between 45%-70%. Additionally, studies report that cardiogenic shock occurs in 0.2%-6% of adult cardiac surgeries, thus highlighting the importance of early diagnosis and appropriate treatment.

II Clinical Classification

1. Based on the Development Process of Cardiogenic Shock

(1) Early stage of cardiogenic shock: The body is in a state of stress with excessive catecholamine secretion and heightened sympathetic activity, often manifesting as restlessness, fear, and nervous tension. Patients are conscious, with pale or mildly cyanotic skin, cold extremities, profuse sweating, rapid heartbeat, rapid and deep breathing, accompanied by nausea and vomiting. Blood pressure may be normal or slightly low, but pulse pressure is reduced, and urine output decreases.

(2) Mid stage of cardiogenic shock: If early shock is not corrected timely, symptoms worsen, characterized by an indifferent expression, sluggish response, confused or unclear consciousness, generalized weakness, feeble and barely palpable pulse, heart rate often exceeding 120 beats per minute, systolic pressure $<$80 mmHg, often immeasurable, pulse pressure $<$20 mmHg, pale

and cyanotic complexion, cold and cyanotic skin, or marbled skin changes, with even less urine output (<17 mL / h) or anuria.

(3) Late stage of cardiogenic shock: Diffuse intravascular coagulation and multi-organ failure may occur, with the former causing extensive bleeding in skin, mucous membranes, and internal organs; the latter manifesting as symptoms of acute kidney, lung, liver, brain, and other vital organ failures.

2. Based on the Severity of Shock

(1) Mild shock: Patients are alert, restless, with pale complexion, dry mouth, sweating, rapid heart rate>100 beats per minute, still strong pulse, warm extremities but slightly cyanotic, cool, systolic pressure<80 mmHg, slightly reduced urine output, pulse pressure<30 mmHg.

(2) Moderate shock: Pale complexion, indifferent expression, cold limbs, cyanotic extremities, systolic pressure 60-80 mmHg, pulse pressure<20 mmHg, significantly reduced urine output (<17 mL / h).

(3) Severe shock: Clouded consciousness, blurred awareness, sluggish response, pale and cyanotic complexion, cold, cyanotic extremities, skin showing marble-like changes, heart rate> 120 beats per minute, muffled heart sounds, weak pulse or disappearing with slight pressure, systolic pressure dropping to 40-60 mmHg, significantly reduced or absent urine output.

(4) Extremely severe shock: Unconscious, comatose, shallow and irregular breathing, cyanotic lips and skin, cold extremities, extremely weak or impalpable pulse, muffled heart sounds or single-tone heart rhythm, systolic pressure<40 mmHg, anuria, widespread subcutaneous, mucosal, and internal organ bleeding, signs of multi-organ failure.

Ⅲ Clinical Presentation

The clinical manifestations of cardiogenic shock are primarily based on the reduced perfusion of vital organs on top of existing heart conditions. Low blood pressure alone is insufficient for diagnosing cardiogenic shock, as many patients may experience severe hypotension (systolic pressure<80 mmHg) shortly after onset. This type of hypotension can often be smoothly corrected, therefore, the presence of shock syndrome is considered only when low blood pressure is accompanied by other signs of circulatory dysfunction.

1. Systemic Circulatory Failure Manifestations. Patients with cardiogenic shock exhibit several characteristics: ① Decreased blood pressure, systolic pressure<90 mmHg or a decrease exceeding 30 mmHg from baseline in patients with hypertension; ② Increased heart rate, weak pulse; ③ Pale complexion, cold limbs, cold, sweaty skin; ④ Disturbances in consciousness; ⑤ Urine output less than 20 mL per hour; ⑥ Pulmonary capillary wedge pressure (PCWP) below 20 mmHg, cardiac index (CI) below 2 L / (min·m^2); ⑦ Excluding the effects of pain, hypoxia, vasovagal reactions, arrhythmias, drug reactions, or hypovolemia.

2. Severe Underlying Cardiac Disease Manifestations. A weakened first heart sound in acute myocardial infarction patients suggests a decline in left ventricular contractility; the presence of gallop rhythm can indicate early left heart failure. New loud systolic murmurs along the left sternal border suggest acute ventricular septal rupture or papillary muscle rupture causing acute mitral regurgitation; if the murmur is accompanied by a thrill or atrioventricular conduction

block, these support the diagnosis of ventricular septal rupture.

3. Hemodynamic Measurements. During cardiogenic shock, hemodynamic measurements indicate severe left ventricular dysfunction; the work per heartbeat decreases, resulting in reduced stroke volume and consequently elevated left ventricular end-diastolic pressure or filling pressure, and a decrease in cardiac output. Additionally, as a general rule, a decrease in cardiac output typically causes a compensatory increase in peripheral resistance. In most myocardial infarction patients, the reduction in cardiac output can be compensated by an increase in systemic vascular resistance, thus not significantly lowering blood pressure. However, in acute myocardial infarction complicated by shock, a considerable portion of patients do not exhibit the expected compensatory increase in systemic vascular resistance but are instead at normal or low levels.

Ⅳ Diagnosis

1. Diagnostic Criteria

(1) Systolic blood pressure $<$90 mmHg lasting $>$30 minutes; or the patient requires vasopressors / IABP to maintain systolic blood pressure $\geqslant$90 mmHg.

(2) Cardiac index (CI) $\leqslant$1.8 L / (min·m^2) without support or $\leqslant$2.2 L / (min·m^2) with support.

(3) Pulmonary capillary wedge pressure (PCWP) $\geqslant$18 mmHg.

(4) Signs of impaired organ perfusion: changes in mental status, cold and clammy skin, oliguria ($<$30 mL / h), elevated serum lactate levels.

2. Laboratory and Additional Examinations

(1) Complete blood count: increased white blood cells, increased neutrophils, decreased or absent eosinophils.

(2) Blood gas analysis: early shock may present with metabolic acidosis and respiratory alkalosis, while late shock often shows combined metabolic and respiratory acidosis, decreased pH, decreased oxygen tension and saturation, and increased carbon dioxide tension and content.

(3) Cardiac enzymes and ECG: essential for diagnosing post-myocardial infarction cardiogenic shock.

(4) Chest X-ray: important findings in cardiogenic shock patients include pulmonary congestion, indicative of acute pulmonary edema or heart failure.

(5) Echocardiography: useful for diagnosing the underlying condition, providing information on ventricular dysfunction; transthoracic color Doppler echocardiography can identify mechanical causes of cardiogenic shock such as ventricular septal defects or free wall rupture. Transthoracic echocardiography can also determine other causes of reduced cardiac output, such as right ventricular infarction and cardiac tamponade.

(6) Invasive hemodynamic monitoring: arterial pressure measurement (via radial, brachial, or femoral artery catheterization), venous catheter monitoring (PCWP, cardiac output, central venous pressure).

(7) Non-invasive hemodynamic monitoring: measures cardiac output, ejection fraction, left ventricular end-diastolic pressure, and PCWP using cardiac impedance graphs.

V Treatment

1. General Management

(1) Treatment of the underlying disease and precipitating factors.

(2) Positioning: supine position with legs elevated during shock; semi-sitting position if there is respiratory distress.

(3) Oxygenation, intubation if necessary.

(4) Monitoring of heart rhythm, blood pressure, and oxygen saturation.

(5) Hemodynamic monitoring if available.

(6) Urine output monitoring: a urine output of 50 mL / h is associated with a better prognosis in shock patients. To ensure accurate measurement, indwelling urinary catheterization is generally recommended.

(7) Establishing intravenous access and fluid resuscitation.

(8) Correction of electrolyte imbalances and acidosis.

2. Vasopressors

(1) Dopamine: The ACC / AHA guidelines recommend dopamine as the vasopressor of choice for hypotensive patients' post-acute myocardial infarction. Dopamine, a precursor of adrenaline, has dose-dependent effects, with minimal increase in heart rate. Starting dose is 1 μg / (kg·min), which can be gradually increased to 15 μg / (kg·min).

(2) Dobutamine: The 2015 French FICS guidelines for adult cardiogenic shock strongly recommend dobutamine for cases of cardiogenic shock with low cardiac output. This catecholamine has positive inotropic effects similar to dopamine and mildly increases heart rate and vasoconstriction. Administration leads to an increase in cardiac index with weak pressor effects. The drug is administered intravenously, with a therapeutic dose of 5-10 μg / (kg·min).

3. Vasodilators. When systolic blood pressure exceeds 85 mmHg and pulmonary capillary wedge pressure (PCWP) surpasses 18 mmHg, the use of vasodilators such as nitrates or sodium nitroprusside to reduce cardiac preload and after-load is beneficial. However, vasodilators can lead to a decrease in blood pressure, necessitating close monitoring of blood pressure changes.

(1) Sodium Nitroprusside: It dilates both arterioles and veins. In cases of cardiogenic shock, it is often used in conjunction with dopamine to increase coronary perfusion pressure. The infusion starts at 10-15 μg / min and can be gradually increased to significantly lower PCWP, although it should not fall below 15 mmHg.

(2) Nitroglycerin: Generally administered intravenously, nitroglycerin dilates the venous system to reduce preload; at higher doses, it reduces after-load and left ventricular end-diastolic pressure while increasing cardiac output. The usual dosage ranges from 10 to 30 μg / min, adjusted according to blood pressure changes.

4. Other Treatments. Glucocorticoids and polarizing solutions have their benefits in treating cardiogenic shock, although their efficacy is uncertain. For acute myocardial infarction patients with concurrent cardiogenic shock, anticoagulation therapy is chosen to reduce the incidence of thromboembolic complications.

5. Mechanical Assistance Treatments

(1) Intra-Aortic Balloon Pump (IABP): IABP, a nearly 50-year-old minimally invasive and safe technique, remains one of the most widely used and effective mechanical circulatory support devices. Post-thrombolytic treatment using IABP can enhance survival rates, improve myocardial perfusion, and reduce myocardial oxygen consumption while increasing cardiac output. However, it lacks active cardiac support and requires residual function in the left ventricle. According to the *2016 European Society of Cardiology Guidelines*, IABP is not routinely recommended for the supportive treatment of cardiogenic shock.

(2) ECMO (Extracorporeal Membrane Oxygenation): ECMO is an effective treatment for severe cardiogenic shock and serves as a bridge to cardiac transplantation and long-term cardiac support. Since its adoption in cardiac surgery by Gibbon in 1953, ECMO has continued to be used, providing substantial cardiopulmonary bypass support with relatively simple operation. Its basic principle involves diverting the patient's venous blood outside the body, where it undergoes gas exchange before being re-infused into the patient's artery or vein, replacing or partially replacing heart and lung functions, and sustaining life for a period to allow recovery from heart and lung pathology. As an extension of extracorporeal life support systems, ECMO significantly improves hemodynamics, providing crucial time for treating the underlying causes of cardiogenic shock. Long-term prognosis for cardiogenic shock patients on ECMO tends to be relatively positive. However, ECMO is not suitable for everyone; exclusion criteria include active bleeding or contraindications to chronic heparin use, uncontrollable malignant tumors, severe neurological damage, age over 80 years, or any severe medical condition that severely impedes rehabilitation and constitutes an absolute contraindication to ECMO use. Technical contraindications include aortic dissection and severe aortic regurgitation.

(3) Ventricular Assist Devices: Ventricular assist devices, such as TandemHeart™ and the Impella system, are used primarily in patients for whom conventional therapy is ineffective, offering better hemodynamic improvement compared to IABP. The Impella 5.0 (Abiomed Inc., Danvers, MA) is a 21F micro-axial pump that is minimally invasive and can generate a flow of 5 L / min, entering the left ventricle at the aortic valve position and exiting at the mid-tubular junction. It actively reduces the load on the left ventricle, enhances coronary perfusion, and thereby improves myocardial oxygen supply. The 2015 FICS Guidelines advise against routine use of IABP following myocardial infarction that has been effectively controlled, recommending ECMO for temporary circulatory support; if experienced in lesion localization, Impella assistance may be used in treating myocardial infarction with cardiogenic shock. Before transferring the patient to a specialized treatment center, establishing arteriovenous ECMO support on site is recommended.

(4) Mechanical Ventilation. In cardiogenic shock, mechanical ventilation through positive airway pressure can improve ventilation, alleviate pulmonary edema, and correct hypoxemia and carbon dioxide retention, thereby relieving respiratory failure.

(5) Blood Purification Therapy. Continuous blood purification encompasses all treatments that continuously and gradually remove fluids and solutes. It is considered a significant advancement in critical care medicine in recent years, swiftly restoring fluid balance and used

in various conditions of fluid overload such as acute heart failure with severe edema, acute pulmonary edema, liver failure, or nephrotic syndrome with uncontrollable edema. Both ACC / AHA and Chinese guidelines list continuous blood purification as a treatment method for refractory heart failure.

Ⅵ Common Questions in Consultations

1. Is a Systolic Blood Pressure $<$90 mmHg Indicative of Cardiogenic Shock? Cardiogenic shock primarily manifests as reduced perfusion to vital organs on the basis of existing cardiac disease. The occurrence of low blood pressure alone is insufficient for a diagnosis of cardiogenic shock. This is because many patients may experience severe hypotension (systolic pressure $<$ 10.7 kPa) shortly after onset, which can often be smoothly corrected. Therefore, shock syndrome is considered present only when low blood pressure accompanies other signs of circulatory dysfunction.

2. Differentiation from Other Types of Shock. Firstly, the etiology should be considered; cardiogenic shock usually has a background of underlying cardiac disease or is secondary to acute myocardial infarction. Treating the primary disease is crucial, and aggressive revascularization is particularly important.

Ⅶ Consultation Process

1. Assess patient vitals and hemodynamics for stability; if signs of instability such as decreased oxygen saturation, rapid shallow breathing, blood pressure drop, malignant arrhythmias are present, immediate interventions like intubation, mechanical ventilation, electrical cardioversion, temporary pacing, anti-arrhythmics, and vasopressors are required.

2. Collect essential historical data, including any underlying cardiac disease such as congenital heart defects, tricuspid regurgitation, right ventricular cardiomyopathy, right ventricular myocardial infarction, thyroid heart disease; respiratory diseases / hypoxia such as COPD, OSAS; chronic pulmonary embolism; idiopathic pulmonary hypertension; connective tissue disease-related pulmonary vascular disease. Also, note any precipitating factors such as fever, exertion, pregnancy, long-duration flights or high-altitude travel.

3. Conduct important physical examinations to check for signs such as cyanosis of the lips, jugular venous distension, enlarged thyroid, barrel chest, reduced breath sounds, wet or dry rales in both lungs, sternal elevation, enlarged cardiac silhouette upon percussion, cardiac murmurs, concomitant hepatomegaly, ascites, joint swelling, deformity, and edema in the limbs (either unilateral or bilateral).

4. Rapidly perform supportive examinations such as blood gas analysis, renal function, electrolytes, ECG (preferably 18 leads), chest X-ray, BNP or NT-proBNP, D-dimer, troponins. If acute pulmonary embolism is suspected, promptly complete a pulmonary artery CTA; swiftly complete cardiac echocardiography to clarify the etiology further. Also, complete a pericardial echocardiography to exclude the possibility of pericardial effusion.

5. Identify whether it is acute or chronic right heart failure. If it is acute, quickly identify the cause and correct it as soon as possible, such as immediate revascularization treatment if the

ECG suggests acute right ventricular myocardial infarction; for pulmonary embolism, evaluate and select thrombolytic therapy, anticoagulation therapy, or pulmonary artery thrombectomy. Administer antibiotics for sepsis, and correct hypoxia, acidosis, etc. If chronic right heart failure is confirmed, refine the diagnosis with right heart catheterization, cardiac MRI, and consider using vasoactive drugs, pulmonary vasodilators, diuretics, etc.

Section 9 Volume Management in Heart Failure

I Importance of Volume Management in Heart Failure

Heart failure (HF) is a clinical syndrome characterized by the inability of the heart to pump blood effectively due to structural or functional cardiac abnormalities, resulting in reduced cardiac output or elevated intracardiac pressures. This leads to classic symptoms such as dyspnea, ankle swelling, and fatigue, as well as signs like elevated jugular venous pressure, pulmonary rales, and peripheral edema.

Heart failure is a progressive condition of pathological damage to the heart, primarily caused by the loss of myocardial cell function or structural abnormalities of the heart. Compensatory responses due to the impaired pumping function of the heart, including the Frank-Starling mechanism and neurohormonal compensation, are significant contributors. In the Frank-Starling mechanism, an increase in left ventricular diastolic pressure can lead to elevated pulmonary capillary wedge pressure, causing severe dyspnea and pulmonary edema. An increase in right ventricular diastolic pressure can lead to elevated venous pressure, resulting in systemic congestion. Neurohormonal mechanisms, which are more complex, typically involve activation of the adrenergic system and the renin-angiotensin system (RAS), leading to fluid and sodium retention and increased peripheral arterial resistance, contributing to cardiac remodeling and worsening heart failure.

Volume overload is a key accompanying feature in the progression of heart failure and a primary reason for hospitalization. Clinically, signs and symptoms of heart failure such as increased volume load often precede overt clinical manifestations. Excessive volume load can increase ventricular wall tension, leading to pulmonary edema or systemic congestion, and contribute to subendocardial ischemia, myocardial necrosis, apoptosis, and activation of neuroendocrine systems, adversely affecting the progression of heart failure. Moreover, decreased renal perfusion and increased renal venous pressure during heart failure can worsen renal function, further complicating and advancing the condition. Thus, management of volume overload, alongside inhibition of neuroendocrine activity and myocardial remodeling, is crucial in the treatment of heart failure, particularly in acute decompensation of chronic heart failure.

II Volume Load Assessment in Heart Failure

1. Historical and Clinical Evaluation. Due to the nonspecific and insen-sitive nature of heart failure symptoms and signs, diagnosing heart failure can be challenging, especially in its early

stages, and in populations such as women, obese individuals, the elderly, or those with chronic obstructive pulmonary disease (COPD) and chronic kidney disease (CKD). Thus, a thorough history and physical examination are crucial for diagnosing and differentiating heart failure.

The principal clinical manifestations of heart failure include dyspnea, fatigue, somnolence, nocturnal cough while lying down, orthopnea, nocturnal paroxysmal dyspnea, increased nocturia, swelling in dependent areas, and loss of appetite. Symptoms like dyspnea, fatigue, and edema are common complaints among heart failure patients; however, these symptoms are also common in patients with other diseases.

Therefore, the specificity and positive predictive value of a single symptom for diagnosing heart failure are low. Among these symptoms, nocturnal paroxysmal dyspnea is a reliable indicator for diagnosing heart failure, but it must also be differentiated from nocturnal awakenings caused by other conditions.

A detailed medical history is foundational for clinical diagnosis. Most heart failure patients have high-risk factors or comorbidities that lead to heart failure, such as hypertension, diabetes, ischemic heart disease, structural heart diseases, arrhythmias, COPD, and CKD. Studies show that prior to being diagnosed with heart failure, 80% of the patients were diagnosed with hypertension, 40% with diabetes, and 45% with ischemic heart disease, occurring on average 8 years, 6 years, and 4 years before the heart failure diagnosis, respectively.

Besides clinical symptoms and medical history, a detailed physical examination and assessment of volume load are crucial for diagnosing heart failure. Physical examination findings in heart failure patients may include tachycardia, arrhythmias, enlarged cardiac silhouette, third heart sound, abnormal blood pressure, jugular venous distention, positive hepatojugular reflux, pulmonary rales, pleural effusion, hepatomegaly, ascites, edema, and weight gain. In physical examinations, assessing volume load is particularly important. Signs like sudden weight gain (2 kg in 2 days or 2.5 kg in one week), lower limb edema, prominent jugular veins, positive hepatojugular reflux, a third heart sound, displaced apical impulse, decreased oxygen saturation, and ascites often indicate excessive volume load. However, excessive volume load does not necessarily indicate the presence of heart failure, as decreased oxygen saturation may be seen in pulmonary diseases, ascites in liver dysfunction or tumors, and lower limb edema in venous valve dysfunction or renal dysfunction. Clinical evaluation often includes measuring jugular venous pressure and checking for pulmonary congestion. Elevated jugular venous pressure not only indicates systemic congestion but is also sensitive (70%) and specific (79%) for suggesting elevated left heart filling pressures, and the degree of decrease in jugular venous pressure correlates well with the decrease in left heart filling pressures. Measuring jugular venous pressure reflects the patient's volume status, and the technique is crucial, usually requiring the patient to be semi-recumbent at 30°-45°, measuring the vertical distance of the jugular pulse to the sternal angle, and adding 5 cm H_2O to estimate right atrial pressure. For pulmonary congestion, the presence of pulmonary rales and pleural effusion are common indicators, and differentiation from pulmonary diseases is necessary. Heart failure-induced pleural effusion typically presents as bilateral, with the right side more commonly affected and only 10% of cases presenting on the left side. Pulmonary rales in heart failure are typically fine, wet rales at the lung bases, but in acute pulmonary edema and cardiogenic asthma, bubbling sounds and wheezing may be present. Although heart failure patients often exhibit signs of volume overload, in patients previously diagnosed with heart failure and currently on diuretic therapy, assessing whether volume overload is excessive is important, along with evaluating for low cardiac output and volume depletion, as indicated by hypotension, fatigue, lethargy, tachycardia, and cold, clammy limbs.

2. Laboratory and Instrumental Assessment

(1) Laboratory Tests: Evaluating volume load in heart failure patients primarily involves measuring biomarkers such as BNP and NT-proBNP (for detailed clinical applications, see the respective sections on BNP and NT-proBNP).

(2) Instrumental Examinations: Instrumental examinations are crucial for diagnosing heart failure, differentiating it from other conditions, treating it, and assessing volume load.

1) Electrocardiogram (ECG): A 12-lead ECG is quick, convenient, and cost-effective, providing essential clues such as atrial fibrillation, myocardial ischemia, atrioventricular block, and intraventricular conduction delay. A 12-lead ECG is also significant for assessing cardiac volume load, such as evaluating left atrial pressure load through P wave morphology in lead V1. While an abnormal ECG can increase the likelihood of diagnosing heart failure, its specificity is low, and patients with a completely normal ECG are less likely to have heart failure (sensitivity 89%).

2) Chest X-Ray: A chest x-ray should be performed for patients suspected of heart failure. It is also quick, convenient, and inexpensive, helping to clarify whether dyspnea is caused by pulmonary diseases or concurrent heart failure, such as COPD, pneumonia, pneumothorax, lung tumors, etc. It also provides information on pulmonary congestion, pulmonary edema, cardiac enlargement, and pleural effusion, which are essential for diagnosing heart failure and assessing the patient's volume load.

3) Routine Ultrasound: Conventional ultrasound has limited diagnostic significance for heart failure but can semi-quantitatively assess the extent of pleural effusion and ascites in patients with heart failure.

4) Echocardiography: Widely used in the evaluation of suspected heart failure patients, echocardiography is risk-free, can be performed bedside if necessary, and provides comprehensive data on cardiac structure, chamber size, wall motion, valve function, intracardiac pressures, and cardiac and diastolic functions. It plays an irreplaceable role in diagnosing heart failure and assessing volume load.

5) Other Examinations: Cardiac MRI is considered the gold standard for measuring left and right ventricular volumes, mass, and ejection fraction, offering diagnostic value for certain types of cardiomyopathies. Single-photon emission computed tomography (SPECT), radionuclide ventriculography, and positron emission tomography (PET) are significant for assessing myocardial ischemia and viability in ischemic heart disease, contributing to the evaluation of the etiology and treatment of heart failure, although they do not assess the volume load in heart failure patients.

(3) Invasive Examinations and Hemodynamic Monitoring

1) Clinical Invasive Examination: Right heart catheterization is commonly used to measure intracardiac pressures, cardiac output, and pulmonary capillary wedge pressure, playing

a significant role in assessing the volume load in heart failure patients. However, with the availability of molecular biomarkers and non-invasive tests meeting the clinical needs of most heart failure patients, the use of invasive tests has declined. Yet, they remain clinically valuable for refractory heart failure, acute heart failure, cardiogenic shock, pump failure, and pre-transplant evaluation in end-stage heart failure.

2) Coronary Angiography (CAG): While CAG does not provide clinical value for assessing volume load in heart failure patients, it has a definitive diagnostic value for ischemic heart disease and guides the etiological treatment of heart failure.

Ⅲ Volume Management in Heart Failure

1. Lifestyle Adjustment and Self-Monitoring. Managing heart failure effectively requires patient understanding and active participation, making education for both patients and their caregivers crucial. Specific measures include:

(1) Daily Weight Monitoring: Patients are encouraged to monitor their weight under consistent conditions. An increase of more than 2 kg in 2 days or more than 2.5 kg in a week may indicate an increase in volume load, necessitating timely adjustments to diuretic therapy.

(2) Fluid Monitoring for Hospitalized Patients: Before heart failure symptoms and signs are controlled, it is vital to record 24-hour fluid intake and output, ensuring that fluid output exceeds intake to alleviate volume load and improve symptoms.

(3) Strict Control of Sodium and Water Intake: Patients exhibiting symptoms and signs of excessive volume load should limit their daily sodium intake to less than 2 g (approximately equivalent to 5 g of sodium chloride); severe heart failure patients should keep their fluid intake between 1,500 and 2,000 mL per day to help reduce volume load.

(4) Enhancing Treatment Adherence: A common cause of increased volume load is patients stopping or altering their medication regimen, particularly with diuretics. Therefore, it is essential that all patients using diuretics to control volume load maintain good compliance.

(5) Prevention and Elimination of Trigger Factors: Common triggers for acute exacerbations of chronic heart failure include various infections (especially respiratory), arrhythmias, and stress responses. Patients who have previously shown signs of excessive volume load must prevent and eliminate these triggers.

(6) Lifestyle Modifications: Encouraging cessation of smoking and alcohol use, along with appropriate exercise, can positively impact health.

2. Volume Management Therapy. Many symptoms of heart failure are due to sodium and water retention and excessive volume load. Thus, volume management is a critical component of heart failure treatment. Clinically, it is important to avoid using drugs that increase sodium and water retention or increase volume load, such as NSAIDs, large volumes of Ⅳ fluids, rapid infusions, and hypertonic solutions. Diuretics play a decisive role in controlling excessive volume load; they are the only medications that can adequately control excessive volume load. Proper use of diuretics is key to successfully managing heart failure volume overload. A Cochrane meta-analysis indicates that diuretics can reduce the risk of death and worsening heart failure and can improve exercise tolerance in patients with chronic heart failure. Depending

on their mechanism of action, diuretics can be categorized as potassium-sparing diuretics, potassium-depleting diuretics, vasopressin V2 receptor antagonists, and recombinant human brain natriuretic peptides.

(1) Loop Diuretics: Loop diuretics, including furosemide, bumetanide, and torsemide, target the thick ascending limb of the loop of Henle in the renal medulla. They are generally suitable for most patients with heart failure, especially those with significant fluid retention or impaired renal function. Furosemide, the most commonly used of these, exhibits a linear dose-response relationship. Its oral bioavailability is around 60%, with an onset of action at approximately 40 minutes, and an intravenous onset of action around 5 minutes. Peak plasma concentrations are reached about 1.5 hours after administration, with a half-life of about 1 hour. The low oral bioavailability of furosemide can be reduced further by food intake, which slows down absorption but does not affect efficacy. In end-stage renal disease and in cases of volume overload with gastrointestinal congestion, the oral bioavailability decreases further, warranting a switch to intravenous administration to enhance effectiveness. Intravenous furosemide can rapidly reduce cardiac preload and increase diuresis, making it suitable for the treatment of acute exacerbations of chronic heart failure or emergency situations. Following intravenous administration, it produces a dose-dependent diuretic effect within 5 minutes. As diuretics can cause electrolyte imbalances, once the volume overload is reduced and clinical symptoms are alleviated, treatment should continue with the lowest effective dose to maintain normal blood volume. Torsemide is almost completely absorbed orally, with a bioavailability of 80%-90%, and bumetanide is significantly more potent than furosemide, being approximately 40 times stronger, with good oral absorption and an approximate bioavailability of 80%. The higher bioavailability of bumetanide and torsemide make them superior in chronic volume overload situations with significant gastrointestinal congestion symptoms.

(2) Thiazide Diuretics: Thiazide diuretics act on the distal convoluted tubule of the kidney and are less potent than loop diuretics. They are suitable for patients with mild fluid retention and high blood pressure with normal renal function. Thiazides include thiazide and thiazide-like diuretics. Hydrochlorothiazide is commonly used clinically, and its diuretic effect is dose-dependent up to a daily dose of 100 mg, beyond which no increase in diuretic effect is seen and adverse effects such as electrolyte imbalances significantly increase. Due to their weak diuretic effect and significant reduction in efficacy in cases of renal insufficiency, thiazides are not recommended for patients with severe volume overload, noticeable edema, or renal insufficiency. However, thiazides can be combined with loop diuretics for resistant cases to produce a synergistic effect.

(3) Potassium-Sparing Diuretics: These include the aldosterone antagonist spironolactone and the drugs amiloride and triamterene. Spironolactone has a weak diuretic effect and is generally not used as a sole agent in patients with significant volume overload. However, it has demonstrated beneficial effects in cardiac remodeling, anti-fibrotic properties, and arrhythmia prevention. Abundant evidence from evidence-based medicine demonstrates that spironolactone improves the prognosis of chronic heart failure and reduces mortality in patients with chronic heart failure. Therefore, the combination of spironolactone with ACEI / ARB and beta-receptor

blockers, known as the "golden triangle" of chronic heart failure drug therapy, forms the foundation of pharmacological treatment for chronic heart failure.

Ambenidine and amiloride both possess mild effects in increasing sodium chloride excretion and countering urinary potassium excretion, with weak diuretic effects. For heart failure patients with excessive volume overload, the use of ambenidine or amiloride alone cannot achieve actual negative sodium balance. Hence, they are not typically used as monotherapy in heart failure patients.

(4) Vasopressin receptor antagonists: Plasma vasopressin levels are elevated in heart failure patients, which can lead to increased systemic vascular resistance and water-sodium retention. Vasopressin mediates its biological activity through three types of receptors: V1a, V2a, and V2. Vasopressin receptor antagonists include selective V2 receptor antagonists and non-selective V1a and V2 receptor antagonists. Currently, the selective vasopressin V2 receptor antagonist tolvaptan is commonly used in clinical practice. It has a strong water excretion effect without significant sodium excretion and is often used in patients with refractory edema accompanied by hyponatremia, or in those with poor response to conventional diuretics, renal insufficiency, or difficult-to-control volume overload.

(5) Recombinant human brain natriuretic peptide (BNP): Brain natriuretic peptide is primarily synthesized and secreted by ventricular cardiomyocytes. The main factors promoting its secretion are ventricular dilation and excessive volume overload. It has effects such as natriuresis, diuresis, reduction of peripheral and pulmonary vascular resistance, antagonism of the renin-angiotensin-aldosterone system and sympathetic nervous system activity, and inhibition of myocardial remodeling. In heart failure, its secretion is compensatorily increased and plays an important role in maintaining cardiac compensatory status. Recombinant human BNP can mimic the action of endogenous BNP, with effects including vasodilation, diuresis and natriuresis, protection of cardiomyocytes, anti-neuroendocrine effects, inhibition of myocardial remodeling, and reduction of pulmonary artery pressure, thereby producing beneficial effects on the cardiovascular system. In 2005, the European Society of Cardiology included it in the standard pharmacological treatment guidelines for heart failure. When using recombinant human BNP to treat heart failure, the antibodies used for detection cannot distinguish between endogenous and exogenous BNP, resulting in elevated BNP levels in the blood, which affects the interpretation of results. However, the influence of recombinant human BNP disappears after 4-5 half-lives (approximately 2 hours). Therefore, when using recombinant human BNP to control volume overload in heart failure patients, if BNP levels need to be measured, it is necessary to discontinue recombinant human BNP for 2 hours before testing. However, NT-proBNP measurement is not affected by recombinant human BNP.

(6) Extracorporeal ultrafiltration: It involves passing the patient's blood through a high-flux membrane, allowing water and sodium to be simultaneously filtered out. It is mainly suitable for patients with refractory edema, end-stage heart failure, diuretic resistance, or concomitant renal failure. Methods of ultrafiltration include continuous hemofiltration, continuous hemodialysis, and continuous hemodiafiltration. During extracorporeal ultrafiltration, it is necessary to maintain a slow fluid flow rate and relatively stable circulating blood volume. A continuous, small-volume

fluid removal approach is often used to prevent excessive activation of the nervous system and the occurrence of hypotension.

3. Precautions for volume management. The use of diuretics should start with a low dose and be adjusted according to the degree of volume overload, recording 24-hour urine output and monitoring weight changes. A daily weight loss of 0.5-1.0 kg is appropriate. Once symptoms are relieved and volume overload is controlled, the minimum effective dose should be maintained long-term to prevent recurrent water-sodium retention, and the dose should be adjusted as needed based on the water-sodium retention status. Diuretics can cause a series of adverse reactions, with common ones including electrolyte disturbances, renal dysfunction, gout and hyperuricemia, hypotension, etc. Patients with refractory heart failure often have diuretic resistance. Therefore, while using diuretics to control volume overload in heart failure patients, it is necessary to monitor for adverse reactions to diuretics.

(1) Diuretic resistance: While diuretics reduce volume overload and decrease water-sodium retention, they can activate internal balancing mechanisms that limit their efficacy. In normal individuals, after administering a certain dose of diuretics, urinary sodium excretion gradually decreases over time, which is known as the "braking phenomenon". In the treatment of heart failure patients, this manifests as diuretic resistance. Diuretic resistance is commonly observed in patients with deteriorating cardiac or renal function, poor medication adherence, concomitant nephrotoxic drug use, or a high-sodium diet. Therefore, a comprehensive assessment of the causes of diuretic resistance is necessary to implement appropriate management strategies.

For patients with poor compliance, it is crucial to enhance patient education about health, encourage a low-sodium diet (less than 2 g of sodium, equivalent to about 5 g of sodium chloride), and control fluid intake strictly to 1,500-2,000 mL daily. It is also important to monitor for medications that may cause fluid and sodium retention, such as NSAIDs, corticosteroids, and thiazolidinediones. In patients with severe volume overload and gastrointestinal congestion, where oral furosemide has low bioavailability, adjusting the medication type, formulation, or timing of administration can increase drug absorption, such as administering on an empty stomach or switching to intravenous formulations of furosemide or using oral agents with higher bio-availability like torsemide or bumetanide. In cases of worsening cardiac function or inadequate renal perfusion, small doses of dopamine [1-3μg / (kg·min)] may be added during continuous intravenous infusion or via an Ⅳ pump to enhance renal perfusion and improve diuretic efficacy. For patients with refractory volume overload, combining loop diuretics with thiazide diuretics is often more effective; thiazides have a longer half-life and can prevent the post-diuretic sodium and water retention, and they inhibit sodium transport in the renal proximal tubule, enhancing the effect of loop diuretics. When using these diuretics in combination, it is vital to monitor blood pressure, renal function, and electrolytes to prevent serious complications. As cardiac and renal functions deteriorate, leading eventually to cardio-renal syndrome and refractory heart failure, a comprehensive treatment approach is required, including continuous infusion of diuretics and dopamine, vasopressor medications, the use of vasopressin V2 receptor antagonists, combination diuretic therapy, and, if necessary, extracorporeal ultra-filtration to reduce volume load.

(2) Electrolyte Disturbances: The most common adverse reactions to diuretic therapy include

hypokalemia and hypomagnesemia, which can lead to malignant arrhythmias and sudden death. Although there is no specific potassium level defined for heart failure patients, clinically, it is advocated to maintain serum potassium levels between 4.0 and 5.0 mmol / L to mitigate the risk of severe arrhythmias and sudden death associated with low potassium and magnesium levels. Regular electrolyte monitoring is necessary when managing volume load in heart failure patients with diuretics. To prevent electrolyte disturbances caused by diuretics, it is often necessary to use potassium-sparing diuretics in combination with potassium-depleting agents, and if required, prophylactic oral potassium and magnesium supplementation may be considered.

(3) Renal Dysfunction: Heart failure often coexists with renal dysfunction, along with common risk factors such as hypertension and diabetes. The interplay between heart failure and renal dysfunction can create a vicious cycle and is a predictor of poor prognosis. Heart failure associated with renal dysfunction is related to common risk factors, inadequate volume, insufficient renal perfusion, the use of nephrotoxic drugs, and the use of ACE inhibitors or ARBs. Regular monitoring of renal function is crucial when managing volume load with diuretics. If renal function deteriorates, re-evaluation of the patient's condition is necessary, discontinuing nephrotoxic drugs, controlling risk factors, reducing volume load if there is excessive volume, reducing diuretic dosage if there is inadequate volume, and if renal perfusion is insufficient, small doses of dopamine [1-3 μg / (kg·min)] may be added to enhance renal perfusion. In cases where serum creatinine increases significantly (>3 mg / dL, an increase>25% or a GFR decrease> 20%), a temporary discontinuation or dose reduction of ACE inhibitors or ARBs is required, and dialysis may be necessary.

(4) Hypotension: Upon initiation of diuretic therapy, symptoms such as decreased blood pressure, reduced exercise tolerance, and increased fatigue often occur. It is essential to distinguish between hypotension caused by inadequate volume and insufficient cardiac output. Clinical symptoms and assessment of volume load are crucial to determine further treatment strategies. In patients with inadequate volume, reducing the diuretic dose often provides relief. However, if the patient's blood pressure drops, urine output is normal, and there is no evidence of inadequate peripheral perfusion, it is usually not necessary to reduce the diuretic dose. Instead, initiating rehabilitation treatment for chronic heart failure patients can improve exercise tolerance and reduce hospitalization and mortality rates in heart failure patients. If heart failure symptoms persist and cardiac output is low after clinical and volume load assessment, positive inotropic agents and vasoactive drugs may be used to maintain blood pressure and cardiac function.

(5) Gout and Hyperuricemia: All heart failure patients undergoing volume load management with diuretics will experience an increase in uric acid levels, and some may develop gout. In patients with hyperuricemia, controlling uric acid levels with uric acid-lowering medications while adhering to a low-purine diet is necessary. For acute gout attacks, colchicine may be used, and corticosteroids should be used sparingly to avoid the use of NSAIDs.

Ⅳ Consultation Process

1. Assess the patient's vital signs and hemodynamic stability. If there are signs of instability such as decreased oxygen saturation, rapid shallow breathing, hypotension, malignant

arrhythmias, etc., immediately initiate emergency treatment such as endotracheal intubation, mechanical ventilation, electrical cardioversion, temporary pacemaker, anti-arrhythmic drugs, vasopressors, etc.

2. Supplement crucial medical history, such as the presence of underlying heart disease: congenital heart disease, tricuspid regurgitation, right ventricular myopathy, right ventricular myocardial infarction, thyrotoxic heart disease; respiratory diseases / hypoxia, such as COPD, OSAS; chronic pulmonary thromboembolism; idiopathic pulmonary arterial hypertension; connective tissue disease-associated pulmonary vascular disease, etc. Also note any potential triggers, such as fever, exertion, pregnancy, long-haul flights, or high-altitude travel.

3. Perform a thorough physical examination, noting cyanosis, jugular venous distension, thyroid enlargement, barrel chest, decreased breath sounds, crackles / wheezes, left sternal heave, cardiomegaly, murmurs, hepatomegaly, ascites, joint swelling / deformities, and unilateral or bilateral edema.

4. Rapidly obtain relevant tests such as arterial blood gas, renal function, electrolytes, ECG (preferably 18-lead), chest X-ray, BNP or NT-proBNP, D-dimer, troponins. If acute pulmonary embolism is suspected, urgently perform CT pulmonary angiography. Promptly obtain echocardiography to further elucidate the etiology. Also rule out pericardial effusion with pericardial ultrasound.

5. Identify acute vs. chronic right heart failure. If acute, rapidly determine the cause, promptly treat the underlying condition (e.g. revascularization for acute RV infarction), evaluate for thrombolysis, anticoagulation or pulmonary thrombectomy for pulmonary embolism, treat sepsis with antibiotics, correct hypoxia and acidosis, etc. For chronic right heart failure, obtain further testing such as right heart catheterization, cardiac MRI to clarify the etiology and guide therapy with vasodilators, pulmonary vasodilators, diuretics, etc.

Section 10 Clinical Application Value of BNP and NT-proBNP

Natriuretic peptides (NP) are a family of hormones with vasodilatory, natriuretic, diuretic, and renin-angiotensin-aldosterone system inhibitory effects. Members include atrial natriuretic peptide (ANP), B-type natriuretic peptide (BNP), C-type natriuretic peptide (CNP), and D-type natriuretic peptide (DNP), of which ANP and BNP are cardiac natriuretic peptides.

BNP and N-terminal pro-BNP (NT-proBNP) are two forms of BNP that not only serve as biomarkers for heart failure diagnosis, but also play crucial roles in clinical diagnosis, prognosis, and potential treatment guidance. The structures and clinical applications of BNP and NT-proBNP are discussed below.

I Structure and Characteristics of BNP and NT-proBNP

BNP / NT-proBNP is initially synthesized by cardiac myocytes as preproBNP, a 134 amino acid precursor. After removal of a 26 amino acid signal peptide from the N-terminus, proBNP (108 amino acids) is formed. Subsequent cleavage by a neutral endoprotease yields the 76 amino acid N-terminal proBNP and the 32 amino acid C-terminal BNP, which are co-secreted in equimolar amounts into the circulation. They have similar diagnostic, monitoring, and prognostic value for cardiovascular disease. BNP is less stable ex vivo, has a short half-life in vivo, low molecular weight, and is cleared by neutral endopeptidase, BNP clearance receptors, and renal metabolism. In contrast, NT-proBNP has a longer half-life, is more stable ex vivo, has a higher molecular weight, and is cleared more slowly by glomerular filtration alone. Its plasma levels are 2-10 times higher than BNP, particularly elevated in heart failure patients, making it better suited for laboratory testing.

BNP is biologically active, while NT-proBNP is not. Their secretion is upregulated by increases in pressure / volume overload. Due to its longer half-life, NT-proBNP levels accumulate higher and more sensitively reflect cardiac function changes, especially early heart failure. NT-proBNP is unaffected by BNP therapy (e.g. nesiritide) and is preferred for monitoring patients on such treatment. Additionally, thyroid hormone, glucocorticoids, ACE inhibitors, diuretics, adrenergic antagonists, and beta-blockers can influence BNP levels.

Ⅱ Clinical Applications

1. BNP and NYHA classification: Research has found that BNP levels in patients with heart failure are positively correlated with NYHA classification (Table 2-2).

Table 2-2 Relationship Between NYHA Class and BNP Levels

NYHA Classification	Ⅰ	Ⅱ	Ⅲ	Ⅳ
BNP Level	83. 1 (49. 1-137) ng / L	235 (137-391) ng / L	459 (200-871) ng / L	1,119 (728-1,300) ng / L

2. BNP / NT-proBNP in Chronic Heart Failure: For suspected chronic heart failure, NT-proBNP < 125 ng / L or BNP < 35 ng / L can exclude the diagnosis, helping differentiate dyspnea due to heart failure. While the Chinese heart failure guidelines suggest monitoring BNP to guide therapy, this remains unsupported by evidence. Comprehensive assessment based on other tests, symptoms and disease course is more advisable.

In one BNP-guided trial aiming for BNP < 100 ng / L, the BNP-guided group had lower hospitalization and cardiovascular event rates compared to clinically guided controls, possibly due to BNP level comparisons influencing clinicians' conservative vs. aggressive treatment decisions. Regarding prognosis, the guidelines state that failure of BNP to decrease by ≥ 30% or increasing levels indicate very high risk of re-hospitalization and death. Reports also show that in chronic heart failure, lack of BNP decline portends high 30-day risk of re-hospitalization / death even if symptoms improve during hospitalization.

3. BNP / NT-proBNP in Acute Heart Failure: BNP plays a more crucial role in detecting and differentiating acute heart failure compared to chronic heart failure. Dual diagnostic and exclusion cutoffs are used, with exclusion cutoffs being more accurate. NT-proBNP < 300 ng / L and BNP < 100 ng / L can exclude acute heart failure. Due to metabolic factors affecting BNP, cutoffs should be adjusted for gender, age, weight, etc.—higher for females, elderly, renal dysfunction,

and lower for obesity, though optimal adjustment requires further study. Diagnostic cutoffs are stratified by age and renal function (Table 2-3). Regarding severity and prognosis, the guidelines suggest NT-proBNP>5,000 ng / L indicates high short-term mortality risk, while>1,000 ng / L indicates higher long-term mortality risk. Post-treatment BNP decrease>30% suggests effective therapy. If BNP rises despite stable symptoms, preemptive advanced therapies like ultra-filtration, vasodilators, inotropes, or synchronized therapy may be warranted.

Table 2-3 Age and Renal Function Stratification for NT-proBNP Diagnostic Cutoffs

Stratum	<50 years	50-75 years	>75 years	Renal Impairment (GFR<60 mL / min)
NT-proBNP Value (Diagnostic Cutoff)	>450 ng / L	>900 ng / L	>1,800 ng / L	>1,200 ng / L

4. BNP / NT-proBNP in Pulmonary Hypertension: Initial BNP research focused on heart failure, but further studies revealed an association between elevated BNP and pulmonary hypertension. BNP and NT-proBNP are now important diagnostic markers for pulmonary hypertension, with some evidence suggesting BNP levels correlate with disease severity. Possible mechanisms include: ① Increased right ventricular pressure from pulmonary hypertension causes myocardial stretch and BNP release. ② Hypoxia and inflammation from underlying conditions like COPD or pulmonary embolism that cause pulmonary hypertension stimulate BNP production. Clinically, elevated BNP does not necessarily indicate heart failure, and pulmonary hypertension should be considered to avoid misdiagnosis. BNP levels in pulmonary hypertension are typically within the gray zone range unless right ventricular hypertrophy is present, necessitating correlation with other findings.

5. BNP / NT-proBNP in Sepsis and Infection: BNP levels are also elevated in severe sepsis or septic shock. Infection induces an inflammatory response, with mediators like TNF-α, IL-1, IL-6 released from inflammatory cells stimulating BNP production by cardiomyocytes. Additionally, ventricular dilation in sepsis leads to increased BNP secretion. Studies suggest higher BNP correlates with greater severity of infection. Clinically, BNP can serve as a marker for assessing infection severity, cardiac dysfunction, and mortality risk in septic patients.

6. BNP / NT-proBNP in Atrial Fibrillation: Studies show that even without overt structural heart disease or heart failure, atrial fibrillation patients have significantly elevated blood NT-proBNP levels and atrial BNP mRNA content. BNP and NT-proBNP levels have clinical value in predicting atrial fibrillation occurrence and recurrence after conversion, with elevated BNP associated with increased thromboembolic risk. In stable heart failure patients, NT-proBNP correlates most closely with atrial fibrillation, suggesting it may be a key factor influencing NT-proBNP in those with structurally normal hearts. To sum up, BNP and NT-proBNP elevations represent atrial and / or ventricular release in response to arrhythmia and have clinical utility in evaluating atrial fibrillation, but caution is warranted in interpreting their elevation in these patients.

7. BNP / NT-proBNP in Coronary Artery Disease: Traditionally considered specific for heart failure, BNP and NT-proBNP are also elevated in acute coronary syndromes. Tuxunguli et al. found higher NT-proBNP in acute coronary syndrome patients versus non-acute coronary syndrome

patients, with levels correlating with extent of coronary disease, suggesting NT-proBNP has early diagnostic value. Other studies show BNP is higher in non-ST elevation myocardial infarction than unstable angina, and increases with number of diseased vessels. Importantly, BNP> 80 pg / mL suggests triple or double vessel disease, and in single vessel disease, BNP is highest with left anterior descending artery involvement. Patients with BNP>80 pg / mL also had higher Gensini scores. BNP inversely correlates with left ventricular ejection fraction and closely relates to myocardial infarct size, allowing clinical estimation of infarct extent.

8. BNP / NT-proBNP in Differentiating Dyspnea: Distinguishing pulmonary from cardiac causes of dyspnea is clinically challenging. Studies indicate rapid, accurate diagnosis and management of acute dyspnea in the emergency department improves patient outcomes, and point-of-care BNP / NT-proBNP measurement facilitates this. Using a 663.2 ng / L BNP cutoff to differentiate acute cardiac from respiratory dyspnea yields 37% sensitivity, 97.2% specificity, 50.7% negative predictive value, and 95.2% positive predictive value. However, applying plasma proBNP for initial diagnosis or serial monitoring to guide therapy in the emergency setting does not improve diagnostic accuracy or treatment efficacy, as BNP levels are affected by gender, age, weight, and renal function. Additionally, compensation in heart failure can cause gradual BNP / NT-proBNP elevation, impacting interpretation. Combined lung-heart-inferior vena cava ultrasound with BNP may be a better approach for determining the etiology of acute dyspnea.

9. BNP / NT-proBNP in Other Diseases: Evaluating plasma NT-proBNP in acute pulmonary embolism and its relationship with adverse outcomes reveals significantly higher levels in patients experiencing adverse events compared to those with an uncomplicated course. An NT-proBNP<500 ng / L had 97% negative predictive value for adverse outcomes. Plasma BNP and NT-proBNP are also elevated in the acute phase of ischemic stroke, gradually declining in the subacute phase, with the degree of elevation closely related to infarct size and location, suggesting prognostic utility. Furthermore, BNP and NT-proBNP increase in diabetic vascular disease, diabetic nephropathy, and primary hypertension. In asymptomatic children with congenital heart disease, plasma BNP and NT-proBNP are typically higher than in those without, indicating potential predicting value in this population.

10. Applications of Recombinant BNP: Recombinant BNP is a drug produced via genetic engineering techniques, essentially a BNP derivative. Its pharmacological effects include: ① Dilating systemic arteries and veins, selectively dilating coronary and pulmonary vasculature to reduce pulmonary vascular resistance; ② Natriuretic and diuretic effects; ③ Inhibition of the renin-angiotensin-aldosterone system; ④ Inhibition of cardiac remodeling. By increasing cardiac output without raising myocardial oxygen demand, promoting natriuresis and diuresis without potassium wasting, preventing remodeling, and lacking pro-arrhythmic effects, recombinant BNP plays an important role in treating refractory heart failure, acute coronary syndromes, and peri-operative management in cardiac surgery. It also shows promise for pulmonary arterial hypertension.

Ⅲ Summary

In summary, BNP not only plays a vital role in the diagnosis, treatment, and prognostic assessment of heart failure, but also has high clinical utility in atrial fibrillation, coronary artery disease, pulmonary hypertension, sepsis, and other conditions. However, due to lack of standardized assay methods, confounding factors influencing results, and unclear diagnostic cutoffs for various diseases, the relationship between BNP / NT-proBNP levels and disease diagnosis, management, and prognosis requires further exploration. As research advances, the applications of BNP are expected to expand significantly.

Ⅳ Consultation Process

1. Assess the patient's vital signs and hemodynamic stability. If unstable with desaturation, rapid shallow breathing, hypotension, malignant arrhythmias, etc., immediately initiate emergency management with endotracheal intubation, mechanical ventilation, cardioversion, temporary pacing, anti-arrhythmics, vasopressors, etc.

2. Supplement key medical history regarding underlying cardiac diseases like coronary artery disease, atrial fibrillation, structural heart disease; pulmonary embolism, pulmonary hypertension, sepsis, ARDS, stroke, renal impairment, etc.

3. Perform a thorough physical examination noting cyanosis, jugular venous distension, barrel chest, decreased breath sounds, crackles / wheezes, heart murmur, arrhythmia, cardiomegaly, hepatomegaly, ascites, peripheral edema (unilateral or bilateral), etc.

4. For diagnosis and differentiation of acute heart failure: BNP $<$100 ng / L or NT-proBNP $<$ 300 ng / L reliably excludes acute heart failure. In renal impairment [eGFR $<$60 mL / (min·1.73 m^2)], use NT-proBNP $<$1,200 ng / L. BNP $>$400 ng / L or NT-proBNP above age-specific cutoffs should raise suspicion for acute heart failure.

BNP / NT-proBNP in the gray zone suggests possible heart failure but necessitates considering other diagnoses like coronary artery disease, atrial fibrillation, pulmonary embolism, pulmonary hypertension, sepsis, ARDS, stroke, etc., requiring careful correlation with clinical history, examination and relevant investigations.

5. For diagnosis and differentiation of chronic heart failure: BNP $<$35 ng / L or NT-proBNP $<$ 125 ng / L excludes chronic heart failure. If above these cutoffs, further testing is required along with clinical correlation, while accounting for non-heart failure causes of BNP / NT-proBNP elevation.

6. If BNP / NT-proBNP is elevated after excluding non-cardiac causes, manage according to heart failure treatment principles.

Section 11 Pulmonary Embolism

Ⅰ Overview

Pulmonary embolism (PE) refers to a group of diseases or clinical syndromes caused by obstruction of the pulmonary arterial system by various emboli, including pulmonary thromboembolism (PTE), fat embolism syndrome, amniotic fluid embolism, and air embolism. PTE is the most common type of PE, with thrombi originating mainly from deep vein thrombosis (DVT), most frequently in the lower extremity and pelvic veins. Acute PTE is a medical emergency with potentially grave consequences. This chapter focuses primarily on acute PTE.

Epidemiological studies indicate the incidence of PE is 100-200 per 100,000 population. International data suggests that 1% of hospitalized patients die from acute PE, accounting for 10% of all in-hospital deaths. U.S. epidemiological data shows that PE is the third most common cardiovascular disease after coronary artery disease and hypertension, with an untreated mortality rate of 25%-30%, ranking third among causes of death after cancer and acute myocardial infarction. There is no definitive epidemiological data from China, though reported cases have increased in recent years, possibly reflecting rising incidence or improved clinician awareness and diagnosis. With timely diagnosis and appropriate treatment, PE mortality can be reduced to around 7%. Therefore, early diagnosis of PE is a critical issue for clinicians.

II Diagnostic Essentials

1. Common clinical presentations include dyspnea, chest pain, syncope, and hemoptysis. Less common are restlessness, impending doom, cough, and abdominal pain. Sometimes the classic triad of dyspnea, chest pain, and hemoptysis (so-called "pulmonary infarction triad") is present, but in less than 30% of patients.

2. Most PE patients have risk factors. Venous stasis, vascular endothelial injury, and hypercoagulability are the three main factors leading to venous thrombosis formation. Common risk factors for venous thromboembolism (VTE) include patient-related (often permanent) and acquired (often transient) factors. Transient or reversible risk factors within 6 weeks to 3 months can precipitate VTE. Different risk factors confer varying relative risk (odds ratio, OR). Among common risk factors, strong risk factors (OR>10) include major trauma, surgery, lower extremity fractures, joint replacements, and spinal cord injury; moderate risk factors (OR 2-9) include knee arthroscopy, autoimmune disorders, hereditary thrombophilia, inflammatory bowel disease, cancer, oral contraceptives, hormone replacement therapy, central venous catheters, stroke with paralysis, chronic heart or respiratory failure, and superficial vein thrombosis; weak risk factors (OR<2) include pregnancy, bedrest>3 days, immobility (e.g. prolonged car / air travel), advanced age, and varicose veins.

3. Diagnostic Tests

(1) D-dimer: High sensitivity, low specificity. Elevated in PE but not specific; normal can exclude PE; elevated requires correlation with typical clinical presentation.

(2) Multidetector CT pulmonary angiography: Very high diagnostic value. Latest multidetector CT can visualize clots in sixth-order pulmonary arterial branches, making it the first-choice confirmatory test for suspected PE and the current "gold standard" for PE diagnosis. Limitation is contraindication in iodine contrast allergy.

(3) MRI: High sensitivity and specificity for detecting clots in lobar or more proximal pulmonary arteries. Disadvantages are longer imaging time and inferior image quality compared to CT.

(4) Ventilation / perfusion lung scan: Infrequently used now, only for patients with CT

contrast allergy.

(5) Echocardiography: Shows indirect signs like right heart dilation, pulmonary hypertension, which are valuable for suggesting diagnosis and excluding other cardiovascular diseases.

(6) Chest X-ray: Non-specific findings like regional oligemia, elevated hemidiaphragm, mediastinal shift, and pleural effusion. Some PE patients may have normal chest X-ray.

(7) Arterial blood gas: Most PE patients have hypoxemia, with hypocapnia from hyperventilation. Hypoxemia refractory to oxygen with typical clinical presentation should raise suspicion for PE. However, some patients have normal blood gases, not excluding PE.

(8) ECG: S wave in lead I, Q wave and T-wave inversion in lead Ⅲ (S1Q3T3 pattern) may be seen in some patients. Other common but non-specific findings include T-wave and ST-segment changes in V1-4, complete or incomplete right bundle branch block, right axis deviation, clockwise rotation, and P pulmonale.

(9) Pulmonary angiography: Previously the gold standard for PE diagnosis but now replaced by CT due to its invasive nature and potential for life-threatening or serious complications. Should be strictly limited to appropriate indications.

(10) Tests for DVT: All suspected or confirmed PE patients should undergo evaluation for DVT to identify the embolic source and prevent recurrence, using modalities like CT, MRI, ultrasound, or venography.

Ⅲ Diagnosis and Differential Diagnosis

The clinical presentation of PE lacks specificity and overlaps with other conditions like acute myocardial infarction, pneumothorax, aortic dissection, and other causes of dyspnea, leading to a historically high rate of missed diagnoses. However, with increased awareness, clinical misdiagnosis rates have declined significantly. Nevertheless, missed diagnoses are associated with higher mortality compared to timely diagnosis and treatment, underscoring the need for vigilance. Patients with risk factors, especially multiple risk factors, should be evaluated for PE. Those presenting with unexplained dyspnea, chest pain, syncope or shock, particularly with unilateral or asymmetric leg swelling / pain, should undergo ECG, chest X-ray, blood gases, echocardiography and lower extremity vascular ultrasound. These results can provisionally suggest or exclude PE. D-dimer testing should be routinely performed, as a negative result essentially rules out PE. For suspected PE after initial testing, CT pulmonary angiography should be urgently pursued for definitive diagnosis. If CT is contraindicated due to contrast allergy or other reasons, MRI or ventilation / perfusion scanning can aid diagnosis.

Once diagnosed, PE requires risk stratification to guide treatment and estimate prognosis. Previously, PE was classified into three groups: ① Non-massive—normotensive without right heart failure; ② Submassive—normotensive with right heart failure; ③ Massive—right heart failure with hypotension or cardiogenic shock, defined as systolic blood pressure $<$90 mmHg or $\geq$40 mmHg drop from baseline for $>$15 minutes. *The 2014 ESC Guidelines* considered this classification unscientific and instead recommended early mortality risk stratification into low, intermediate-low, intermediate-high, and high-risk groups based on presence of hypotension /

shock, pulmonary embolism severity index (PESI) score, right ventricular dysfunction, and cardiac biomarker levels. PESI is complex, so the 2014 ESC guidelines proposed a simplified PESI scoring 1 point each for age, cancer, heart failure / chronic lung disease, heart rate≥110 bpm, systolic blood pressure<100 mmHg, and oxygen saturation<90%. The 2015 Chinese Expert Consensus also recommends using the ESC risk stratification scheme (Table 2-4).

Table 2-4 2014 ESC Guidelines for Early Mortality Risk Stratification in Acute PE

Early Mortality Risk	Risk Stratification Criteria and Score			
	Shock / Hypotension	Simplified PESI≥1	Right Ventricular Dysfunction	Cardiac Biomarker
High risk	+	+	+	+
Moderate risk				
Moderate-high risk	-	+	+	
Moderate-low risk	-	+	One positive or both negative	
Low risk	-	-	-	-

Ⅳ Treatment Principles

1. General Measures: Oxygen therapy, mechanical ventilation for severe hypoxemia. Morphine analgesia unless in shock. Treatment of heart failure and shock with vasopressors like dopamine and dobutamine as indicated.

2. Anticoagulation: The classic treatment for PE is anticoagulation, with most patients achieving good results with aggressive, effective anticoagulation. Standard therapy duration is at least 3-6 months, or lifelong for unprovoked PE. Initial treatment options include unfractionated heparin, low molecular weight heparin, or fondaparinux for 5-10 days parenterally. Warfarin should overlap with par-enteral therapy for 4-5 days, targeting an INR of 2-3. Once INR is therapeutic for two consecutive readings, par-enteral therapy can be stopped. Warfarin requires regular INR monitoring and dose adjustment. Newer oral anticoagulants like dabigatran, rivaroxaban, apixaban and edoxaban have predictable pharmacokinetics without need for monitoring. Rivaroxaban and apixaban can be started directly or after 1-2 days of par-enteral bridging, while dabigatran and edoxaban are started after completing a par-enteral lead-in. These agents are contraindicated in severe renal impairment.

3. Thrombolysis: First-line therapy for high-risk patients. Agents, dosing, and contraindications are identical to those for acute ST-elevation myocardial infarction thrombolysis. For life-threatening high-risk PE, especially at centers without surgical / interventional capabilities, there are essentially no absolute contraindications to thrombolysis. For intermediate-risk PE, guidelines do not recommend routine thrombolysis but rather aggressive anticoagulation with close monitoring for clinical deterioration requiring rescue thrombolysis.

4. Surgery and Interventional Therapy: Select high-risk patients with contraindications to thrombolysis or failed thrombolysis may undergo surgical pulmonary thrombectomy or catheter-directed treatment. If local surgical / interventional options are unavailable but safe transfer is feasible, the patient should be transferred to an experienced center.

5. Vena Cava Filters: It is not recommended to routinely insert inferior vena cava filters in patients with acute PE. In patients with absolute contraindications to anticoagulant drugs and those who still experience recurrence after receiving adequate intensity anticoagulant therapy, the option of inserting a venous filter may be considered.

V Common Questions in Cardiology Consultations

1. How to Avoid Missing a Diagnosis of Pulmonary Embolism (PE). PE can occur across various departments such as orthopedics, obstetrics, surgery, oncology, hematology, geriatrics, and neurology. Patients in these departments presenting with chest pain, shock, or respiratory distress typically require a cardiology consultation. The consulting cardiologist should conduct a thorough medical history review. If there are high-risk factors for deep vein thrombosis (DVT), prompt testing for D-dimer levels and pulse oximetry should be performed. If oxygen saturation does not improve despite oxygen therapy, a high suspicion of PE should be maintained, and immediate CT pulmonary angiography should be performed to aid in diagnosis.

2. Differentiating Between Acute Coronary Syndrome (ACS) and PE in the Presence of Precordial Lead T-wave Changes and ST-Segment Abnormalities with Chest Pain. First, inquire about the history to assess for DVT high-risk factors. If present, PE should be suspected, and appropriate investigations should be undertaken. If an echocardiogram shows segmental contraction abnormalities, ACS is more likely. If it shows enlargement of the right atrium or ventricle and pulmonary hypertension, PE is more likely. Multiple electrocardiogram reviews are crucial; if there is dynamic evolution of changes, ACS is likely, whereas a lack of such evolution should raise suspicions of PE.

3. Whether to Administer Thrombolytic Therapy. If PE is confirmed, immediate risk stratification must be performed. High-risk patients should be assessed for contraindications; if none are present, thrombolytic therapy should be initiated without delay. For some hemodynamically unstable high-risk patients with relative contraindications, the risk-benefit ratio of bleeding versus therapeutic benefit should be evaluated. If the potential benefit outweighs the risks, thrombolytic therapy may be considered after thorough discussion with the patient's family.

4. Prevention of PE. Prevention of PE is more significant than its treatment. During external consultations, cardiologists should thoroughly inquire about the patient's medical history and past medical conditions. Departments with patients having high-risk factors for DVT should be alerted to the risks. With increasing recognition of PE, surgical departments, particularly orthopedics, have heightened their focus on DVT and PE prevention. Adhering to guidelines and expert consensus, if awareness is maintained, these departments will implement appropriate preventive measures.

VI Consultation Process

1. Assess the patient's vital signs and hemodynamic stability. If signs of hemodynamic instability such as decreased blood oxygen levels, rapid and shallow breathing, hypotension, or shock are present, immediate interventions like intubation, mechanical ventilation, and vasopressors should be administered.

2. Collect essential historical data, including any recent surgeries, trauma / fractures, prolonged bed rest, long-distance air or road travel, malignancies, certain chronic diseases (e.g., antiphospholipid syndrome, nephrotic syndrome, inflammatory bowel disease, myeloproliferative disorders), pregnancy, and genetic factors.

3. Perform crucial physical examinations, checking for consciousness, cyanosis of the lips, respiratory rate, diminished breath sounds, and whether there is edema in the legs (unilateral or bilateral).

4. Rapidly conduct necessary diagnostic tests such as arterial blood gas analysis, electrocardiogram, chest X-ray, BNP or NT-proBNP levels, D-dimer, and troponin levels. If acute pulmonary embolism is suspected, expedite the completion of a CT pulmonary angiogram (CTA).

5. For patients with unstable hemodynamics and suspected high-risk pulmonary thromboembolism (PTE), promptly complete a pulmonary artery CTA to confirm the diagnosis. If the CTA is positive, consider thrombolytic (interventional or surgical) treatment.

For stable patients suspected of non-high-risk PTE, complete a D-dimer test; if elevated and arterial blood gases indicate hypoxemia, further investigation with a pulmonary artery CTA is warranted. If CTA is contraindicated (e.g., due to contrast allergy, severe renal failure, pregnancy), consider alternative diagnostics like nuclear lung ventilation / perfusion scans or lower limb venous ultrasound. If non-high-risk PTE is confirmed, initiate anticoagulation therapy.

Section 12 Cardiomyopathies

In China, the definition and classification of cardiomyopathies adopted are those from the World Health Organization and the joint working group of the International Society and Federation of Cardiology. Considering the current situation, the terms "hypertensive cardiomyopathy" and "inflammatory cardiomyopathy" are not used for the time being under the category of specific cardiomyopathies. In recent years, cardiomyopathy induced by rapid arrhythmias, known as "tachycardia-induced cardiomyopathy", and cardiomyopathy associated with obesity, termed "obesity cardiomyopathy," have drawn increasing clinical attention. Based on their pathophysiological features, cardiomyopathies are classified into five types.

1. Dilated Cardiomyopathy (DCM): Characterized by left ventricular or biventricular dilatation accompanied by impaired contractile function. It can be idiopathic, familial / genetic, viral and / or immune-mediated, alcoholic / toxic, or occur in the presence of known cardiovascular diseases, but the degree of myocardial dysfunction cannot be explained by abnormal loading conditions or the extent of myocardial ischemic injury.

2. Hyper-trophic Cardiomyopathy (HCM): Characterized by left ventricular and / or right ventricular hypertrophy, often with asymmetric hypertrophy involving the inter-ventricular septum. Typical features include normal or decreased left ventricular volume and a systolic pressure gradient across the left ventricular outflow tract. Familial cases are often autosomal dominant inherited.

3. Restrictive Cardiomyopathy (RCM): Characterized by impaired ventricular filling and

reduced diastolic volume in one or both ventricles, while systolic function and wall thickness remain normal or near-normal.

4. Arrhythmogenic Right Ventricular Cardiomyopathy (ARVC): Progressive replacement of the right ventricular myocardium by fibro-fatty tissue, initially presenting as a regional process and later involving the entire right ventricle and, to a lesser extent, the left ventricle and interventricular septum. Autosomal dominant inheritance with incomplete penetrance is typical, but recessive forms have also been reported.

5. Unclassified Cardiomyopathies: Include cases that do not entirely fit into any of the above categories (e.g., fibro-elastic deficiency, non-compacted cardiomyopathy, impaired systolic function with only mild ventricular dilatation, mitochondrial disorders). Some patients may exhibit features of more than one type of cardiomyopathy (e.g., amyloidosis, systemic hypertension).

Dilated Cardiomyopathy

I Definition and Disease Characteristics

The clinical presentation of dilated cardiomyopathy includes dilatation of one or both ventricles, reduced ventricular contractile function, with or without congestive heart failure. Ventricular and atrial arrhythmias are common, and the disease progressively worsens, with the possibility of death occurring at any stage. The etiology is considered to be related to viral infections, genetic factors, fluid and cellular immunity, autonomic nervous system dysregulation and endocrine abnormalities, chemical or toxic exposure, and myocardial energy metabolism disturbances.

II Diagnostic Essentials

In combination with the clinical presentation of heart failure, chest X-ray, echocardiography, and other examinations, it is not difficult to establish the diagnosis.

1. Clinical Presentation: Cardiac enlargement, reduced ventricular contractile function with or without congestive heart failure, arrhythmias, and the possibility of thromboembolism and sudden death.

2. Cardiac Enlargement: Chest X-ray suggests a cardio-thoracic ratio>0.5, and echocardiography reveals overall cardiac enlargement, especially of the left ventricle. A left ventricular end-diastolic diameter>2.7 cm, generally>55 mm in males and>53 mm in females, should raise suspicion of left ventricular dilatation, which should be evaluated in conjunction with regional wall motion abnormalities and other echocardiographic parameters.

3. Reduced Ventricular Contractile Function: Echocardiography demon-strates diffuse hypokinesis, and the ejection fraction is below normal.

4. Exclusion of Other Specific (Secondary) Cardiomyopathies and Localized Myocardial Diseases (Keshan Disease): This includes ischemic cardiomyopathy, peripartum cardiomyopathy, alcoholic cardiomyopathy, metabolic and endocrine diseases such as hyperthyroidism, hypo-

thyroidism, amyloidosis, diabetes mellitus, hereditary neuromuscular disorders, systemic diseases like systemic lupus erythematosus, rheumatoid arthritis, and toxic cardiomyopathies. Only after excluding these conditions can a diagnosis of idiopathic dilated cardiomyopathy be made.

5. Endomyocardial Biopsy: Pathological examination is not specific for this disease but can help differentiate it from specific cardiomyopathies and acute myocarditis. Performing polymerase chain reaction (PCR) or in situ hybridization on endomyocardial biopsy specimens can assist in diagnosing infectious etiologies or analyzing specific cellular genetic abnormalities.

Ⅲ Differential Diagnosis

1. Coronary Heart Disease: In middle-aged and older individuals presenting with cardiac enlargement, arrhythmias, or heart failure without apparent cause, coronary heart disease and cardiomyopathy should be considered. The presence of risk factors such as hypertension, hyperlipidemia, or diabetes mellitus, along with segmental wall motion abnormalities, favors the diagnosis of coronary heart disease. Diffuse impairment of myocardial contractility supports the diagnosis of dilated cardiomyopathy. Chronic extensive myocardial ischemia and fibrosis due to coronary artery disease can lead to heart failure, termed "ischemic cardiomyopathy", which presents with heart failure and arrhythmias. In the absence of angina pectoris or myocardial infarction, it may be indistinguishable from cardiomyopathy. Additionally, cardiomyopathy can also present with pathological Q waves and angina pectoris. At this time, identification must rely on coronary angiography or coronary artery CTA examination.

2. Rheumatic Heart Disease: Cardiomyopathy can also present with systolic murmurs in the mitral or tricuspid valve areas, but generally without diastolic murmurs. These murmurs are louder during heart failure and diminish or disappear with improved heart failure control, contrary to rheumatic heart disease. In cardiomyopathy, multiple cardiac chambers are often dilated, whereas in rheumatic heart disease, the left atrium, left ventricle, or right ventricle is predominantly affected. Echocardiography can aid in differentiating these conditions.

3. Congenital Heart Disease: In congenital displacement of the tricuspid valve, a murmur in the tricuspid area may be present, along with a gallop rhythm, muffled heart sounds, right ventricular enlargement, and heart failure. These features should be distinguished from cardiomyopathy, and echocardiography can provide a definitive diagnosis.

4. Left Ventricular Non-Compaction (LVNC): A relatively rare congenital disorder with a familial tendency. Its characteristics include left ventricular dilatation, reduced systolic and diastolic function, and the presence of prominent trabeculations and deep intertrabecular recesses within the left ventricular cavity, forming a meshwork with blood flow through the recesses. The right ventricle may or may not be involved. Pathological examination reveals progressive thinning of the compacted myocardium from the base to the apex, with the thinnest region at the apex having almost no compacted myocardium. The affected ventricular cavity displays multiple, abnormally prominent trabeculations and deep intertrabecular recesses, with a ratio of non-compacted to compacted myocardium greater than 2 : 1. In dilated cardiomyopathy, the left ventricular cavity lacks such prominent trabeculations and a meshwork of recesses. Echocardiography or cardiac MRI can aid in the diagnosis.

5. Secondary Cardiomyopathies: Systemic diseases such as systemic lupus erythematosus, scleroderma, hemochromatosis, amyloidosis, glycogen storage disorders, and neuromuscular diseases often present with their primary manifestations, which can help differentiate them from cardiomyopathy. An important distinction is from myocarditis. Acute myocarditis often occurs during or shortly after a viral infection, making it less challenging to differentiate. However, chronic myocarditis without a clear history of acute myocarditis can be indistinguishable from cardiomyopathy. In clinical practice, many cases of dilated cardiomyopathy evolve from myocarditis, known as "myocarditis-associated cardiomyopathy".

Ⅳ Treatment Principles

As the etiology is often unclear, prevention and treatment are challenging. Some cases of dilated cardiomyopathy evolve from viral myocarditis, making the prevention of viral infections, such as enteric Coxsackie B virus and respiratory viruses, crucial. Since dilated cardiomyopathy manifests as heart failure, respiratory infections can trigger or exacerbate heart failure episodes and should be prevented and promptly treated. Treatment primarily targets the clinical manifestations.

1. General Management: Emphasis should be placed on rest and avoidance of exertion, especially for individuals with cardiac enlargement and reduced cardiac function, who may require prolonged rest to prevent disease progression. Respiratory infections should be avoided, and influenza vaccination is currently recommended during the winter and spring seasons to prevent exacerbation of heart failure due to influenza.

2. Treatment of Heart Failure: The principles are the same as for general heart failure management, incorporating the cornerstone "triple therapy" for heart failure: angiotensin-converting enzyme inhibitors (ACEIs) / angiotensin receptor blockers (ARBs) + beta-blockers + aldosterone receptor antagonists, along with diuretics, inotropes, and vasodilators for symptomatic relief. Commonly used ACEIs include perindopril and benazepril. If intolerance or cough occurs, ARBs such as candesartan, losartan, and valsartan can be substituted, as recommended by guidelines. Beta-blockers frequently used include sustained-release metoprolol and carvedilol. The aldosterone receptor antagonist of choice is spironolactone. Attention should be paid to fluid management, electrolyte imbalances (e.g., hypokalemia), and management of concomitant liver or kidney dysfunction.

3. Management of Arrhythmias: Symptomatic arrhythmias require anti-arrhythmic drug treatment, with aggressive management for rapid ventricular arrhythmias and high-degree atrioventricular block due to the risk of sudden cardiac death.

4. Metabolic Modulators: Agents such as trimetazidine, vitamin C, adenosine triphosphate, coenzyme A, and coenzyme Q10 can be used as adjunctive therapies. Antiviral and immunomodulatory drugs may also have potential benefits in improving left ventricular function.

5. Anticoagulation Therapy: Anticoagulation with warfarin can be considered for patients with significant ventricular dilatation and low ejection fraction, New York Heart Association (NYHA) functional class Ⅲ-Ⅳ, prolonged bedrest, history of thromboembolic events, or deep vein thrombosis formation. Regular monitoring of prothrombin time is necessary to maintain the

international normalized ratio (INR) between 2 and 3.

6. Cardiac Resynchronization Therapy (CRT / D): Primarily indicated for patients with sub-optimal response to medical therapy, QRS duration$>$120 ms, ejection fraction$\leqslant$0.35, and complete left bundle branch block or intraventricular conduction delay. Biventricular, triple-chamber, or quadruple-chamber pacing can be considered to improve cardiac function and alleviate symptoms in refractory heart failure. For patients with persistent rapid ventricular arrhythmias, implantable cardioverter-defibrillators (ICDs) may be considered.

7. Left Ventricular Assist Devices (LVADs): LVADs divert blood from the left ventricle into the aorta using a mechanical device, reducing the workload on the left ventricle. They are an effective treatment option for maintaining systemic circulation in end-stage dilated cardiomyopathy patients awaiting heart transplantation or for those ineligible for heart transplantation. However, the widespread use of LVADs is currently limited by their high cost.

8. Left Ventricular Reconstruction Surgery: This procedure involves excising a portion of the dilated left ventricle and replacing the mitral valve to reduce left ventricular end-diastolic volume and regurgitation, aiming to improve cardiac function. It is considered an option for refractory cases. However, high mortality rates due to worsening heart failure and arrhythmias after ventricular reconstruction have hindered the clinical application of this procedure.

9. Heart Transplantation: Should be considered for patients with long-standing refractory heart failure unresponsive to medical therapy. Aggressive infection control, optimized immunosuppression, and rejection management are crucial post-transplantation, with 1-year survival rates exceeding 85%. However, the severe shortage of donor organs remains a significant limitation.

V Common Questions in Consultation

1. Confirming the Diagnosis of Dilated Cardiomyopathy: Echocardio-graphy, BNP, and 24-hour Holter monitoring can provide crucial clues. The diagnosis of dilated cardiomyopathy is not difficult with echocardiography, which reveals myocardial involvement, abnormal cardiac structure and function, and the "four cardinal features" ("one large" "two small" "three thin" "four weak"). "One large" refers to overall or left ventricular dilatation; "two small" indicates a relatively small valve annulus compared to the dilated chamber, resembling a "large room with a small window"; "three thin" signifies thinned ventricular walls; and "four weak" describes diffuse hypo-kinesis with impaired contractile function. The etiology of myocardial involvement requires further investigation by the clinician, considering whether it is primary or secondary cardiomyopathy. Secondary causes, such as ischemia, endocrine disorders, toxicity, alcohol, and the increasingly prevalent cardio-toxicity from cancer chemotherapy and radiation therapy (the emerging field of "onco-cardiology"), should be excluded. After ruling out secondary causes, primary cardiomyopathy can be considered. BNP testing is a crucial indicator for evaluating heart failure, and 24-hour Holter monitoring assesses the presence of malignant arrhythmias, ventricular tachycardia, ventricular fibrillation, or long pauses. Echocardiography, BNP, and 24-hour Holter monitoring are essential for evaluating, diagnosing, treating, and monitoring patients.

2. Treatment Principles: Improving myocardial metabolism, correcting heart failure and arrhythmias. Metabolic modulators such as trimetazidine, vitamin C, adenosine triphosphate, coenzyme A, and coenzyme Q10 can be used as adjunctive therapies. Antiviral and immunomodulatory drugs may also have potential benefits in improving left ventricular function.

The cornerstone of heart failure treatment is the "triple therapy": angiotensin-converting enzyme inhibitors (ACEIs) / angiotensin receptor blockers (ARBs) + beta-blockers + aldosterone receptor antagonists, along with diuretics, inotropes, and vasodilators for symptomatic relief.

Symptomatic arrhythmias require anti-arrhythmic drug treatment, with aggressive management for rapid ventricular arrhythmias and high-degree atrioventricular block due to the risk of sudden cardiac death. Commonly used beta-blockers include sustained-release metoprolol, carvedilol, or bisoprolol. The aldosterone receptor antagonist of choice is spironolactone. Attention should be paid to fluid management, electrolyte imbalances (e.g., hypokalemia), and management of concomitant liver or kidney dysfunction.

3. Comprehensive Evaluation: Based on the current stage of the patient's condition, the next step in treatment, precautions, and follow-up monitoring depend on the compensatory state, stability, and degree of deterioration of left ventricular function and hemodynamics. This generally parallels the New York Heart Association (NYHA) functional classification. According to international data, the 1-year mortality rate for dilated cardiomyopathy patients with NYHA Class Ⅰ is 10%, Class Ⅱ is 10%-15%, Class Ⅲ is 20%-25%, and Class Ⅳ reaches 50%. A LVEF$<$ 25% portends a very poor prognosis. Left ventricular internal diameter, right ventricular function, and BNP levels are also associated with prognosis. Overall, the disease course varies, with some patients succumbing within a year of onset, while others can survive for 20 years or more.

Therefore, chronic patients should be enrolled in chronic disease management programs, with monitoring of treatment adherence and regular follow-up.

Hyper-trophic Cardiomyopathy

Ⅰ Definition and Disease Characteristics

Hyper-trophic cardiomyopathy (HCM) is characterized by myocardial hypertrophy. Typically, the left ventricle is hypertrophied, particularly the inter-ventricular septum, although concentric hypertrophy can occasionally occur. The left ventricular cavity volume is usually normal or reduced, and occasionally, the right ventricle is involved. HCM is a hereditary cardiomyopathy, typically with autosomal dominant inheritance. Clinical symptoms and electrocardiographic findings are non-specific, making clinical diagnosis and management challenging. The prognosis is poor, with a high risk of severe arrhythmias and approximately 50% of patients experiencing sudden cardiac death.

Ⅱ Classification

Based on the presence or absence of left ventricular outflow tract obstruction, HCM can be classified as obstructive or non-obstructive. According to the location of ventricular wall hypertrophy, Maron et al. further divided HCM into four types: Type Ⅰ, hypertrophy of the anterior inter-ventricular septum; Type Ⅱ, hypertrophy of the anterior and posterior inter-ventricular septum; Type Ⅲ, hypertrophy of the inter-ventricular septum and the anterior left ventricular wall, potentially involving the posterior septum and / or lateral wall, or confined to the apical region; Type Ⅳ, no hypertrophy of the anterior inter-ventricular septum or the left ventricular posterior (inferior) wall. Type Ⅲ is the most common, accounting for 52% of cases.

Ⅲ Diagnostic Essentials

Patients with left ventricular outflow tract obstruction typically present with characteristic clinical manifestations, facilitating diagnosis. Echocardiography and cardiac magnetic resonance imaging are crucial non-invasive diagnostic modalities, aiding in the evaluation of both obstructive and non-obstructive forms. Echocardiographic findings include:

1. Typical Obstructive Hyper-trophic Cardiomyopathy: ① Asymmetric septal hypertrophy, with the ratio of inter-ventricular septal thickness to left ventricular posterior wall thickness > (1.3-1.5) : 1, and septal thickness of at least 15 mm; ② Systolic anterior motion of the mitral valve anterior leaflet, with a "dagger-shaped" configuration of the CD segment; ③ Reduced left ventricular cavity size and outflow tract narrowing; ④ Left ventricular diastolic dysfunction, including decreased compliance, prolonged rapid filling time, and prolonged isovolumic relaxation time. Doppler studies can identify the origin of murmurs and quantify the pressure gradient across the obstruction.

2. Non-Obstructive Hyper-trophic Cardiomyopathy: Marked inter-ventricular septal hypertrophy, with a ratio to the left ventricular wall thickness < 1.3 : 1. Hypertrophy of the anterior free wall may also be present.

3. Apical Hyper trophic Cardiomyopathy: A subtype accounting for approximately 25% of HCM cases. The left ventricle has a "spade-like" configuration at end-diastole, with apical hypertrophy > 12 mm.

Ventriculography can also contribute to the diagnosis.

Ⅳ Differential Diagnosis

Clinically, when a systolic murmur is detected at the left sternal border's lower segment, this disease should be considered. Physiological maneuvers or pharmacological interventions that alter hemodynamics and cause changes in the murmur can aid in diagnosis. Additionally, the following differential diagnoses must be made:

1. Hypertensive heart disease: Patients with hypertension may also present with symmetric or even asymmetric left ventricular hypertrophy, making differentiation from this disease challenging. However, primary hypertension patients generally do not have left ventricular outflow tract obstruction. The presence or absence of a family history of hypertrophic cardiomyopathy is also a key differentiating factor.

2. Ventricular septal defect: The location of the systolic murmur is similar, but it is pansystolic. There is usually no murmur at the apex. Echocardiography, cardiac catheterization, and cardiovascular angiography can differentiate between the two conditions.

3. Aortic valve stenosis: The symptoms and murmur characteristics of this disease resemble those of hypertrophic cardiomyopathy. However, the murmur is located higher, and there is often an ejection click at the aortic valve area that may radiate to the neck. An early diastolic murmur may also be present. X-ray examination shows dilation of the ascending aorta. Left heart catheterization reveals a systolic pressure gradient across the aortic valve. Echocardiography can clearly identify the lesion site.

4. Rheumatic mitral regurgitation: The cardiac murmur is similar to that of hypertrophic cardiomyopathy, but it is usually pansystolic. Atrial fibrillation is often present, and the left atrium is enlarged. Echocardiography can clearly determine the extent of valve lesions.

5. Coronary heart disease: Compared to hypertrophic cardiomyopathy, angina pectoris, ST-T changes, and abnormal Q waves on the electrocardiogram are common to both conditions. However, coronary heart disease does not have characteristic murmurs and is often associated with hypertension and hyperlipidemia. Echocardiography shows no interventricular septal thickening but may reveal segmental wall motion abnormalities. Tc myocardial perfusion imaging demonstrates exercise-induced myocardial ischemia, which cannot distinguish between hypertrophic cardiomyopathy and coronary heart disease. Definitive diagnosis often relies on coronary angiography.

V Treatment Principles

The main objectives in the treatment of HCM are to alleviate symptoms, prevent complications, and reduce the risk of death.

1. General Management: Strenuous activity, emotional excitement, and sudden vigorous exercise should be avoided. Medications that enhance myocardial contractility and reduce cardiac workload, such as digitalis preparations, beta-adrenergic agonists (e.g., isoproterenol), and nitrates, should be avoided as they may exacerbate left ventricular outflow tract obstruction.

2. Beta-Blockers: These agents reduce myocardial contractility, alleviating outflow tract obstruction and myocardial oxygen consumption, while increasing ventricular diastolic dimensions and stroke volume through bradycardia. Current guidelines advocate achieving complete beta-blockade. Studies have shown that beta-adrenergic receptor blockade can prevent sudden death and reduce mortality in HCM, even in asymptomatic patients, although the precise benefit remains to be further clarified. Commonly used beta-blockers include metoprolol and bisoprolol. However, the response to beta-blockers varies considerably, with symptomatic improvement occurring in only *one-third to two-thirds* of the patients.

3. Calcium Channel Blockers: For patients unresponsive to beta-blockers, calcium channel blockers can effectively improve symptoms by reducing the left ventricular outflow tract gradient, enhancing diastolic filling, and improving regional myocardial blood flow. Verapamil is the most commonly used agent, with a typical daily dose of 120-480 mg divided into 3-4 doses and can provide long-term symptomatic relief. Caution is advised in patients with hypotension, sinus node dysfunction, or atrioventricular conduction disturbances. Diltiazem can improve diastolic function and alleviate ischemia, with a typical dose of 30-60 mg three times daily. Nifedipine can be used to relieve angina in HCM patients. Combination therapy with beta-blockers and calcium

channel blockers can produce synergistic effects, reducing adverse effects while enhancing therapeutic efficacy.

4. anti-arrhythmic Drugs: These agents are primarily used to control rapid ventricular arrhythmias and atrial fibrillation. Commonly used drugs include amiodarone and sotalol. In cases of refractory arrhythmias, electrical cardioversion may be considered, which can reduce recurrence rates following successful cardioversion.

5. Other Medications: The use of digitalis preparations should gene-rally be avoided, unless atrial fibrillation or systolic dysfunction is present. Previously, diuretics were thought to exacerbate outflow tract gradients and were contraindicated. However, studies have shown that judicious use of diuretics can help alleviate pulmonary congestion, particularly when used in combination with beta-blockers or calcium channel blockers. Patients with atrial fibrillation and no contraindications should receive anticoagulation therapy. Approximately 5% of the patients develop infective endocarditis, especially in the presence of mitral regurgitation, commonly involving the aortic or mitral valve, and should receive prompt antimicrobial treatment.

6. Dual-Chamber DDD Pacemaker Implantation: DDD pacemakers may assist in the management of some patients with outflow tract gradients and severe symptoms, particularly in the elderly. Symptoms are often improved, with an average reduction in the pressure gradient of approximately 25%. However, only a small proportion (less than 10%) of the patients are suitable candidates for this treatment, and the long-term benefits remain unclear.

7. Implantable Cardioverter-Defibrillator (ICD) Implantation: ICDs should be considered in high-risk patients, particularly those with sustained monomorphic ventricular tachycardia or at risk of sudden cardiac death, as they can effectively prevent sudden death.

8. Alcohol Septal Ablation: This treatment is effective for patients with outflow tract gradients at rest or during exercise. It involves selectively injecting alcohol into the septal perforator arteries via a cardiac catheter, inducing a localized septal infarction, thinning the inter-ventricular septum, and thereby reducing the outflow tract gradient, mitral regurgitation, and improving ventricular diastolic function, potentially reversing myocardial hypertrophy and alleviating symptoms.

9. Surgical Treatment: The aim is to reduce the outflow tract pressure gradient. Patients with a resting gradient > 50 mmHg, sub-optimal response to medical therapy, and significant symptoms are the most suitable candidates. However, this subset comprises less than 5% of all HCM patients. Typical procedures include septal myectomy and partial resection of the hypertrophied septal myocardium to relieve symptoms. The operative mortality rate is 2%-3% or lower. Surgery can reduce obstruction and mitral regurgitation, with long-term symptomatic and functional improvement in 70%-90% of patients.

Ⅵ Common Questions in Consultation

1. Confirming the Diagnosis of Hyper-trophic Cardiomyopathy: Echo-cardiography, MRI, and 24-hour Holter monitoring can provide crucial clues. Patients with left ventricular outflow tract obstruction typically present with characteristic clinical features, facilitating diagnosis. Echocardiography is an essential non-invasive diagnostic modality, aiding in the evaluation of

both obstructive and non-obstructive forms. Marked septal hypertrophy, systolic anterior motion of the mitral valve leaflet or chordae tendineae, and continuous-wave Doppler measurement of the left ventricular outflow tract gradient (≥30 mmHg) support the diagnosis of obstructive HCM. To differentiate obstructive from non-obstructive cases, if the resting left ventricular outflow tract (LVOT) gradient is<30 mmHg, patients can be instructed to perform a squat maneuver. If they experience mild chest discomfort and the post-exercise LVOT gradient is≥30 mmHg, occult obstructive HCM should be considered. These patients require heightened vigilance for the risk of exercise-induced sudden death and early intervention. Additionally, MRI plays a crucial role in diagnosing HCM, while cardiac catheterization demonstrating an LVOT pressure gradient can establish the diagnosis. Ventriculography can also aid in the diagnosis. Echocardiography and 24-hour Holter monitoring are essential for evaluating, diagnosing, treating, and monitoring patients.

2. Treatment Principles: The primary goal is to reduce the LVOT gradient, coupled with correcting arrhythmias that may exacerbate the obstruction. Pharmacological options include beta-blockers and calcium channel blockers, while non-pharmacological treatments involve alcohol septal ablation and surgical myectomy (Morrow procedure) to alleviate the outflow tract pressure gradient.

Beta-blockers can prevent sudden cardiac death and reduce mortality in Hyper-trophic cardiomyopathy, even in asymptomatic patients, although their precise efficacy warrants further elucidation. Clinically, metoprolol and bisoprolol are commonly used. However, the response to beta-blockers varies considerably, with only one-third to two-thirds of the patients experiencing symptomatic improvement. In patients' refractory to beta-blocker therapy, calcium channel blockers are often effective in alleviating symptoms, as they can reduce LVOT obstruction and improve diastolic filling and regional myocardial perfusion.

To correct arrhythmias and control rapid ventricular arrhythmias and atrial fibrillation, anti-arrhythmic drugs such as amiodarone and sotalol are frequently used. When pharmacological management fails, electrical cardioversion can be considered. These agents can reduce the recurrence rate after successful cardioversion.

3. Follow-up: Echocardiographic assessment of LVOT, 24-hour Holter monitoring, guidance for subsequent treatment and precautions. The disease course is slow and indeterminate. Stability may persist for years, but once symptoms manifest, gradual deterioration can occur. Sudden cardiac death and malignant arrhythmias are the leading causes of mortality. Sudden death is more common in children and young adults and is associated with physical exertion, with a close link to "athlete's sudden death". Unexplained syncope, hypotension during upright exercise testing (treadmill or bicycle), significant myocardial hypertrophy (>30 mm), family history of sudden death, and sustained or non-sustained ventricular tachycardia are risk factors for sudden death. Potential mechanisms include rapid ventricular arrhythmias, sinus node dysfunction and conduction disturbances, myocardial ischemia, diastolic dysfunction, LVOT obstruction, and hypotension, with the first two being the most important. The occurrence of atrial fibrillation can promote heart failure. A minority of patients develop complications such as infective endocarditis or embolism. To sum up, chronic patients should be enrolled in chronic disease management programs, with monitoring of adherence and regular follow-up.

Restrictive Cardiomyopathy

I Definition and Disease Characteristics

The hallmark of this type is primary myocardial and / or endocardial fibrosis or infiltrative myocardial lesions, leading to diastolic dysfunction due to impaired cardiac filling. This type mainly occurs in tropical and subtropical regions, including Africa, South Asia, and South America. In China, most cases have been found in the south, with a sporadic distribution. The onset is relatively slow. In the early stage, fever may be present, and gradually, fatigue, dizziness, and shortness of breath develop. When the lesions primarily involve the left ventricle, signs of left heart failure and pulmonary hypertension, such as dyspnea, cough, hemoptysis, basal lung rales, and accentuated second heart sound in the pulmonary valve area, may be observed. When the lesions mainly affect the right ventricle, manifestations of right ventricular inflow obstruction, such as jugular venous distension, hepatomegaly, lower limb edema, and ascites, may be present. Cardiac pulsations are often weakened, the cardiac dullness is slightly enlarged, heart sounds are low, heart rate is rapid, and diastolic gallop rhythm and arrhythmias may occur. Pericardial effusion can also be present, and visceral embolism is not uncommon.

II Classification

Among the restrictive cardiomyopathies caused by infiltrative lesions, there are types such as amyloidosis (accumulation of amyloid substances in the interstitium), sarcoidosis (infiltration of sarcoid-like substances in the myocardium), hemochromatosis (deposition of hemosiderin in the myocardium), and glycogen storage disease (excessive accumulation of glycogen in the myocardium). Among the non-infiltrative restrictive cardiomyopathies, there are two types: endomyocardial fibrosis, which is seen in the tropics, and Löffler endocarditis, which is seen in temperate regions. In fact, the pathological changes of the two are similar.

III Diagnostic Considerations

Since the early clinical manifestations of this type are not obvious, diagnosis is difficult. Once clinical symptoms appear, a definitive diagnosis can be made based on various examinations. Echocardiography is a non-invasive and effective examination method. Endomyocardial biopsy, if positive for specific findings, can aid in diagnosis and may also reveal infiltrative lesions.

Echocardiography may show significantly dilated inferior vena cava and hepatic veins, and abnormal ultrasound echo density of the endomyocardial structure. The left and right atria are enlarged, and the endocardium at the apex of the right ventricle is thickened, or even the cardiac cavity is occluded, forming a rigid, deformed abnormal echo area that distorts the entire cardiac cavity. The myocardial wall may be thickened, normal, or of uneven thickness, and the ventricular wall contractility is weakened. When the lesions involve the atrioventricular valves, mitral and tricuspid regurgitation may occur. The pericardium is generally not thickened. Cardiac catheterization shows a gradual increase in ventricular end-diastolic pressure, resulting in a dip-and-plateau waveform. In cases where the left ventricle is primarily affected, pulmonary artery pressure may be elevated. In cases where the right ventricle is primarily affected, right atrial pressure is high, and the right atrial pressure curve shows a prominent v wave replacing the a wave. The systolic time interval measurement is abnormal.

Ⅳ Differential Diagnosis

Clinically, it is necessary to differentiate this condition from constrictive pericarditis, especially in restrictive cardiomyopathy with predominantly ventricular lesions, as the clinical manifestations of the two are similar. A history of acute pericarditis, X-ray findings of pericardial calcification, and chest CT or MRI showing pericardial thickening support the diagnosis of pericarditis. Electrocardiographic evidence of atrial or ventricular hypertrophy, bundle branch block, and abnormal systolic time intervals support the diagnosis of cardiomyopathy. Echocardiography is of great help in differentiating between the two conditions. The presence of apical cavity obliteration and endocardial thickening establishes the diagnosis of cardiomyopathy. For cases with diagnostic difficulties, ventricular angiography and endomyocardial biopsy can be performed.

Ⅴ Treatment Principles

Treatment is mainly symptomatic. Prevention is limited to avoiding complications. Patients should avoid overexertion and prevent infections. For those with atrial fibrillation, digitalis drugs can be given. For those with edema and ascites, diuretics are appropriate. When using diuretics or vasodilators, care should be taken not to excessively reduce ventricular filling pressure, which may affect cardiac function. Anticoagulants can be used to prevent embolism. In recent years, surgical resection of the fibrotic and thickened endocardium, combined with artificial valve replacement in cases of atrioventricular valve involvement, has shown better results.

Ⅵ Considerations During Consultation

This type mainly occurs in tropical and subtropical regions, including Africa, South Asia, and South America. In China, most cases have been found in the south, with a sporadic distribution. Therefore, the patient's residential history is crucial for diagnosis. Echocardiography is a non-invasive and effective examination method. Endomyocardial biopsy, if positive for specific findings, can aid in diagnosis and may also reveal infiltrative lesions. Clinically, it is necessary to differentiate this condition from constrictive pericarditis, especially in restrictive cardiomyopathy with predominantly ventricular lesions, as the clinical manifestations of the two are similar. In actual clinical practice, this type of cardiomyopathy is not very common. The course of the disease varies in its progression. In the past, due to incomplete treatment, once symptoms appeared, patients gradually lost their ability to work and eventually died. Cases with predominantly left ventricular lesions have a slightly better prognosis than those with predominantly right ventricular lesions. In recent years, surgical treatment has brought some hope.

Arrhythmogenic Right Ventricular Cardiomyopathy

I Definition and Disease Characteristics

Arrhythmogenic right ventricular cardiomyopathy (ARVC, also known as right ventricular cardiomyopathy, arrhythmogenic right ventricular dysplasia, or idiopathic right ventricular myocardial dysplasia) is a disease of unknown etiology predominantly affecting the right ventricular myocardium. The myocardium is replaced by fibrous or fatty tissue, leading to various arrhythmias, particularly malignant ventricular arrhythmias, or chronic right heart failure. Some patients present with malignant arrhythmias like sustained ventricular tachycardia, ventricular flutter, or ventricular fibrillation, with cardiac arrest or sudden death as the first manifestation—an important cause of sudden death in youth. Early physical examination is often unremarkable, though various arrhythmias may be detected.

II Diagnostic Considerations

Histopathological evidence is the gold standard for diagnosing ARVC, with endomyocardial biopsy confirming myocardial replacement by fibrous or fatty tissue. However, as right ventricular involvement may be segmental, patchy, or non-transmural, and the inter-ventricular septum is often spared or small fatty infiltrates may be present in normal hearts, endomyocardial biopsy cannot objectively and accurately reflect the disease, and its value should be interpreted cautiously (Table 2-5).

Table 2-5 Diagnostic Criteria for Arrhythmogenic Right Ventricular Cardiomyopathy (McKenna, 1994)

Global and Regional Functional and Structural Alterations	Depolarization / Conduction Abnormalities
Major Criteria:	Major Criteria:
Severe dilatation and reduction of right ventricular ejection fraction	Epsilon waves or localized prolongation (>110 ms) of QRS complex in right precordial leads (V1-V3)
With normal or only mild left ventricular involvement	Minor Criteria:
Localized right ventricular aneurysms	Late potentials on signal-averaged ECG
Severe segmental dilatation of the right ventricle	Arrhythmias
Minor Criteria:	Minor Criteria:
Mild global right ventricular dilatation and / or ejection fraction reduction with normal left ventricle	Left bundle branch block type ventricular tachy-cardia (sustained or paroxysmal) (ECG, Holter monitoring, exercise testing)
Mild segmental dilatation of the right ventricle	
Regional Right Ventricular Akinesia, Dyskinesia or Aneurysm	>1,000 premature ventricular contractions / 24 hours (Holter)
Tissue Characterization of Right Ventricular Wall	
Major Criteria:	Family History
Endomyocardial biopsy demonstrating fibro-fatty replacement of myocardium	Major Criteria:
	Familial disease confirmed at necropsy or surgery
Repolarization Abnormalities	Minor Criteria:
Minor Criteria:	Suspected familial ARVC with sudden death (<35 years)
Inverted T waves in right precordial leads (V1-V3) in individuals>12 years of age without right bundle branch block	Family history of ARVC based on present criteria

Diagnosis can be made by presence of 2 major criteria, or 1 major plus 2 minor criteria in Table 2-5.

Ⅲ Differential Diagnosis

1. Idiopathic Dilated Cardiomyopathy: The 1995 WHO / ISFC classified ARVC as a distinct cardiomyopathy, separate from Hyper-trophic, dilated, and restrictive types. However, ARVC presenting predominantly with heart failure requires differentiation from idiopathic dilated cardiomyopathy. Frequent right ventricular premature contractions / tachycardias on ECG, and echocardiographic / MRI findings aid diagnosis.

2. Isolated Myocarditis: Some myocarditis cases develop fatty infiltration during healing, manifesting with arrhythmias. However, these fatty deposits are scattered rather than localized as in ARVC.

Ⅳ Treatment Principles

Medical management of ARVC is primarily symptomatic. For isolated right heart failure or biventricular failure, diuretics, vasodilators, inotropes (digoxin, dobutamine, phosphodiesterase inhibitors), beta-blockers, and ACE inhibitors may be used (as for chronic heart failure). For predominant arrhythmias, anti-arrhythmic drugs like amiodarone or sotalol can be tried. If drug therapy is ineffective, CRT / D or ICD is preferred. Some may benefit from radiofrequency ablation. For end-stage heart failure, cardiac transplantation may be considered.

Ⅴ Common Questions in Consultation

The non-specific clinical presentation and wide age range make diagnosis challenging, relying on imaging (echocardiography, MRI) and 24-hour Holter monitoring. The disease broadly follows 3 stages:

(1) Concealed Phase: Patients may have "benign arrhythmias" or be asymptomatic. Some present with syncope or sudden death. Young patients are prone to electrical instability during exercise, risking malignant arrhythmias and sudden death, underscoring the importance of early diagnosis and exercise restriction.

(2) Overt Arrhythmic Phase: Patients experience severe arrhythmias and recurrent syncope, with high risk of sudden cardiac death.

(3) Right Heart Failure Phase: Manifestations mimic dilated cardiomyopathy with biventricular failure. Some end-stage patients may require heart transplantation.

To sum up, while the precise prognosis is unclear, ARVC is often a malignant progressive disease with a guarded outlook.

Specific Cardiomyopathies

Specific cardiomyopathies refer to myocardial diseases associated with specific cardiac disorders or systemic diseases. Management primarily targets the underlying etiology.

I Classification

There are several diseases in this category, mainly including the following:

1. Ischemic cardiomyopathy: It presents similarly to dilated cardiomyopathy, with contractile dysfunction that cannot be explained by the extent of coronary artery disease or ischemic injury.

2. Valvular cardiomyopathy: It manifests as ventricular dysfunction inconsistent with the abnormal loading conditions.

3. Hypertensive heart disease: It presents with left ventricular hypertrophy, accompanied by features of dilated or restrictive cardiomyopathy, and heart failure.

4. Inflammatory cardiomyopathy: Myocarditis associated with cardiac dysfunction. Myocarditis is an inflammatory disorder of the myocardium, with histological, immunological, and immunohistochemical diagnostic criteria. It can be idiopathic, autoimmune, or caused by infections. Inflammatory myocardial diseases are also related to the pathogenesis of dilated cardiomyopathy and other cardiomyopathies, such as South American trypanosomiasis (Chagas disease), HIV, enterovirus, adenovirus, and cytomegalovirus-induced cardiomyopathies.

5. Hypersensitivity and toxic reactions: These include reactions to alcohol, catecholamines, anthracyclines, radiation, and other insults. In alcoholic cardiomyopathy, there may be a history of heavy alcohol consumption, but it is currently unclear whether alcohol is a direct cause or merely a conditional factor. Alcoholic cardiomyopathy is relatively common in clinical practice, and in some patients, cardiac structure and function may improve after alcohol abstinence.

6. Peripartum cardiomyopathy: It refers to cardiomyopathy with onset during the peripartum period and may represent a mixed group of diseases. After 6 months of follow-up with standard anti-heart failure treatment and medications to improve myocardial metabolism, some patients' cardiac size and left ventricular ejection fraction return to normal. Some patients have a better prognosis after termination of pregnancy.

7. Obesity cardiomyopathy: A recently proposed condition where heart failure is entirely or partially caused by obesity, seen in morbidly obese patients. The cardiomyopathy in obese patients cannot be explained by diabetes, hypertension, coronary heart disease, or other causes. Cardiac structural changes include left ventricular wall thickening, increased mass, left atrial and ventricular dilation, concentric and eccentric left ventricular hypertrophy, right ventricular hypertrophy, increased volume, and significantly reduced left ventricular diastolic function. Obesity is an independent risk factor for heart failure and myocardial dysfunction, surpassing the effects of hypertension, diabetes, and coronary heart disease. Being overweight or obese, especially with increased abdominal fat, increases the risk of heart failure. Obesity cardiomyopathy is preventable, and myocardial changes have the potential for reversibility.

8. Metabolic cardiomyopathy: ① Endocrine: such as toxic goiter, hypothyroidism, adrenal cortical insufficiency, pheochromocytoma, acromegaly, and diabetes mellitus; ② Familial storage or infiltrative diseases: such as hemochromatosis, glycogen storage diseases, Hurler syndrome, Refsum syndrome, Niemann-Pick disease, Hand-Schuller-Christian disease, Fabry-Anderson disease, Morquio-Ullrich disease; ③ Nutritional deficiencies: such as metabolic abnormalities, selenium deficiency, nutritional abnormalities (e.g., Kwashiorkor, anemia, vitamin B deficiency,

selenium deficiency); ④ Amyloidosis: primary, secondary, familial, hereditary cardiac amyloidosis, familial Mediterranean fever, senile amyloidosis, etc.

9. Systemic diseases: These include connective tissue diseases, such as systemic lupus erythematosus, rheumatoid arthritis, scleroderma, dermatomyositis, etc.

10. Muscular dystrophies: These include Duchenne, Becker, and rigid muscular dystrophies.

11. Neuromuscular diseases: These include Friedreich's ataxia, Noonan syndrome, and neurofibromatosis.

12. Keshan disease: It belongs to the category of idiopathic dilated cardiomyopathy and is named after Keshan County of Heilongjiang Province, China, where it was discovered as an endemic cardiomyopathy. The disease is mostly concentrated in a belt spanning the cold climate of Northeast China (also found in Japan and Korea) and the hot and humid climate of Southwest China, more common in middle-aged and young people, and more frequent in females than males. Although the etiology is unknown, it may be related to the involvement of multiple comprehensive factors: peripheral environment (especially water, soil, grain, etc.), personal hygiene habits, nutritional status, deficiency of certain trace elements (selenium), and viral infections (Coxsackie virus, ECHO virus). The main pathological changes are myocardial degeneration, necrosis, and scar formation, leading to left ventricular enlargement, global heart enlargement, and heart failure. According to the clinical course, it is divided into acute, subacute, chronic, and latent types, eventually developing into clinical manifestations similar to those of idiopathic dilated cardiomyopathy. Based on epidemiological characteristics, population incidence, clinical manifestations, and related examinations, and after excluding the presence of other heart diseases, the diagnosis is not difficult. In addition to symptomatic treatment, other methods for managing heart failure can be adopted. Due to improvements in the environment and living conditions, attention to nutrition (supplementation of trace elements such as selenium), changes in lifestyle habits, and the implementation of active comprehensive preventive measures, early detection, and early treatment, the disease has become rare.

13. Stress cardiomyopathy: Also known as apical ballooning syndrome or broken heart syndrome, also called Tako-Tsubo syndrome. There are currently no accurate statistics on the incidence rate. The disease is more common in postmenopausal women. Most clinical manifestations are similar to acute coronary syndrome (ACS), such as ischemic-like chest pain and ECG changes; severe psychological stress is reported in about 27% of all reported cases. ECG abnormalities are present in 90% of patients, with anterior ECG abnormalities, but the degree of ST-segment elevation is lower than that of STEMI; deep inverted symmetrical T waves and QT interval prolongation often appear within 24-48 hours of onset; transient Q waves in the anterior septum are present in one third of the patients; there are no reliable ECG criteria to distinguish stress cardiomyopathy from STEMI. In most patients, the ECG manifestations are transient and completely recover within months. Myocardial enzymes, troponin, or CK-MB are mildly elevated, and the degree of elevation is not proportional to the extent of wall motion abnormalities. Cardiac catheterization shows negative coronary angiography results or mild coronary atherosclerosis in most patients. Left ventriculography may reveal segmental wall motion abnormalities beyond the perfusion territory of a single coronary artery, most

commonly apical wall motion abnormalities, and a small proportion may present with segmental motion abnormalities in the mid-left ventricle. There are many types of left ventricular motion abnormalities, including apical and mid-left ventricular abnormalities, mid-septal or basal abnormalities, etc. Echocardiography or MRI shows apical ballooning, with markedly abnormal systolic and diastolic function; it may also indicate septal motion abnormalities without apical abnormalities in systole.

In patients with stress cardiomyopathy, the left ventricular motion disorder is predominantly apical. The Mayo Clinic diagnostic criteria are: ①Transient apical and regional wall motion abnormalities beyond the perfusion territory of a single coronary artery; ②No evidence of coronary stenosis or acute plaque rupture; ③ECG changes (ST-segment elevation in precordial leads and / or T-wave inversion) or troponin elevation. Left ventricular function recovers rapidly in this disease, often requiring only supportive treatment during hospitalization. In the vast majority of cases, left ventricular function recovers within 1-3 months, and a few may fully recover during hospitalization. Complications are rare, but a small number of patients may develop hemodynamic instability, atrial and ventricular arrhythmias, heart failure, and cardiogenic shock. A few patients may develop outflow tract obstruction due to apical and mid-septal motion abnormalities. The main causes of death are cardiogenic shock and systemic embolism.

Currently, there is no standard treatment regimen guided by clinical trials, and supportive treatment is the mainstay: ① Remove triggering factors (acute infection or physical stress events) and treat primary diseases (pheochromocytoma, upper gastrointestinal bleeding, cerebrovascular accidents, etc.); ② Acute phase treatment mainly targets congestive heart failure, and severe hemodynamic disorders require vasopressors or intra-aortic balloon pump assistance; ③ Long-term use of ACEIs or ARBs and beta-receptor blockers is recommended; ④ For those with severe left ventricular dysfunction, consider warfarin anticoagulation. Data on recurrence are relatively lacking, with a recurrence rate of 2%-10% within a few years after the first episode. Theoretically, taking beta-receptor blockers may reduce the recurrence rate.

Ⅱ Common Questions in Consultation

As specific cardiomyopathies are often associated with specific cardiac disorders, systemic diseases, or myocardial involvement following psychological trauma, interventions should actively target the underlying etiology. In the presence of heart failure or arrhythmias, appropriate management with heart failure and anti-arrhythmic therapies should be considered. Additionally, psychological treatment is equally important.

Ⅲ Consultation Process

1. Assess the patient's vital signs and hemodynamic stability. If life-threatening conditions such as hypoxemia, respiratory distress, hypotension, or malignant arrhythmias are present, promptly initiate emergency measures like endotracheal intubation, mechanical ventilation, cardio-version, temporary pacing, anti-arrhythmic drugs, and vasopressors.

2. Obtain critical medical history, including family history, genetic disorders, prior episodes of sudden death or syncope, pregnancy, obesity, and endocrine disorders like hyperthyroidism,

hypothyroidism, or diabetes mellitus.

3. Perform a thorough physical examination, focusing on signs of heart failure, arrhythmias (cyanosis, jugular venous distention, thyroid enlargement, pulmonary rales, apical impulse, cardiac borders, murmurs, rhythm irregularities, hepatomegaly, ascites, edema, etc.).

4. Rapidly obtain essential investigations like arterial blood gas, renal function, electrolytes, electrocardiogram, chest X-ray, BNP or NT-proBNP. In emergencies, expedite bedside echocardiography to assess cardiac status and pericardial effusion to exclude constrictive pericarditis.

5. Identify risk factors for sudden cardiac death: dilated cardiomyopathy with significant cardiac enlargement, ejection fraction<30%, heart failure or malignant arrhythmias; Hypertrophic cardiomyopathy with unexplained syncope, hypotension on upright exercise testing, severe hypertrophy (>30 mm), family history of sudden death, sustained or non-sustained ventricular tachycardia. Patients with arrhythmogenic right ventricular cardiomyopathy are prone to recurrent syncope, increasing the risk of sudden cardiac death.

6. In stable patients, pursue comprehensive evaluations like echocardiography, transesophageal echocardiography, left ventriculography, cardiac MRI, and genetic testing to establish the cardiomyopathy subtype. Early recognition of concealed cardiomyopathies like arrhythmogenic right ventricular cardiomyopathy is crucial, necessitating vigilance for subtle electrocardiographic changes and differentiation of early myocardial hypertrophy from Hypertrophic cardiomyopathy or other etiologies. Based on the underlying cause, initiate targeted interventions. For heart failure or arrhythmias, provide appropriate heart failure and antiarrhythmic therapies. Consider ICD or CRT / D in eligible patients.

Chapter 3

Arrhythmia

Section 1 Causes and Management of Sinus Tachycardia

I Confirming Sinus Tachycardia

The key characteristics of sinus tachycardia are: ① The P waves are sinus in origin (upright in leads I, Ⅱ, Ⅲ, aVF, V; inverted in aVR), and may fuse with the preceding T wave at high rates; ② In adults, the sinus rate exceeds 100 beats/min but rarely exceeds 160 beats/min, while in adolescents it can occasionally reach 200 beats/min; ③ The PR interval ≥ 0.12 seconds, and the PP intervals do not vary by more than 0.12 seconds. Sinus tachycardia indicates intact sinoatrial node function.

Ⅱ Major Causes and Clinical Clues

1. Normal physiological responses: Exercise, emotional stress, smoking, alcohol, tea, or coffee consumption.

2. Internal medicine's medical conditions

(1) Cardiovascular diseases: Heart failure, hypotension and shock, cardiomyo-pathy, myocarditis, acute blood loss, pericarditis, arteriovenous fistula, acute myocardial infarction, and other structural heart diseases.

(2) Other diseases: Anemia (iron deficiency, megaloblastic), bleeding (e.g., gastrointestinal), shock, respiratory failure, fever, hyperthyroidism, and neurogenic disorders.

(3) Drug-induced: Sympathomimetic drugs like ephedrine, epinephrine; anticholinergic agents like caffeine, thyroid hormone, atropine, amphetamines can precipitate sinus tachycardia.

3. Surgical conditions: Postoperative bleeding, pain, shock, infection.

4. Inappropriate sinus tachycardia: Characterized by resting or dispropor-tionately elevated heart rate with minimal exertion; a relatively uncommon clinical entity that requires exclusion of other causes. Severe cases may require treatment with beta-blockers, calcium channel blockers, or digoxin.

Ⅲ Management

Sinus tachycardia generally does not require specific treatment beyond addressing the underlying cause. Symptomatic cases may benefit from sedatives or beta-blockers. Inappropriate sinus tachycardia can be considered for catheter ablation.

Ⅳ Inpatient Cardiology Consultation Approach

1. Carefully analyze the ECG to distinguish from other tachycardias like paroxysmal supraventricular tachycardia, atrial tachycardia, and atrial flutter.

2. Obtain a detailed history regarding recent strenuous activity, emotional stress, smoking, alcohol, tea / coffee consumption; symptoms like dyspnea, cough, sputum, fever, dizziness, abdominal pain, melena, weight loss, tremors; use of sympathomimetics, anticholinergics; and past medical history of heart disease, chronic lung disease, renal impairment, etc.

3. Perform a thorough physical exam, assessing for goiter, exophthalmos, asymmetric breath sounds, barrel chest, cyanosis, cardiac enlargement, murmurs, crackles, jugular venous distention, and edema.

4. Rapidly obtain relevant investigations like arterial blood gas, complete blood count, renal function, electrolytes, calcium, ECG, chest X-ray, BNP / NT-proBNP, D-dimer, thyroid function tests.

5. Actively treat the precipitating condition. Symptomatic cases may require sedation or beta-blockade.

Section 2 Diagnosis and Management of Narrow QRS Complex Tachycardias

Narrow QRS complex tachycardia refers to a tachyarrhythmia with a QRS duration < 120 ms and a rate > 100 beats/min. It includes sinus tachycardia, sinoatrial node re-entrant tachycardia, atrial flutter, atrial fibrillation, atrial tachycardia, atrioventricular node re-entrant tachycardia, atrioventricular re-entrant tachycardia, and junctional tachycardia.

Ⅰ Clinical Presentation Should Not Be Ignored

Before analyzing the ECG, a thorough history and physical examination are essential. The paroxysmal nature of certain tachycardias and their potential termination by vagal maneuvers, such as atrioventricular node re-entrant tachycardia or atrioventricular re-entrant tachycardia, should raise suspicion for re-entrant mechanisms. Long-standing hypertension, chronic obstructive pulmonary disease, or Hyper-trophic cardiomyopathy predisposing to atrial enlargement increases the likelihood of atrial tachyarrhythmias like atrial tachycardia or atrial fibrillation. An irregular first heart sound, absolute arrhythmia, and pulse deficits on examination suggest atrial fibrillation. Hemodynamic instability warrants prompt cardioversion, irrespective of the tachycardia mechanism.

Ⅱ Analysis of the Surface ECG

1. Regularity of the rhythm: An absolutely irregular ventricular response, where no two RR intervals are equal, indicates atrial fibrillation. However, an irregular ventricular response can also occur with atrial flutter, atrial tachycardia, or even atrioventricular node re-entrant tachycardia, albeit with some discernible pattern.

At rates around 150 beats/min, the possibility of 2 : 1 atrial flutter conduction should be carefully evaluated (Figure 3-1).

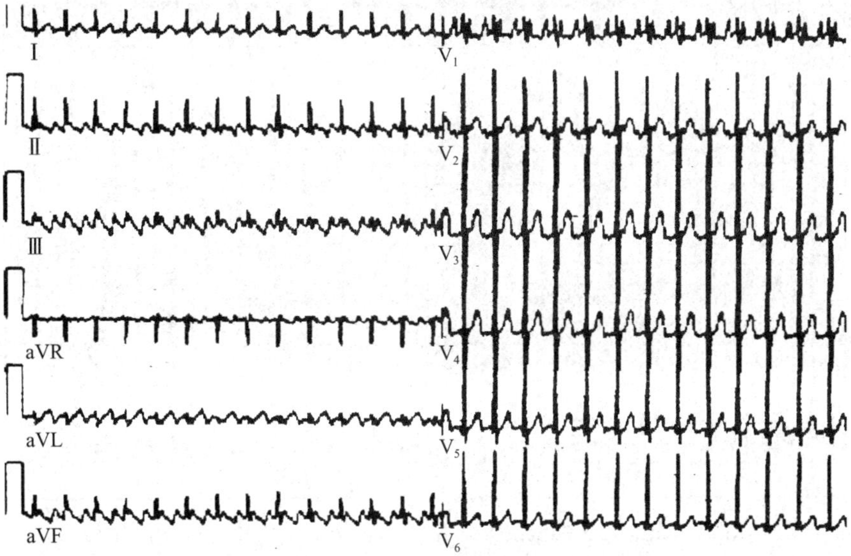

Figure 3-1 An Example of a Patient with Atrial Flutter, with a Rate of Approximately 150 Beats/min, Confirmed as 2 : 1 Atrial Flutter Conduction by Intracardiac Electrography

2. Comparison with the sinus rhythm ECG: The presence of pre-excitation during sinus rhythm suggests atrioventricular re-entrant tachycardia.

Comparing the tachycardia ECG with the sinus rhythm ECG can further identify the presence of retrograde P waves. If RP<PR, atrioventricular node re-entrant tachycardia or atrioventricular re-entrant tachycardia should be considered. If RP>PR, the possibilities include atrial tachycardia, atypical atrioventricular node re-entrant tachycardia, and atrioventricular re-entrant tachycardia involving a slow bystander pathway.

Pseudo S waves and pseudo r' waves are suggestive of atrioventricular node re-entrant tachycardia. Pseudo S waves refer to the appearance of S waves in leads Ⅱ, Ⅲ, and aVF during tachycardia but not during sinus rhythm. Pseudo r' waves refer to the presence of an rSr' pattern in lead V1 during tachycardia but not during sinus rhythm (Figure 3-2).

3. QRS Alternans is a phenomenon in which the QRS amplitude differs by>0.1 mV in at least one lead (Figure 3-3). The study by Kalbfleisch et al. found that 27% of patients with atrioventricular re-entrant tachycardia exhibited QRS alternans, while the incidence was significantly lower in those with atrioventricular nodal re-entrant tachycardia. The potential mechanism is that atrioventricular re-entrant tachycardia requires the involvement of both atrial and ventricular myocardium, and the non-uniform refractory periods of the myocardium result in the shorter refractory periods participating in each excitation, while the longer ones participate in excitation every other cycle.

4. ST-Segment Changes: During tachycardia, atrioventricular re-entrant tachycardia has a higher frequency and greater magnitude of ST-segment depression compared to atrioventricular

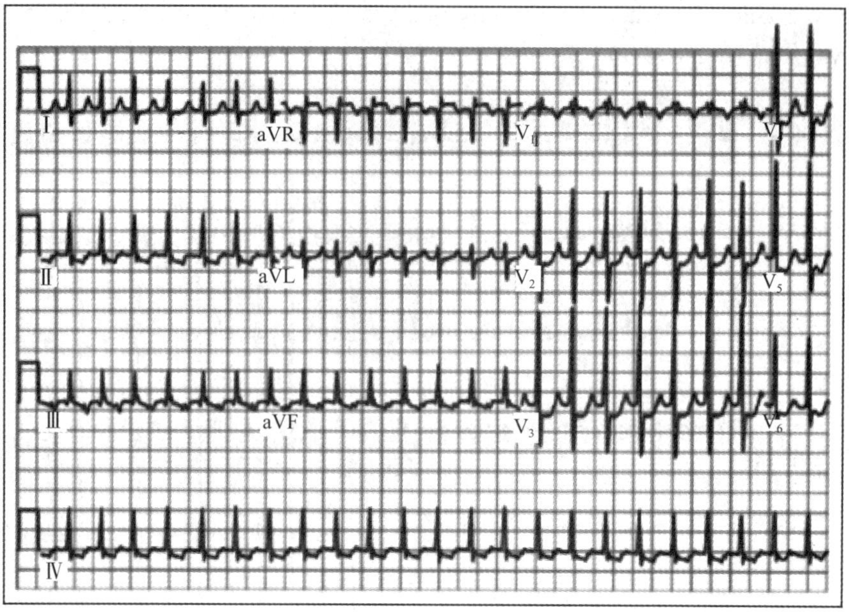

Figure 3-2 An Example of a Patient with Atrioventricular Node Re-entrant Tachycardia, Demonstrating Pseudo S Waves in the Inferior Leads and a Pseudo r' Wave in Lead V_1

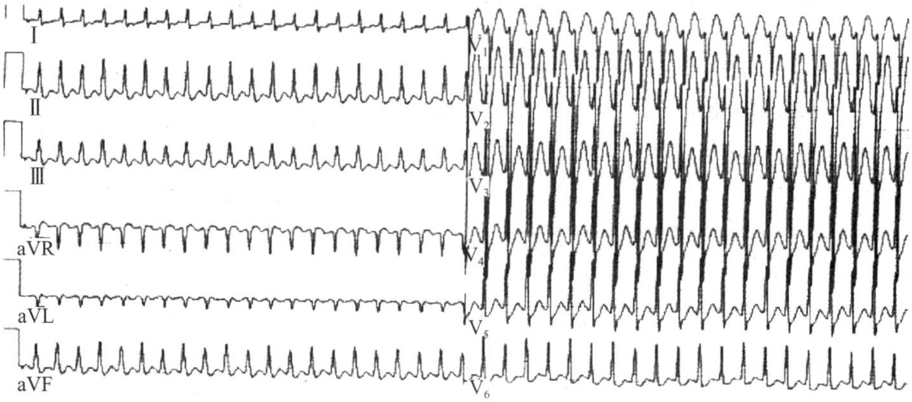

Figure 3-3 A Patient with Atrioventricular Reciprocating Tachycardia. Varying Degrees of Electrical Alternans Are Present in Each Lead, Especially Prominent in the Inferior Leads

nodal re-entrant tachycardia. ST-segment depression of $>$0.2 mV can occur in one or more leads, and T-wave inversion may even be observed (Figure 3-4). This is possibly due to the retrograde P wave initiating excitation at the atrial end of the bypass tract during atrioventricular re-entrant tachycardia, with conduction occurring primarily through the myocardial cells at a relatively slow speed, resulting in the retrograde P wave overlapping the ST segment.

Ⅲ Other Methods

For narrow QRS tachycardia, the primary observation is the relationship between the P wave and QRS complex. When this cannot be clearly discerned on the surface ECG, trans-esophageal

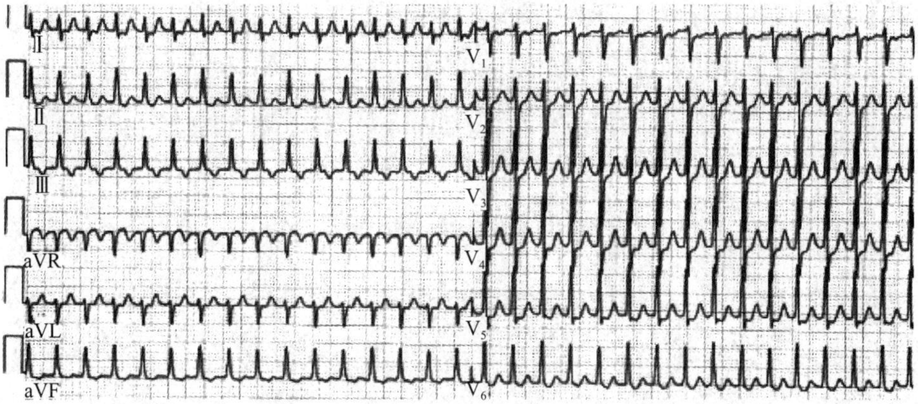

Figure 3-4 A Case of Atrioventricular Reciprocating Tachycardia. Except for the aVR Lead, Each Lead Shows Varying Degrees of ST-segment Depression, Which Is Particularly Prominent in the Precordial Leads

atrial pacing ECG can be considered, as it provides a better visualization of the P wave, aiding in the differentiation between supra-ventricular and ventricular tachycardias, as well as between atrioventricular re-entrant and atrioventricular nodal re-entrant tachycardias. This method requires simple equipment, is convenient to perform, and is safe and reliable, making it suitable for use in primary care settings. If necessary, intracardiac electrophysiological studies can be considered for a definitive diagnosis.

Ⅳ Characteristics of Various Narrow QRS Tachycardias

1. Inappropriate Sinus Tachycardia: Heart rate persistently > 100 bpm at rest or the increase in sinus rate is disproportionate to the degree of exertion, emotion, pathology, or drug effect. P waves are sinus in morphology (upright in leads Ⅰ, Ⅱ, Ⅲ, aVF, V_5-V_6; inverted in aVR). The onset and termination of tachycardia exhibit a gradual acceleration or deceleration pattern. Often seen in females without structural heart disease.

2. Atrial Tachycardia: ECG features: P wave morphology differs from sinus P waves; PR interval is normal or prolonged; as the atrioventricular node and ventricles are not involved in the tachycardia, Wenckebach or 2 : 1/3 : 1 atrioventricular conduction may be observed (Figure 3-5), which is an important characteristic of atrial tachycardia. Mechanistically, it can be classified as macro-reentrant or focal atrial tachycardia, with the former often associated with structural heart disease or prior cardiac surgery, and the latter originating from specific atrial sites such as the crista terminalis, coronary sinus ostium, or pulmonary veins. If the mechanism is automatic, a "warm-up" phenomenon with gradually increasing rate may be observed at the onset.

3. Atrioventricular Re-entrant Tachycardia: In narrow QRS atrioventricular re-entrant tachycardia, ante-grade conduction occurs through the atrioventricular node, while retrograde conduction occurs through the bypass tract. During sinus rhythm, ECG features of preexcitation may be present; tachycardia onset is abrupt, with rates of 150-250 bpm; RP interval > 110 ms; appropriately timed atrial or ventricular premature beats can induce or terminate the tachycardia;

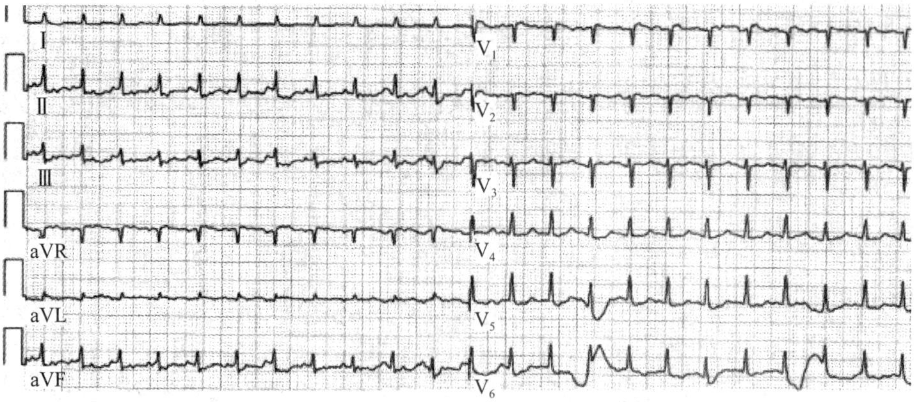

Figure 3-5 A Case of Atrial Tachycardia with 2 : 1 Atrioventricular Conduction, with Prominent P Waves in the Inferior and V_1 Leads

vagal maneuvers (e.g., carotid sinus massage) can terminate the tachycardia; QRS alternans may be observed; functional bundle branch block may occur at the onset of tachycardia, with RR interval prolongation of >30 ms if the block occurs on the same side as the bypass tract, or no change in RR interval if the block occurs on the opposite side; the atria, ventricles, atrioventricular conduction system, and bypass tract are all required components of the re-entrant circuit, with 1 : 1 atrioventricular conduction maintained during tachycardia; if P waves are not discernible, trans-esophageal ECG may be considered for differentiation.

4. Atrioventricular Nodal Re-entrant Tachycardia: This is caused by reentrant excitation due to the presence of two pathways with different conduction velocities within or around the atrioventricular node. The right posterior extension near the tricuspid annulus and coronary sinus ostium serves as the functionally slow pathway, while the anterior-superior aspect of the atrioventricular node (the apex of the Koch's triangle) is the fast pathway. It often occurs without structural heart disease. In typical (slow-fast) atrioventricular nodal re-entrant tachycardia, the R wave and P wave appear nearly simultaneously or the P wave occurs at the terminal portion of the QRS complex; RP interval<70 ms; a pseudo-S wave may be observed in lead V_1 (rSr' pattern); pseudo-Q waves may be present; appropriately timed atrial premature beats can induce and terminate the tachycardia, and ventricular premature beats can also induce it, with the atrial premature beat initiating tachycardia conducting over the slow pathway, resulting in a prolonged PR interval for the first beat ("jump" phenomenon), indicating dual pathway properties. In atypical (fast-slow) atrioventricular nodal re-entrant tachycardia, the ECG features include RP interval>70 ms, and RP interval>PR interval; definitive diagnosis requires electrophysiological study to differentiate from atrial tachycardia.

5. Atrial Flutter: This is caused by re-entrant excitation within the atria due to intra-atrial conduction block, with the wavefront circulating around the area of block. The most common form is counterclockwise reentry around the tricuspid annulus, but clockwise reentry can also occur (Figure 3-1). Atrial scarring, such as after atrial septal defect repair surgery, can lead to intra-atrial conduction delays and cause reentry within the left atrium, right atrium, or atrial septum, resulting in atrial flutter. On the ECG, normal sinus P waves disappear and are replaced

by flutter waves (termed F waves), which have a sawtooth appearance and are most prominent in leads Ⅱ, Ⅲ, aVF, and V_1; the ventricular rate depends on atrioventricular conduction, with 2 : 1 to 5 : 1 atrioventricular conduction often observed due to concealed atrioventricular nodal conduction; when the ventricular rate is around 150 bpm and regular, 2 : 1 atrioventricular conduction is likely; increased sympathetic tone can even result in 1 : 1 atrioventricular conduction.

6. Atrial Fibrillation is a supra-ventricular rapid arrhythmia characterized by rapid, disorganized atrial electrical activity (Figure 3-6). The ECG manifestations include disappearance of P waves, replaced by variably sized and shaped fibrillatory (f) waves; absolutely irregular PP intervals; absolutely irregular ventricular rate, typically 60-100 beats per minute (bpm), with the rate determined by the electrophysiological properties of the atrioventricular node, autonomic tone, and drug effects. If the RR intervals are regular during atrial fibrillation, other possibilities such as atrioventricular nodal re-entrant tachycardia, ventricular tachycardia, and third-degree atrioventricular block should be considered. If associated with flutter waves, it is termed impure atrial fibrillation or atrial flutter-fibrillation.

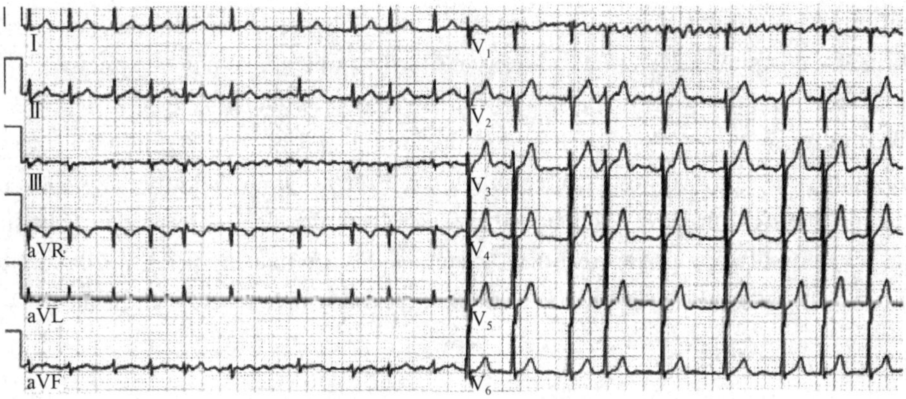

Figure 3-6 A Case of Atrial Fibrillation, with Absence of P Waves and Presence of Fine Fibrillatory (f) waves

Atrioventricular Junction (Junctional) Tachycardia is generally considered to arise from enhanced automaticity of the atrioventricular node or the proximal His bundle. It can be seen after cardiac surgery, with a structurally normal heart, or following radio-frequency ablation of the fast pathway in the atrioventricular junction region. The ECG features include a regular supra-ventricular rhythm, rate 150-200 bpm, with an absolutely regular rhythm; retrograde junctional P' waves may appear before, within, or after the QRS complex, but the RP interval is $<$120 ms; the onset and termination are gradual rather than abrupt.

V Principles of Treatment

1. Acute Termination

(1) If tachycardia is accompanied by hemodynamic instability, such as hypotension or shock, or acute heart failure, direct current cardioversion should be considered, with an energy selection

of 100-150 J. Vagal maneuvers, such as the Valsalva maneuver, ocular pressure, or carotid sinus massage, can also be attempted during tachycardia.

(2) Anti-arrhythmic drug therapy: Intravenous administration of medications such as procainamide, verapamil, and adenosine may be used. However, drug selection should be tailored to the specific tachycardia type. For atrial flutter patients, ventricular rate control should precede the use of procainamide, as procainamide can slow the atrial flutter rate, but its vagolytic effect may enhance atrioventricular conduction, leading to 1 ∶ 1 atrioventricular conduction of flutter waves. Adenosine can terminate narrow-complex tachycardias and also aid in differentiating atrial arrhythmias, but it should be administered rapidly with close monitoring of the heart rate. For atrial fibrillation with preexcitation, only procainamide or amiodarone can be used. In patients with heart failure, Class ⅠC anti-arrhythmic drugs should be avoided.

(3) If drugs fail to terminate the tachycardia, trans-esophageal or intracardiac programmed electrical stimulation may be considered.

2. Prevention of Recurrence

(1) Pharmacological control: For atrial flutter, atrial fibrillation, and atrial tachycardia, Class ⅠC anti-arrhythmic drugs such as procainamide or Class Ⅲ drugs like amiodarone can be used. In patients with heart failure, amiodarone or similar medications should be the choice. For other types of narrow-complex tachycardias, various anti-arrhythmic drugs may be effective.

(2) Catheter ablation: For all types of narrow-complex tachycardias, except permanent atrial fibrillation, catheter ablation is recommended as a first-line treatment strategy. The electrophysiological study during catheter ablation not only aids in definitive diagnosis but also offers the potential for cure; even if a cure is not achieved, the electrophysiological findings can guide the selection of appropriate treatment strategies. For permanent atrial fibrillation, catheter ablation can be considered if drug therapy is ineffective, or symptoms are significant.

Ⅵ Consultation Process

1. A thorough medical history should be obtained, and a physical examination should be performed. Clinically, if the tachycardia has an abrupt onset and termination, and vagal maneuvers can abruptly terminate it, re-entrant tachycardias such as atrioventricular nodal re-entrant tachycardia or atrioventricular re-entrant tachycardia are likely. Long-standing hypertension, chronic obstructive pulmonary disease, or hyper-trophic cardiomyopathy can lead to atrial enlargement, increasing the likelihood of atrial tachycardias or atrial fibrillation. On physical examination, varying intensity of the first heart sound, absolutely irregular rhythm, and a deficient pulse suggest atrial fibrillation.

2. Pay attention to important physical examination findings, such as thyroid enlargement, exophthalmos, asymmetric breath sounds (suggesting unilateral lung pathology), barrel chest deformity, cyanosis, enlarged cardiac borders on percussion, murmurs in valve areas, presence of rales, jugular venous distension, and edema (unilateral or bilateral).

3. Carefully analyze the ECG and compare it with previous ECGs to establish the diagnosis and type of arrhythmia.

4. Observe the patient's vital signs and mental status. If hemodynamic instability, such as

hypotension or shock, or acute heart failure is present, direct current cardioversion should be considered, with an energy selection of 100-150 J. For hemodynamically stable patients, vagal maneuvers and anti-arrhythmic drug therapy can be employed. For atrioventricular nodal re-entrant tachycardia and atrioventricular re-entrant tachycardia, verapamil or adenosine are the preferred agents for termination. For atrial flutter, atrial fibrillation, and atrial tachycardia, pharmacological control can involve Class ⅠC anti-arrhythmic drugs such as procainamide or Class Ⅲ agents, such as amiodarone. In patients with heart failure, amiodarone should be the choice.

Section 3 Diagnosis and Management of Wide QRS Complex Tachycardias

Wide QRS complex tachycardia refers to a tachycardia with a QRS duration≥120 ms and a rate≥100 bpm. It is a challenging problem frequently encountered in cardiology consultations, with approximately 80% of cases being ventricular tachycardia, which carries a higher mortality rate. The remaining cases include supra-ventricular tachycardias with bundle branch block, supra-ventricular tachycardias with intraventricular conduction delays, atrioventricular re-entrant tachycardias with preexcitation (e.g., Mahaim fibers), and atrial arrhythmias (including atrial fibrillation and atrial flutter) with preexcitation. Accurate diagnosis not only guides treatment but also aids in prognostic evaluation.

Ⅰ Determining the Indication for Cardioversion

If the patient's hemodynamic status is compromised, including altered mental status, inadequate perfusion leading to chest discomfort or pain, or acute heart failure, immediate cardioversion should be performed. A biphasic defibrillator with a maximum energy of 200 J can be used. If ventricular flutter or fibrillation occurs, rendering synchronized cardio-version ineffective, the non-synchronized mode should be selected. In cases of unsuccessful cardio-version attempts, electrolyte or acid-base disturbances should be considered, and continuous cardiopulmonary resuscitation should be maintained.

Ⅱ If Hemodynamics Are Stable

(i) Obtain a Detailed Medical History

Inquire about the presence of structural heart disease, such as a history of myocardial infarction or heart failure, as these conditions increase the likelihood of ventricular tachycardia.

(ii) Record a 12-Lead ECG

1. Absolutely Irregular Ventricular Rhythm: The 12-lead ECG should ideally be recorded simultaneously. An absolutely irregular ventricular rhythm may suggest atrial fibrillation with preexcitation or bundle branch block, with the former typically having a minimum RR interval< 250 ms and a larger RR interval difference>50 ms (Figure 3-7). If the QRS rate is around 150 bpm, consider the possibility of atrial flutter with 2 : 1 conduction.

2. Evidence of Ventricular Tachycardia: If the rhythm is relatively regular, as 80% of wide

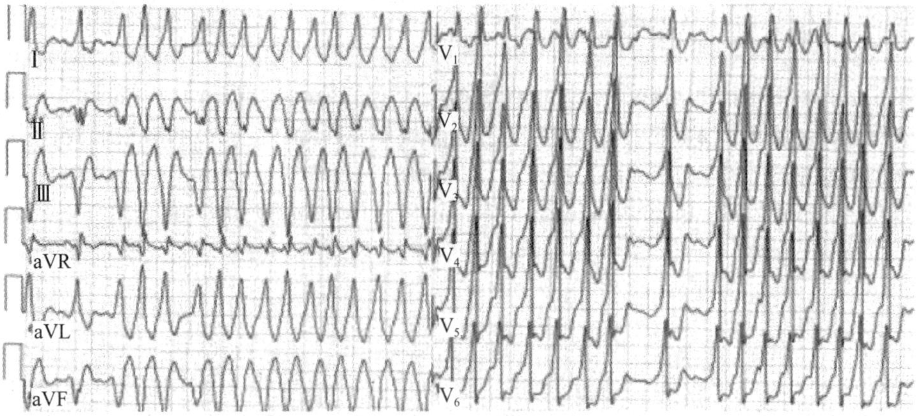

Figure 3-7 A Case of Atrial Fibrillation with Preexcitation, with a Minimum RR Interval of 200 ms, Confirmed as a Left-sided Accessory Pathway by Intracardiac Electrocardiogram

QRS complex tachycardias are ventricular tachycardias, seek evidence supporting this diagnosis.

(1) Atrioventricular Dissociation: This is 100% specific but only 20%-50% sensitive for ventricular tachycardia. During ventricular tachycardia, the atrial activation site (often the sinus node) controls the atria, while the ventricular tachycardia activation site controls the ventricles, leading to dissociated atrial and ventricular rates. Ventriculoatrial Wenckebach conduction may also be observed.

(2) Sinus Capture or Fusion Beats: This occurs when a sinus impulse competes with and captures the ventricles during ventricular tachycardia. If both the sinus and ventricular tachycardia impulses activate part of the ventricles simultaneously, the resulting QRS morphology appears intermediate between sinus and ventricular tachycardia.

(3) QRS Axis and Morphology: A right bundle branch block-like QRS morphology with a duration$>$140 ms or a left bundle branch block-like QRS with a duration$>$160 ms suggests ventricular tachycardia. A QRS axis in the "no-man's land" (i. e., negative complexes in limb leads Ⅰ, Ⅱ and Ⅲ) is nearly 100% specific for ventricular tachycardia.

(4) Precordial QRS Progression: Negative QRS complexes across the precordial leads (Figure 3-8), with leads V_1-V_6 showing predominantly negative deflections, are 100% specific for ventricular tachycardia. However, if the precordial QRS complexes are all positive, the specificity is only 80%, and supra-ventricular tachycardia with complete right bundle branch block or preexcitation via a left-sided accessory pathway should be excluded. Reverse or irregular precordial QRS progression (Figure 3-9) can also suggest ventricular tachycardia.

(5) QRS Morphology in Leads V_1 and V_6:

1) In lead V_1, a right bundle branch block pattern (left rabbit ear, biphasic qR or Rs morphology, or a single R wave) or, in lead V_6, an R/S ratio $<$1 or QRS, QS, or QR morphology suggests ventricular tachycardia.

2) In lead V_1, a left bundle branch block pattern (r wave duration $>$30 ms, S wave descending limb, or RS interval $>$70 ms from the onset of the r wave to the peak of the S wave) or the presence of Q or q waves in lead V_6 suggests ventricular tachycardia.

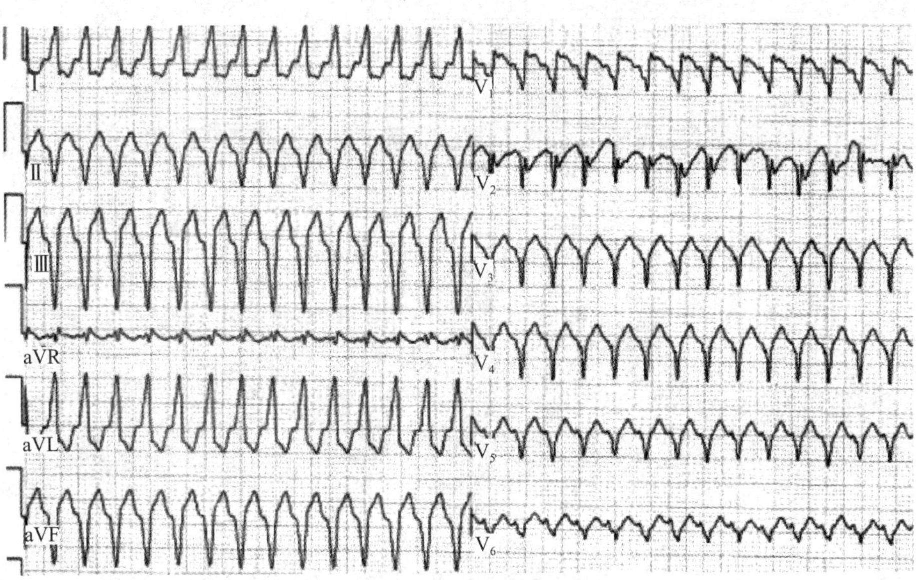

Figure 3-8 A Case of Ventricular Tachycardia with Negative Precordial QRS Complexes

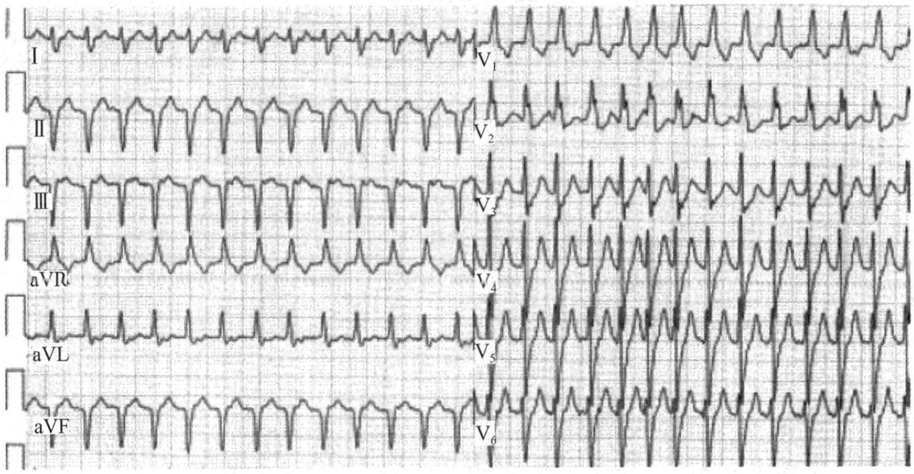

Figure 3-9 A Case of Ventricular Tachycardia with a QRS Axis in the "No-man's Land" (Negative Complexes in Leads Ⅰ, Ⅱ and Ⅲ) and Reverse Precordial QRS Progression

Ⅲ Brugada's Diagnostic Algorithm

Brugada's diagnostic algorithm involves four steps, with the fourth step being as described in (5) above. However, this method has low sensitivity and specificity, particularly for patients with pre-existing intraventricular conduction delays (Figure 3-10).

Ⅳ Vereckei's Diagnostic Algorithm

Although Brugada's algorithm is convenient, it has low sensitivity and specificity, especially for patients with pre-existing intraventricular conduction delays. In 2007, Vereckei proposed a new four-step algorithm (Figure 3-11), with the fourth step involving the calculation and

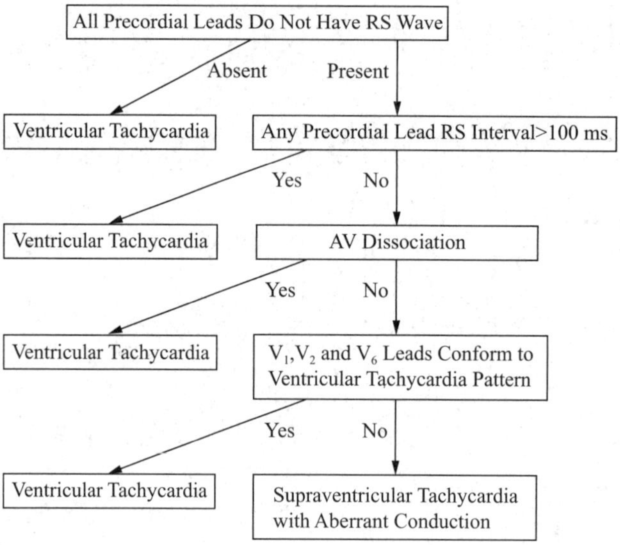

Figure 3-10 Brugada Diagnostic Algorithm

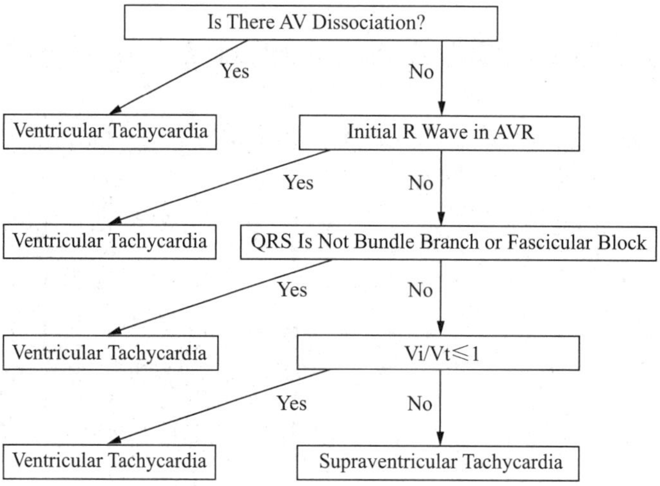

Figure 3-11 Vereckei Differential Diagnosis Flowchart

comparison of Vi and Vt values.

If the Vi value (the initial 40 ms of the QRS complex's depolarization rate) ≤Vt value (the terminal 40 ms of the QRS complex's depolarization rate), it is positive for ventricular tachycardia, i. e., a Vi / Vt ratio≤1 suggests ventricular tachycardia, while a Vi / Vt ratio> 1 suggests supra-ventricular tachycardia (Figure 3-12). The rationale is that normal conduction occurs through the Purkinje fibers, whereas in ventricular tachycardia, the depolarization begins in the myocardium and later activates the Purkinje network.

V aVR Lead-Specific Identification Process

The first two identification processes are quite complex. In 2008, Vereckei introduced a new aVR lead-specific identification process (Figure 3-13), based on the following theory:

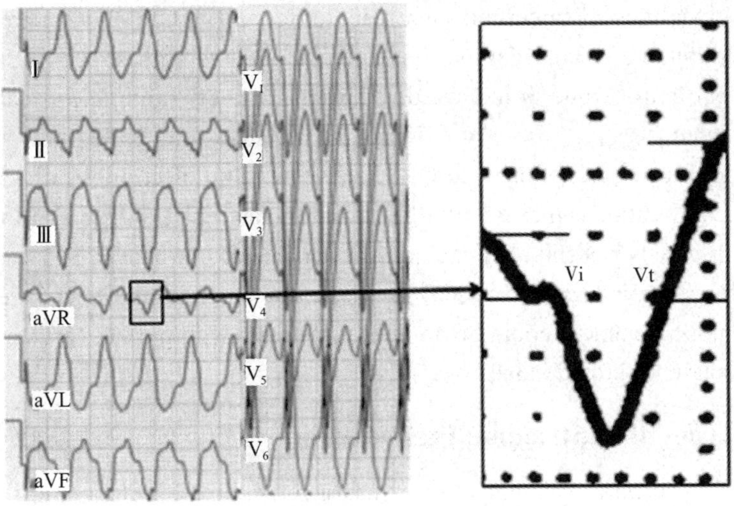

Figure 3-12 In Lead aVR, a Vi/Vt Ratio of <1 (Vi=1 mV, Vt=2.5 mV) Suggests Ventricular Tachycardia

Excitations originating from supra-ventricular sources move away from the aVR lead, thus typically beginning with a Q wave and displaying Qr, Qs, or qr configurations. On the other hand, ventricular tachycardias originating from the apex, left ventricular side wall, or inferior wall begin with an R wave due to the initial depolarization vector facing the aVR lead. Ventricular tachycardias from other regions can start with a Q wave in aVR, where slow intramyocardial conduction causes a q wave duration>40 ms; even in QS configurations, the slow onset of depolarization results in a notched start of the QRS complex.

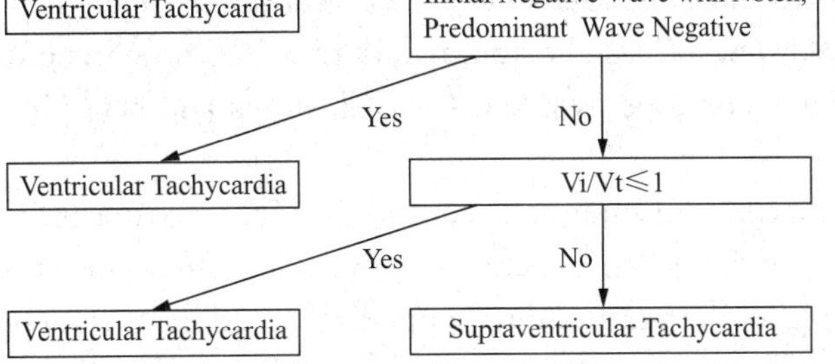

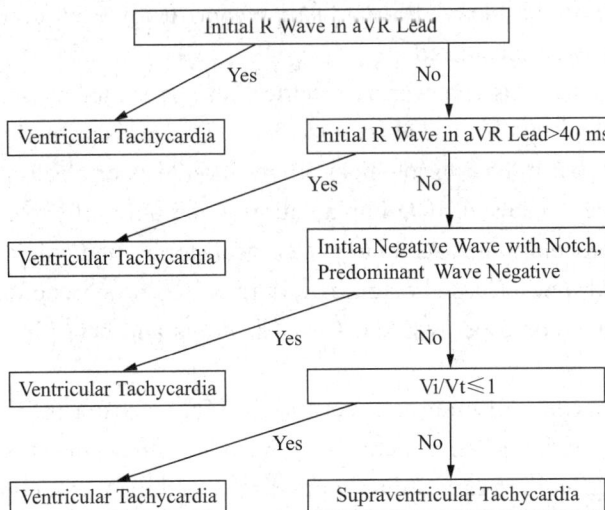

Figure 3-13 aVR Single-lead Differentiation Flowchart

Ⅵ Treatment Principles

1. Terminating Tachycardia. If diagnosis is confirmed, treatment should follow the

corresponding guidelines. If uncertain, pharmacologic termination may be considered, using intravenous propafenone or amiodarone; however, in patients with structural heart disease or heart failure, only amiodarone is indicated. If drugs are ineffective, electrical cardioversion should be considered.

2. Preventing Recurrence. For wide QRS tachycardia, an electrophysiological study may be considered, and treatment may involve radio-frequency ablation based on the findings. If structural heart disease is present, after excluding reversible or transient causes such as electrolyte imbalances or drugs, implantation of an ICD may be considered. For those who are not candidates for ICD, amiodarone treatment could be an option; patients with normal cardiac function might be treated with sotalol or propafenone.

Ⅶ Special Types of Ventricular Tachycardia

1. Long QT Syndrome. This condition is characterized by a prolonged QT interval on the electrocardiogram (QTc≥450 ms for males, ≥460 ms for females) and can lead to ventricular arrhythmias such as Torsades de Pointes, causing syncope and sudden death. It is classified into congenital and acquired types. The latter can be caused by electrolyte imbalances (hypo-kalemia, hypo-calcemia, hypo-magnesemia), medications (quinidine, disopyramide, amiodarone, and other antiarrhythmics, phenothiazines, tricyclic antidepressants), or intracranial lesions. Treatment for acquired Long QT Syndrome involves identifying and eliminating the underlying cause and may include intravenous magnesium sulfate and avoiding Class Ⅰa and Class Ⅲ antiarrhythmics. Isoproterenol, atropine, or temporary pacing might be used to increase the heart rate. Lidocaine and mexiletine are generally ineffective. For congenital Long QT Syndrome, beta-blockers are recommended; for those with a baseline slow heart rate, pacemaker insertion combined with β-blocker therapy may be considered. If drug therapy is ineffective, left cervical sympathectomy or ICD implantation may be considered.

2. Brugada Syndrome. This is a primary electrical disease caused by ion channel mutations, placing individuals at high risk for sudden cardiac death. Diagnosis primarily relies on ECG and, if typical features are absent, pharmacological provocation tests or electrophysiological studies may be required. Once diagnosed, ICD implantation is the only effective measure to prevent sudden death. Isoproterenol can be used to treat electrical storms, and quinidine may be effective against Brugada Syndrome. Class Ⅰc antiarrhythmics like propafenone, which can induce ventricular fibrillation, should be avoided; Class Ⅲ drugs and beta-blockers do not prevent sudden death.

3. Catecholaminergic Polymorphic Ventricular Tachycardia (CPVT). It is a genetic arrhythmia that occurs during physical activity or emotional stress, manifesting as bidirectional and polymorphic ventricular tachycardias, potentially leading to syncope or sudden death; typically without structural heart disease. Diagnosis is primarily based on exercise stress tests, Holter monitoring, or implantable Holter monitors. beta-blockers are recommended for prevention and treatment, proven effective clinically; verapamil and flecainide may also be used. If optimized pharmacotherapy fails, left cervical sympathectomy or an implantable cardioverter-defibrillator may be considered.

4. Short QT Syndrome. It is a rare ion channelopathy characterized by a QTc≤ 330 ms, QTc<360 ms, and may include pathogenic mutations, a family history of Short QT Syndrome, or a family history of sudden death at age≤40. Individuals with a history of cardiac arrest and/or spontaneous sustained ventricular tachycardia, and those with a family history of sudden cardiac death, should consider an implantable cardioverter-defibrillator. Asymptomatic individuals with a family history of sudden cardiac death may consider using quinidine or sotalol.

Ⅷ Consultation Process

1. It is crucial to monitor the patient's hemodynamic status. Should shock, consciousness impairment, or insufficient perfusion causing chest tightness or pain, or acute cardiac failure occur, immediate electrical cardioversion is required.

2. Inquire about the patient's medical and family history to identify diagnostic clues.

3. Carefully analyze the electrocardiogram (ECG); the aVR lead-specific identification process may be employed for diagnostic differentiation.

4. Treat patients with paroxysmal supra-ventricular tachycardia with aberrant conduction as cases of paroxysmal supra-ventricular tachycardia; use propafenone or amiodarone for atrial fibrillation with pre-excitation; opt for amiodarone in cases of ventricular tachycardia.

5. Comprehensive auxiliary examinations are necessary, such as blood gas analysis, complete blood count, renal function, electrolytes, BNP or NT-proBNP, D-dimer, thyroid function, ECG, chest X-ray, echocardiography, and coronary angiography / CT to ascertain the causes and triggers of the tachycardia, guiding further treatment.

Section 4 Long QT Syndrome

Ⅰ Definition

The congenital long QT syndrome (LQTS) is a group of disorders caused by mutations in genes encoding cardiac ion channels. Despite normal cardiac structure, these syndromes are characterized by QT interval prolongation, abnormal T-wave morphology, and episodes of torsade de pointes (TdP), a polymorphic ventricular tachyarrhythmia that can lead to syncope, seizures, and sudden cardiac death.

Ⅱ Genotypes

The genotypes of LQTS are shown in Table 3-1.

Table 3-1 Genotypes of LQTS

Items	LQT1	LQT2	LQT3
Triggering factors	Exercise and emotional excitement, such as swimming	Emotional excitement, auditory stimulation	Rest or sleep
T-wave morphology	Broad T-wave, prolonged T-wave interval	Notched T-wave, low amplitude	Late-onset tall, peaked, and narrow T-wave

(Continued)

Items	LQT1	LQT2	LQT3
T-wave changes during exercise testing	QT prolongation	Normal QT	QT shortening
Treatment	beta-blockers (+++)	beta-blockers (+)	Mexiletine

Ⅲ Clinical Manifestations

The clinical manifestations include arrhythmic events and electrocardiographic abnormalities. Arrhythmic events typically present as TdP, which, if sustained, can lead to syncope, cardiac arrest, or ventricular fibrillation and sudden death.

Untreated patients may experience recurrent syncope, ultimately progressing to sudden death. As the first presentation can be sudden death in some patients, treatment is warranted even in asymptomatic individuals. LQTS patients may also experience atrial arrhythmias, such as atrial fibrillation.

The triggers for arrhythmic events are largely genotype-dependent. LQT1 patients often experience events during exercise or emotional stress, LQT2 patients during sudden auditory stimuli while sleeping, and LQT3 patients during resting or sleeping.

Electrocardiographic abnormalities are varied. QT prolongation is the hallmark but may not always be apparent. Up to 10% of genotype-positive LQT3 and 37% of LQT1 patients have a normal QT interval at rest. In addition to prolonged ventricular re-polarization, other morphological abnormalities are common, some with genotype specificity. T-wave alternans is highly characteristic and indicates electrical instability. T-wave notching is typical of LQT2 and suggests a higher arrhythmic risk. Prolonged sinus pauses are relatively common in LQT3 patients. The clinical manifestations in Chinese patients are generally consistent with those reported globally.

Ⅳ Diagnosis

The recommended diagnostic criteria for LQTS are as follows:

1. A definite diagnosis can be made if any of the following are present: ① No secondary causes for QT prolongation, Schwartz score ≥3.5; ② Presence of a definite pathogenic mutation in at least one LQTS gene; ③ No secondary causes for QT prolongation, 12-lead QTc ≥500 ms.

2. A diagnosis can be made under the following circumstances: Unexplained syncope, no secondary causes for QT prolongation, no identified pathogenic gene mutation, 12-lead QTc 480-599 ms (Table 3-2).

Table 3-2 Schwartz Scoring System for Congenital LQTS

Diagnostic Criteria	Score
Electrocardiographic Findings	
QTc (ms)	
>480	3.0

(Continued)

Diagnostic Criteria	Score
460-470	2.0
>450	1.0
Torsades de pointes*	2.0
T-wave alternans	1.0
Notched T-wave (in 3 or more leads)	1.0
Resting heart rate below the 2nd percentile for age	0.5
Clinical presentation	
Syncope	
With stress	2.0
Without stress	1.0
Congenital deafness	0.5
Family history	
Definite LQTS in family members	1.0
Unexplained sudden cardiac death <30 years in immediate family	0.5

Note: Excluding secondary causes of torsade de pointes; Score >4: Definite LQTS; Score 2-3: Possible LQTS.

V Treatment

The treatment plan is determined by the risk factors for potentially life-threatening arrhythmias. Lifestyle modifications are routinely recommended: LQT1 patients should avoid strenuous exercise, particularly swimming, when unaccompanied; LQT2 patients should avoid sudden auditory stimuli (e.g., alarm clocks, telephone rings); and all LQTS patients should avoid medications that may prolong the QT interval. There is no consensus on whether LQTS patients should participate in competitive sports. For some low-risk patients with genetic evidence, borderline QTc values, asymptomatic status, and no family history of sudden cardiac death, participation in limited sports activities may be considered after comprehensive clinical evaluation, appropriate treatment, and training in basic life support under supervised conditions. However, high-risk patients and those with exercise-induced symptoms should avoid competitive sports.

1. beta-Blockers are first-line pharmacotherapy, recommended for patients without contraindications like active asthma, including those with normal QTc but positive genotype. There is insufficient evidence to preferentially recommend highly cardiac-selective beta-blockers, except in patients with asthma, where this class is preferred. Most LQTS patients are initially treated with propranolol; for those unable to tolerate or adhere to propranolol, long-acting formulations such as nadolol, metoprolol succinate, carvedilol, or atenolol can be used. Immediate-release metoprolol should be avoided in adults. Age and weight-adjusted maximum tolerated doses are recommended, with gradual upward titration and avoidance of abrupt discontinuation.

2. Implantable Cardioverter-Defibrillator (ICD): ICD therapy should be considered for patients with prior cardiac arrest or recurrent syncope despite beta-blocker therapy; prophylactic ICD is recommended for Jervell and Lange-Nielsen syndrome (LQTS with congenital deafness) and symptomatic patients with ≥2 mutations. As ICD therapy is lifelong with potential complications, a thorough risk-benefit assessment is warranted before implantation in young patients. For LQT1 patients with prior cardiac arrest but not yet on beta-blockers, beta-blocker or left cardiac sympathetic denervation (LCSD) should be the initial treatment, especially in infants and young children where ICD implantation carries higher risks.

3. LCSD can reduce arrhythmic events and is an option for patients intolerant or refractory to beta-blockers. It can be performed via a supraclavicular or minimally invasive approach in experienced centers. Reported efficacy in drug-refractory LQTS patients in China ranges from 81%-90%. LCSD is commonly used in high-risk infants too small for ICD implantation, recurrent syncope despite beta-blockers, contraindications or intolerance to β-blockers like asthma.

4. Other Treatments: For high-risk LQTS patients refractory to beta-blockers, ICDs, and LCSD, mexiletine, flecainide, and ranolazine can be considered. Sodium channel blockers, particularly mexiletine which inhibits late sodium current, are primarily used in LQT3. While their use is based on clinical observations of efficacy in some patients, long-term follow-up data are lacking.

Ⅵ Common Questions in Consultation

What precautions should congenital LQTS patients take?

1. Avoid strenuous exercise and emotional stress.

2. Avoid medications that prolong the QT interval.

3. Prevent hypokalemia, adhere to prescribed medications, and avoid abrupt discontinuation.

Ⅶ Consultation Process

1. Monitor vital signs like heart rate and blood pressure; if sinus rhythm is not restored, anti-arrhythmic treatment with beta-blockers as the first choice can be initiated. If hemodynamic instability, altered mental status, inadequate perfusion with chest discomfort / pain, or acute heart failure occurs, immediate cardioversion should be performed.

2. Obtain a detailed personal and family history to identify diagnostic clues.

3. Rapidly perform relevant investigations like arterial blood gas, complete blood count, renal function, electrolytes, calcitone, ECG, chest X-ray, BNP / NT-proBNP, D-dimer, thyroid function, and echocardiography.

Section 5 Brugada Syndrome

Ⅰ Definition and Pathogenesis

Brugada syndrome is a hereditary cardiac ion channel disorder, characterized by: ① Normal cardiac structure; ② Characteristic coved or saddle-back ST-segment elevation in the right precordial leads (V_1-V_3), with or without right bundle branch block; ③ Clinical manifestations of recurrent syncope or even sudden cardiac death due to ventricular fibrillation or polymorphic ventricular tachycardia. This condition was first proposed by the Brugada brothers in 1992 and officially named Brugada syndrome in 1996.

The syndrome predominantly affects males, with a male-to-female ratio of approximately 8 : 1, and typically presents between 30 and 40 years of age. It is most prevalent in Asia, particularly Southeast Asia, but has been reported globally in recent years, with sporadic cases and a familial inheritance pattern in 50% of cases. Brugada syndrome is an autosomal dominant inherited disorder. Mutations in the SCN5A gene, encoding the cardiac sodium channel, have been identified as the causative gene, leading to a loss of sodium channel function.

Ⅱ Classification

In August 2002, the European Society of Cardiology (ESC) summarized the electrocardiographic features of Brugada syndrome and classified it into three types, based on the characteristic J-wave, T-wave, and ST-segment morphologies (Figure 3-14).

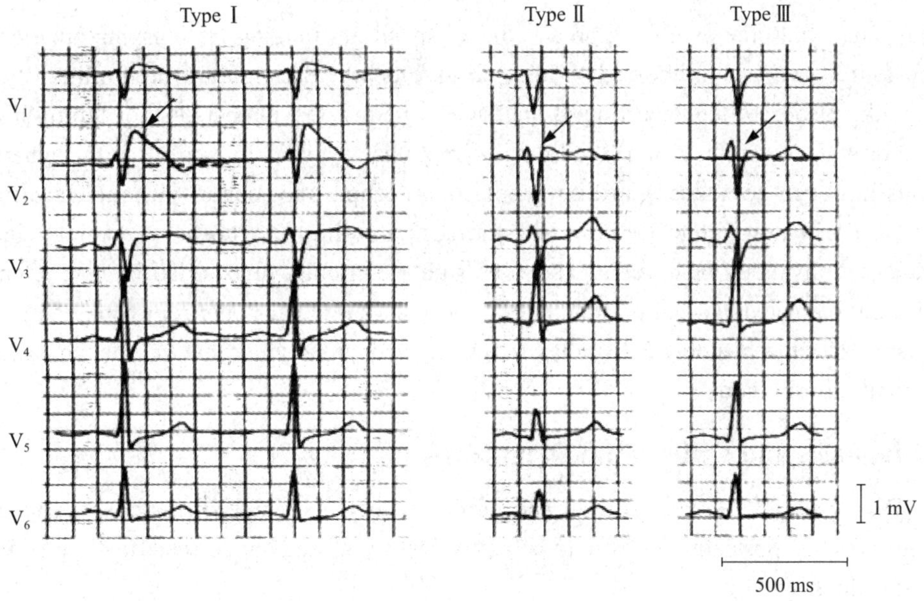

Figure 3-14 Electrocardiographic Features of Brugada Syndrome

Type Ⅰ: Characterized by a prominent coved ST-segment elevation, with a J-wave or ST-segment peak amplitude ≥2 mm, followed by a negative T-wave, with little or no isoelectric separation between the ST-segment and T-wave.

Type Ⅱ: Characterized by a saddle-back appearance, with a J-wave amplitude ≥ 2 mm, giving rise to a ST-segment elevation ≥1 mm above the baseline, followed by a positive or biphasic T-wave.

Type Ⅲ: Characterized by a saddle-back or coved ST-segment elevation < 1 mm, with or without a positive T-wave (Table 3-3).

Table 3-3 ESC Consensus Definition and Classification of Brugada ECG Patterns

Classification	Type Ⅰ	Type Ⅱ	Type Ⅲ
J-wave amplitude	≥2 mm	≥2 mm	≥2 mm
T-wave	Negative	Positive or Biphasic	Positive
ST-T configuration	Coved	Saddle-back	Saddle-back
Terminal ST-segment	Gradually descending	Elevated ≥1 mm	Elevated <1 mm

Note: 1 mm = 0.1 mV; Terminal ST-segment refers to the latter half of the ST-segment.

Brugada ECG patterns may also exhibit the following special characteristics: ① Intermittent normalization in >40% of the patients; ② Variability, with spontaneous or provoked transitions between Types Ⅰ, Ⅱ and Ⅲ in the same patient; ③ Concealed pattern, with a normal ECG despite carrying an SCN5A mutation, even after sodium channel blocker challenge; ④ Non-classical lead locations, with reported cases of inferolateral ECG manifestations. These features can make diagnosis challenging based solely on the ECG, leading to potential underdiagnosis.

Ⅲ Clinical Manifestations

Brugada syndrome exhibits a broad clinical spectrum, ranging from asymptomatic carriers to recurrent syncope and aborted sudden cardiac death. Patients are predominantly young males, with episodes often occurring during sleep, and may have a personal or family history of syncope or sudden cardiac death. Prodromal symptoms are typically absent, with asymptomatic intervals between episodes. Cardiac events or syncope may occur without warning, with ventricular fibrillation frequently observed during monitoring. Diagnostic evaluations, including echocardiography, ventriculography, and even right ventricular myocardial biopsy, often reveal no structural cardiac abnormalities, although mild left ventricular hypertrophy may be present in some cases. Electrophysiological studies frequently induce polymorphic ventricular tachycardia or ventricular fibrillation.

Ⅳ Diagnosis and Differential Diagnosis

1. Diagnosis: A detailed personal and family history is crucial for diagnosis. Unexplained syncope, presyncope, palpitations, and a family history of sudden cardiac death are important diagnostic clues.

In the presence of a typical Type Ⅰ ECG pattern and any of the following clinical features, after excluding other causes of ECG abnormalities, a diagnosis of Brugada syndrome can be made: ① Documented ventricular fibrillation; ② Self-terminating polymorphic ventricular tachycardia; ③ Family history of sudden cardiac death (<45 years); ④ Family members with a typical Type Ⅰ ECG pattern; ⑤ Inducible ventricular fibrillation on electrophysiological study; ⑥ Syncope or nocturnal agonal respiration.

For patients with Type Ⅱ or Type Ⅲ ECG patterns, a diagnosis of Brugada syndrome can be made if they have a positive drug challenge test or positive electrophysiological study, in addition to the aforementioned clinical features. In the absence of these clinical symptoms and with only characteristic ECG changes, the condition should be termed an "idiopathic Brugada

ECG pattern" rather than Brugada syndrome. If the ECG criteria are not completely met (e.g., a J-point elevation of only 1 mm in Type Ⅰ), but one or more of the clinical features are present, the diagnosis should be made with caution.

2. Differential Diagnosis: In diagnosing Brugada syndrome, all potential causes of ST-segment elevation in the right precordial leads should be excluded. Differentiating from arrhythmogenic right ventricular cardiomyopathy or dysplasia is particularly important, as these conditions share many clinical similarities. The following conditions can also mimic Brugada ECG patterns and should be considered in the differential diagnosis: ① Acute anterior myocardial infarction; ② Right or left bundle branch block; ③ Left ventricular hypertrophy; ④ Right ventricular infarction; ⑤ Left ventricular aneurysm; ⑥ Cocaine intoxication; ⑦ Acute pulmonary embolism; ⑧ Inherited neuromuscular disorders.

V Treatment

The goal of treatment for Brugada syndrome is to prevent ventricular fibrillation and reduce the risk of sudden cardiac death.

1. Non-pharmacological Treatment

(1) Implantable Cardioverter-Defibrillator (ICD): ICD therapy has proven efficacy in preventing sudden cardiac death in Brugada syndrome, compared to no treatment, beta-blocker therapy, or quinidine. The Second International Consensus on Brugada Syndrome recommends ICD implantation for symptomatic patients with a Type Ⅰ Brugada ECG pattern and a history of cardiac arrest, without the need for an electrophysiological study. For patients with relevant symptoms such as syncope, seizures, or nocturnal agonal respiration, after excluding non-cardiac causes, ICD implantation is also recommended.

For asymptomatic patients with a Type Ⅰ Brugada ECG pattern and a family history of sudden cardiac death suspected to be caused by Brugada syndrome, an electrophysiological study should be performed. If the Type Ⅰ pattern is spontaneous and the family history is negative, electrophysiological testing can provide diagnostic clarity. If ventricular arrhythmias are inducible, the patient should receive an ICD.

(2) Pacemakers: The occurrence of ventricular tachyarrhythmias or ventricular fibrillation in Brugada syndrome may exhibit rate-dependence, suggesting a potential role for dual-chamber pacing. However, large-scale studies and long-term follow-up data are currently lacking to draw definitive conclusions regarding the efficacy of this approach.

(3) Radio-frequency Catheter Ablation: Limited case reports have described radio-frequency catheter ablation targeting the triggers for ventricular tachycardia or ventricular fibrillation in Brugada syndrome. However, the number of cases treated with this approach is still limited, and the long-term efficacy remains to be evaluated through larger studies and extended follow-up.

ICD implantation remains the only proven effective therapy for preventing sudden cardiac death in Brugada syndrome. Pharmacological treatments and catheter ablation can only serve as adjunctive therapies to reduce the frequency of ICD shocks and improve the patient's quality of life, but they are not recommended as standalone treatments.

2. Pharmacological Treatment

(1) Quinidine: It is currently the only drug that can significantly inhibit the Ito current. Experimental evidence suggests that quinidine can correct ECG abnormalities and prevent the occurrence of ventricular fibrillation.

(2) Isoproterenol: During the acute phase of ventricular tachyarrhythmias or after electrical cardioversion for ventricular fibrillation, isoproterenol can be used to prevent ventricular fibrillation storms. Isoproterenol enhances calcium influx through L-type calcium channels, leading to the normalization of elevated ST-segments in patients.

(3) Cilostazol: It is a phosphodiesterase Ⅲ inhibitor that can normalize elevated ST-segments by increasing the ICa^{2+} current.

Currently, there is limited evidence-based medical data on the efficacy of these pharmacological treatments, and their precise effects remain to be determined. Class Ⅰ antiarrhythmic drugs, which inhibit sodium influx and relatively increase the Ito current, are contraindicated in Brugada syndrome patients as they can induce ventricular fibrillation. Class Ⅲ antiarrhythmic drugs (amiodarone) and beta-blockers are ineffective in preventing sudden cardiac death.

To sum up, Brugada syndrome is a primary electrical heart disease caused by ion channel gene abnormalities and is a high-risk factor for cardiac-related sudden death, with a severe prognosis. Therefore, prompt identification is crucial in clinical practice to allow for early intervention. For asymptomatic patients with a normal ECG, provocation testing, or electrophysiological studies can be performed to establish the diagnosis. Once the diagnosis is confirmed, immediate ICD implantation is the only effective measure to prevent sudden cardiac death.

Ⅵ Common Questions in Consultation

What factors can influence the Brugada pattern?

1. Slow Rate Dependence: In general, both the Brugada pattern and the occurrence of malignant arrhythmias exhibit slow rate dependence. The Brugada pattern becomes less typical as the heart rate increases and more pronounced as the heart rate slows down. This phenomenon can explain why life-threatening arrhythmias in Brugada syndrome patients often occur at night. However, a minority of patients exhibit the opposite pattern, with the Brugada pattern becoming more evident following an increase in heart rate or exercise, potentially leading to syncope or sudden death during the daytime.

2. Autonomic Influence: Increased vagal tone can slow the heart rate, accentuate the Brugada pattern, and increase the spontaneous occurrence and inducibility of ventricular tachycardia and ventricular fibrillation. The effects of sympathetic stimulation are generally opposite to those of vagal stimulation.

3. Effects of Antiarrhythmic Drugs: Different classes of antiarrhythmic drugs have varying effects on the Brugada pattern. Class Ⅰ drugs, which block the sodium channels in cardiac myocytes, can accentuate the Brugada pattern. Similarly, vagal stimulants, alpha-adrenergic antagonists, beta-blockers, and tricyclic antidepressants can also exacerbate the Brugada pattern.

Ⅶ Consultation Process

1. Closely monitor the patient's vital signs, including heart rhythm and blood pressure. If sinus rhythm has not been restored, antiarrhythmic treatment can be initiated, with beta-blockers as the preferred initial choice. In the event of shock, altered mental status, or acute heart failure with inadequate perfusion leading to chest discomfort or pain, immediate electrical cardio-version should be performed.

2. Obtain a detailed medical and family history to identify diagnostic clues.

3. Promptly perform ancillary investigations, such as blood gas analysis, complete blood count, renal function tests, electrolytes, parathyroid hormone, electrocardiogram, chest radiography, B-type natriuretic peptide (BNP) or N-terminal pro-BNP, D-dimer, thyroid function tests, and echocardiography.

4. Actively treat and prevent the occurrence of ventricular fibrillation to reduce the risk of sudden cardiac death. Simultaneously, ensure that the patient and their family members are informed about the condition and the proposed treatment plan.

Section 6 Syncope

Ⅰ Overview

Syncope refers to a transient loss of consciousness due to global cerebral hypo-perfusion, causing the patient to collapse or be unable to maintain an upright posture due to a loss of muscle tone. It is characterized by a sudden onset, short duration, and spontaneous recovery.

Syncope is a common clinical presentation, accounting for 0.9%-1.7% of emergency department visits and 1%-3% of hospital admissions. It can lead to injuries or disabilities and may be the only warning sign of impending sudden cardiac death. Most syncopal events occur in isolation and do not prompt medical attention as patients often do not seek medical care. The age distribution of syncope is bimodal, with the first peak occurring in the 10-30 age group, reaching its highest incidence around 15 years of age, and the second peak occurring in individuals over 65 years old. The prognosis of syncope patients varies significantly depending on the underlying etiology. Patients with structural heart diseases have a higher risk of sudden cardiac death and overall mortality. The mortality rate in orthostatic hypotension syncope can be significantly increased, and the prognosis largely depends on the patient's comorbidities. In contrast, neurally mediated syncope in younger individuals generally has a more favorable prognosis.

Ⅱ Classification

1. Neurally Mediated Syncope (Reflex Syncope): This type of syncope is caused by an abnormal reflex arc leading to increased vagal tone and/or decreased sympathetic tone, resulting in bradycardia and vasodilation. When the underlying mechanism is predominantly vasodilation-induced hypotension, it is termed vasodepressor syncope. When bradycardia or impaired cardiac contractility is the predominant mechanism, it is termed cardio-inhibitory syncope. The

coexistence of both mechanisms is referred to as mixed syncope.

2. Orthostatic Hypotension Syncope: This syncope occurs when transitioning from a supine or squatting position to an upright position. It is related to impairment of the baroreceptor reflex arc during postural changes and a reduction in venous return.

3. Cardiac Syncope: This is the most dangerous and prognostically unfavorable type of syncope, with a high risk of sudden cardiac death. It is caused by an acute reduction in cardiac output, leading to a sudden decrease in cerebral perfusion. The most common etiology is arrhythmia, where various diseases or adverse drug reactions can induce bradycardia, tachycardia, or inherited arrhythmia syndromes, resulting in hemodynamic impairment, acute reduction in cardiac output, and decreased cerebral perfusion pressure, leading to syncope. In patients with structural cardiovascular diseases, syncope is related to the circulatory load exceeding the compensatory capacity of the heart, and the mechanism of increased vagal tone may also contribute (Table 3-4).

Table 3-4 Classification of Syncope

Neurally Mediated Syncope (Reflex Syncope)
Vasovagal Syncope
Emotional stress: fear, pain, heat exposure, fatigue
Orthostatic position mediated
Situational Syncope
Coughing, sneezing
Gastrointestinal tract stimulation (swallowing, defecation, abdominal pain)
Urination
Post-exercise
Postprandial
Others (such as laughter, weight lifting, and Valsalva maneuver)
Carotid Sinus Syncope
Atypical Syncope (no clear triggers or atypical symptoms)
Orthostatic Hypotension Syncope
Primary Autonomic Failure
Pure autonomic failure, Multiple System Atrophy, Parkinson's Disease without autonomic dysfunction, Lewy Body Dementia
Secondary Autonomic Failure
Diabetes, Amyloidosis, Uremia, Spinal cord injury
Drug-induced Orthostatic Hypotension
Alcohol, vasodilators, diuretics, antidepressants
Hypovolemia
Bleeding, diarrhea, vomiting, Addison's disease
Cardiogenic Syncope
Arrhythmic Syncope
Bradycardia
Sinus node dysfunction (including tachy-brady syndrome)
AV nodal dysfunction
Device dysfunction (pacemakers, ICDs)
Tachycardia
supra-ventricular (including pre-excitation syndromes like Wolff-Parkinson-White Syndrome)
Ventricular (idiopathic, secondary to structural heart disease)

(Continued)

Drug-induced bradycardia and tachycardia
Genetic Arrhythmia Syndromes
Long QT Syndrome, Brugada Syndrome, Short QT Syndrome, Catecholaminergic Polymorphic Ventricular Tachycardia, etc.
Structural Cardiovascular Disease-Related Syncope
Cardiac Causes: Valvular heart disease, Acute myocardial infarction / ischemia, Hypertrophic cardiomyo-pathy, Cardiac tumors (atrial myxoma, other tumors), Pericardial diseases / cardiac tamponade, Congeni-tal coronary artery anomalies, Prosthetic valve dysfunction
Others: Pulmonary embolism / pulmonary hypertension, Acute aortic dissection, Cyanotic congenital heart disease

Ⅲ Diagnosis and Assessment

1. Taking a diagnostic history is extremely important for diagnosing syncope. By inquiring about the rapidity of onset, duration of unconsciousness, and residual symptoms after the attack, syncope can be clearly diagnosed and differentiated from cerebrovascular diseases and epilepsy. By asking about the triggering factors, emotional state, environmental context, body position during the attack, as well as prodromal symptoms, cardiovascular disease history, and medication history, syncope can be broadly classified.

(1) Neurally Mediated Syncope

1) Vasovagal Syncope: There are often obvious triggers before onset, commonly pain, fear, anxiety, heat, fatigue, etc. Attacks almost always occur in the standing or sitting position, rarely in the supine position. Prodromal symptoms of autonomic dysfunction such as pallor, nausea, sweating, dizziness, tinnitus, etc. are present. The main diagnostic and differential diagnostic method are the tilt table test.

2) Situational Syncope: Occurs in certain specific situations, including micturition, coughing, swallowing, and exercise.

3) Carotid Sinus Syncope: Caused by carotid sinus hypersensitivity reflex, commonly due to atherosclerosis, arteritis, carotid body tumors, etc.

(2) Orthostatic Hypotensive Syncope: This type of syncope usually occurs after standing up, with insignificant prodromal symptoms, abrupt blood pressure drop, and symptom relief upon lying down. Notably, unless hypovolemia causes a reflex tachycardia, there is generally no significant heart rate change during the attack. Orthostatic blood pressure testing can assist diagnosis.

(3) Cardiac Syncope

1) Arrhythmic Syncope: Persistent bradycardia $<$40 bpm while awake, or recurrent sinoatrial block or sinus pause $\geqslant$3s; second-degree Type Ⅱ or third-degree atrioventricular block; alternating left and right bundle branch block; ventricular tachycardia or paroxysmal supra-ventricular tachycardia; non-sustained polymorphic ventricular tachycardia, long QT or short QT syndrome, Brugada syndrome, etc.

2) Structural Cardiovascular Syncope: Syncope occurs with acute myocardial infarction, obstructive hypertrophic cardiomyopathy, obstructive valvular heart disease, atrial myxoma, pulmonary embolism, etc.

2. Auxiliary Examinations

(1) Carotid Sinus Massage: For patients>40 years old with unexplained syncope, carotid sinus massage is recommended. A positive test is diagnosed if carotid sinus massage causes cardiac pause>3s and/or systolic blood pressure drop>50 mmHg; if syncope occurs, it is diagnosed as carotid sinus syncope.

(2) Tilt Table Test: For suspected reflex syncope, a tilt table test is recommended, with the endpoint being hypotension / bradycardia or delayed orthostatic hypotension, accompanied by syncope or presyncope. A negative result cannot rule out reflex syncope: a cardio-inhibitory response has high predictive value for syncope caused by cardiac pause, while a vasodepressor, mixed, or even negative response cannot rule out syncope caused by cardiac pause.

(3) Cardiac Monitoring: Includes in-hospital ECG monitoring, Holter monitoring, external or implantable loop recorders [implantable Holter, implantable loop recorder (ILR)], and remote ECG monitoring.

(4) Electrophysiological Study: Has low sensitivity and specificity for diagnosing suspected intermittent bradycardia, bundle branch block (near-complete AV block), and suspected tachycardia causing syncope. However, it is not recommended for patients with severely reduced left ventricular ejection fraction, who should receive an ICD without investigating the mechanism of syncope.

(5) Echocardiography and Other Imaging: Echocardiography is important for diagnosing structural heart disease and identifying rare causes of syncope such as aortic stenosis, atrial myxoma, cardiac tamponade, etc. Some patients may need trans-esophageal echocardiography, CT, and MRI for conditions like aortic dissection, hematoma, pulmonary embolism, cardiac tumors, pericardial and myocardial diseases, and coronary artery anomalies.

(6) Exercise Testing: For patients with syncope during or shortly after exercise, an exercise test should be performed with close ECG and blood pressure monitoring during exercise and recovery. Syncope during exercise is likely cardiac, while post-exercise syncope is almost always due to a reflex mechanism. Exercise-induced second- or third-degree AV block after tachycardia suggests disease at the AV node level and potential progression to permanent AV block.

(7) Cardiac Catheterization: For suspected myocardial ischemia or infarction, coronary angiography should be performed to rule out ischemia-induced arrhythmia.

Ⅳ Treatment Principles

1. General Principles

The treatment principles for syncope are to prolong survival, prevent physical injury, and prevent recurrence. Identifying the cause of syncope is crucial for selecting the treatment plan. Appropriate treatment should be based on risk stratification.

2. Treatment of Neurally Mediated Syncope aims primarily to prevent recurrence, related injuries, and improve quality of life.

(1) Education: For most patients, especially those with infrequent attacks and clear triggering factors, education and psychological counseling are the main treatments. Avoiding triggers like heat, fatigue, etc., cautious use of alcohol, diuretics, and vasodilators, and increasing salt intake to expand blood volume are recommended.

(2) Isometric Counter-Pressure Maneuvers: Including tilt training, head-up tilt sleeping (> 10°), isometric leg and arm counter-pressure maneuvers, and moderate aerobic and isometric exercise.

(3) Pharmacotherapy: Many drugs attempted for reflex syncope have poor efficacy, including beta-blockers, pindolol, disopyramide, theophylline, ephedrine, midodrine, clonidine, and selective serotonin re-uptake inhibitors. Long-term treatment is not recommended for occasional patients.

(4) Cardiac Pacing: Rarely used for reflex syncope unless severe bradycardia is found. Pacing may benefit carotid sinus syncope.

3. Orthostatic Hypotensive Syncope

(1) Non-Pharmacological Treatment: Lifestyle changes can significantly improve orthostatic hypotension symptoms; even a 10-15 mmHg blood pressure increase can produce functional improvement within the body's self-regulatory range. For non-hypertensive patients, adequate salt and fluid intake (2-3 L fluid and 10 g sodium chloride daily) is recommended. Elevating the head of the bed (10°) during sleep can prevent nocturnal polyuria and maintain proper fluid distribution and nocturnal blood pressure. Abdominal binders or compression stockings can treat venous pooling in the elderly.

(2) Pharmacotherapy: The alpha-agonist midodrine is a first-line drug, with variable efficacy and significant benefit in some patients. Midodrine raises supine and standing blood pressures, alleviating orthostatic hypotension symptoms. Fludrocortisone promotes sodium retention and expands fluid volume, reducing symptoms and raising blood pressure.

4. Cardiac Syncope

(1) Arrhythmic Syncope: Factors affecting this type of syncope include ventricular rate, left ventricular function, and vascular compensatory ability. The treatment principle is to address the underlying cause.

1) Sinoatrial Node Dysfunction: If bradycardia or abnormal sinus node recovery time (CSNRT>525 ms) is recorded during syncope, a pacemaker should be implanted. An atrial-based, minimally ventricular paced mode is recommended over a conventional dual-chamber rate-adaptive pacemaker. radio-frequency ablation can be used for sick sinus syndrome presenting mainly as tachycardia-bradycardia syndrome.

2) Atrioventricular Conduction System Disease: AV block associated with syncope should be treated with cardiac pacing. For patients with reduced left ventricular ejection fraction and complete left bundle branch block, or QRS≥150 ms without left bundle branch block, bi-ventricular pacing should be performed.

3) Paroxysmal supra-ventricular Tachycardia and Ventricular Tachycardia: For syncope patients related to atrioventricular nodal re-entrant tachycardia, atrioventricular re-entrant tachycardia, and typical atrial flutter, catheter ablation is the first-line treatment. Pharmacotherapy is limited to pre-ablation preparation or failed ablation cases. Treatment for syncope related to atrial fibrillation or atypical left atrial flutter should be individualized. For patients with normal or mildly impaired cardiac function, ventricular tachycardia causing syncope can be treated with catheter ablation and/or antiarrhythmic drugs.

For syncope patients with ventricular tachycardia or ventricular fibrillation due to impaired cardiac function from irreversible causes, an implantable cardioverter-defibrillator (ICD) should be implanted. Although ICD implantation cannot prevent syncope episodes, it can reduce the risk of sudden cardiac death.

(2) Cardiac Implantable Electronic Device Malfunction: In rare cases, syncope is triggered by pacemaker malfunction. Syncope related to implanted devices may be caused by pulse generator battery depletion or failure, or lead dislodgement, requiring lead replacement or device re-implantation. For pacemaker syndrome patients with ventriculoatrial conduction, pacemaker reprogramming should be performed, and some patients may need pacemaker replacement, such as switching from single-chamber ventricular to dual-chamber pacing. Syncope related to ICDs is often due to the ICD intervening too late to prevent loss of consciousness. For patients where ICD reprogramming (more aggressive anti-tachycardia pacing and/or earlier shock delivery) cannot resolve the issue, anti-arrhythmic drugs or catheter ablation may be effective.

(3) Structural Cardiovascular Disease-Related Syncope: For syncope patients secondary to structural heart diseases, including congenital heart defects or cardiopulmonary diseases, the treatment goal is not only to prevent syncope recurrence but also to treat the underlying disease and reduce the risk of sudden cardiac death. However, the presence of heart disease does not necessarily indicate syncope is related, as some patients have typical reflex syncope, while in others, such as inferior wall myocardial infarction or aortic stenosis, the underlying disease may play an important role in triggering or inducing the reflex mechanism. For syncope caused by severe aortic stenosis and atrial myxoma, surgical intervention is recommended. For syncope secondary to acute cardiovascular diseases like pulmonary embolism, myocardial infarction, or cardiac tamponade, treatment should target the primary disease. For hyper-trophic cardiomyopathy-related syncope, most patients should receive an ICD to prevent sudden cardiac death, while surgical intervention or chemical ablation of hypertrophied vessels should be considered for patients with left ventricular outflow tract obstruction.

V Common Questions in Consultation

1. How to Differentiate Syncope from Epilepsy

Epilepsy can cause brief loss of consciousness, with patients experiencing unresponsiveness, falling, and amnesia in sequence; this only occurs during tonic, clonic, tonic-clonic, and generalized seizures. In children's absence seizures and adults' complex partial seizures, there is a change in consciousness rather than loss of consciousness; compared to brief loss of consciousness, these patients experience symptom onset while standing. Complete body limpness during unconsciousness does not support epilepsy, with the sole exception of the rare "atonic seizure". The differential diagnosis of epilepsy and syncope is shown in Table 3-5.

Table 3-5 Differential Diagnosis Between Epilepsy and Syncope

Clinical Manifestations of Suggesting Diagnosis	Epilepsy	Syncope
Pre-seizure Symptoms	Odd smells (such as unusual odors)	Nausea, vomiting, abdominal discomfort, cold sweats, dizziness, and blurred vision

(Continued)

Clinical Manifestations of Suggesting Diagnosis	Epilepsy	Syncope
Manifestations During Unconsciousness	Prolonged tonic-clonic seizures starting; with loss of consciousness; Unilateral clonic movements; Distinct automatisms such as chewing, smacking lips, or frothing at the mouth (seen in partial seizures); Tongue biting; Facial cyanosis;	Brief tonic-clonic seizures (<15 seconds), occurring after loss of consciousness
Post-seizure Symptoms	Prolonged postictal confusion; Muscle pain;	Short postictal confusion Nausea, vomiting, and facial pallor

2. How to Assess Risk in Syncope Patients

After establishing the syncope diagnosis, the patient's risk of major cardiovascular events and sudden cardiac death should be assessed. Patients with life-threatening risk in the near-term (7-30 days) should be hospitalized. Those with one major risk factor should undergo urgent (within 2 weeks) cardiac evaluation, and those with one or more minor risk factors should also be considered for urgent cardiac evaluation. Risk factor assessment is shown in Table 3-6.

Table 3-6 Short-Term Risk Factors for Syncope

Risk Factors	Manifestations
Main: Abnormal ECG	Bradycardia, tachycardia or conduction system disease New-onset myocardial ischemia or old myocardial infarction
History of heart disease	Myocardial ischemia, arrhythmia, myocardial infarction, valvular disease
Hypotension	Systolic BP <90 mmHg
Heart failure	History or current occurrence
Secondary: Age > 60 years	
Dyspnea	
Anemia	Hematocrit <0.30
Hypertension	
Cerebrovascular disease	
Family history of premature sudden death	Sudden death age <50 years
Special circumstances	Syncope in supine position, during exercise, or without prodrome

3. How to Differentiate Orthostatic Hypotensive Syncope, Vasovagal Syncope, and Idiopathic Orthostatic Hypotension. Orthostatic hypotensive syncope typically occurs after standing up, with insignificant presyncope symptoms, abrupt blood pressure drop, and symptom relief upon lying down. Notably, unless hypovolemia causes a reflex tachycardia, there is generally no significant heart rate change during the attack. Vasovagal syncope has obvious triggers, and the three stages of syncope symptoms are more typical, with marked bradycardia in addition to the rapid blood pressure drop during attacks. In addition to manifesting as orthostatic hypotensive syncope, idiopathic orthostatic hypotension also presents with various symptoms of autonomic dysfunction.

4. How to Manage Syncope of Unknown Cause. For some syncope patients whose mechanism remains unclear even after comprehensive examination, disease-specific treatment should still be provided for those at high risk of sudden cardiac death to reduce mortality or life-threatening adverse events. However, even with effective treatment of the underlying disease, patients still have a risk of syncope recurrence. For example, after ICD implantation, patients may still experience loss of consciousness because the ICD prevents sudden cardiac death but does not treat the cause of syncope. Indications for ICD implantation in patients with syncope of unknown cause at high risk of sudden cardiac death include: ① Ischemic cardiomyopathy with LVEF ≤35% or heart failure; ② Non-ischemic cardiomyopathy with LVEF ≤35% or heart failure; ③ High-risk hyper-trophic cardiomyopathy; ④ High-risk arrhythmogenic right ventricular cardiomyopathy; ⑤ Spontaneous type Ⅰ ECG changes in Brugada syndrome; ⑥ Long QT syndrome with high-risk factors, for which combined beta-blocker and ICD therapy should be considered.

Ⅵ Consultation Process

1. Carefully inquire about the patient's medical history: Onset triggers such as psychological stimuli, fever, hunger, poisoning, positional changes, recent medication history, etc. Understand changes in the patient's living and working environment. Changes in accompanying symptoms before and after syncope attacks, such as headache, dizziness, chest pain, chest tightness, shortness of breath, diarrhea, abdominal pain, etc. Detailed history of underlying diseases, especially cardiovascular and cerebrovascular diseases.

2. Detailed physical examination, including the patient's vital signs, mental status, pupil size, lung sounds, heart rhythm, muscle strength, and pathological signs, as well as presence of neurological localizing signs.

3. Rapid auxiliary examinations are needed, such as blood tests, renal function, electrolytes, cardiac enzymes, bedside troponin, electrocardiogram, chest X-ray, cranial CT scan, etc.

4. Cause-specific treatment after diagnosis, e.g., acute cerebrovascular accident indicated on cranial CT requires prompt neurological hospitalization; acute myocardial infarction on ECG requires urgent revascularization; bradyarrhythmia treated with isoprenaline to increase heart rate or temporary cardiac pacing; tachyarrhythmia treated with anti-arrhythmic drugs, with cardio-version if necessary.

Section 7 Pharmacotherapy for Atrial Fibrillation

Ⅰ Antithrombotic Therapy

(i) Thromboembolism and Bleeding Risk Assessment in Atrial Fibrillation Patients

Atrial fibrillation is an independent risk factor for stroke, and thromboembolism risk should be regularly assessed.

1. CHADS2 Score: Based on recent congestive heart failure (1 point), hyper-tension (1 point), age ≥75 years (1 point), diabetes (1 point), and prior stroke / thromboembolism (2 points) to

stratify stroke risk. Anti-coagulation is recom-mended for CHADS2 score ⩾2.

2. CHA2DS2-VASc Score: Congestive heart failure / left ventricular dysfunction (C, 1 point), hypertension (H, 1 point), age⩾75 years (A, 2 points), diabetes (D, 1 point), prior stroke / TIA / thromboembolism (S, 2 points), vascular disease (V, 1 point), age 65-74 years (A, 1 point), female sex (Sc, 1 point). Anti-coagulation is recommended for score⩾2; score of 1, anticoagulant or aspirin or no antithrombotic is acceptable; score of 0, no antithrombotic needed (Table 3-7).

Table 3-7 CHA2DS2-VASc Stroke Risk Stratification in Non-Valvular Atrial Fibrillation

Risk Factor	Score (Point)
Congestive heart failure / LV dysfunction (C)	1
Hypertension (H)	1
Age ⩾75 years (A)	2
Diabetes mellitus (D)	1
Stroke / TIA / Thromboembolism (S)	2
Vascular disease (V)	1
Age 65-74 years (A)	1
Sex category (female) (Sc)	1
Total score	9

3. HAS-BLED Score (Bleeding Risk Assessment): Hypertension (H, 1 point), abnormal renal / liver function (A, 1 point each, 1 or 2 points), stroke (S, 1 point), bleeding (B, 1 point), labile INRs (L, 1 point), elderly (E, age >65 years, 1 point), drugs or alcohol (D, 1 point each, 1 or 2 points). Score ⩽2 is low bleeding risk, ⩾3 indicates high risk.

(ii) Selection of Antithrombotic Drugs

Medications for preventing thromboembolic events in patients with atrial fibrillation include anticoagulants and antiplatelet agents. General medication selection: Patients with atrial fibrillation and a CHA2DS2-VASc score ⩾2 require warfarin or novel oral anticoagulants (NOACs). Those with a score of 0 do not need Anti-coagulation or antiplatelet therapy, while those with a score of 1 are recommended to take warfarin / NOACs or aspirin, or may forgo antithrombotic treatment.

1. Antiplatelet drugs: Aspirin 100 mg orally once daily, clopidogrel 75 mg orally once daily are far less effective than warfarin in preventing stroke in patients with atrial fibrillation. The advantage is that INR monitoring is not required. Clopidogrel combined with aspirin is also less effective than warfarin in preventing stroke.

2. Vitamin K antagonist—Warfarin

(1) Cardioversion: For paroxysmal or persistent atrial fibrillation, if cardio-version is planned and atrial fibrillation duration is <48 hours, anti-coagulation is not required pre-cardioversion. If duration is uncertain or ⩾48 hours, there are two anti-coagulation strategies clinically:

1) Start warfarin Anti-coagulation to achieve INR 2.0-3.0, then cardio-vert after 3 weeks.

2) Perform trans-esophageal echocardiography; if no atrial thrombus, give intravenous heparin and cardio-vert. Post-cardio version, continue heparin and warfarin until INR⩾2.0, then stop

heparin and continue warfarin. After cardioversion, anti-coagulate for at least 4 weeks; decision on long-term Anti-coagulation depends on the patient's stratified thromboembolism risk.

(2) Routine: Initial warfarin dose 2-3 mg/day, onset 2-4 days, peak therapeutic effect at 5-7 days. Therefore, INR should be monitored 1-2 times weekly initially. Once stable (3 consecutive INRs within therapeutic range), monitor every 1-2 months and adjust warfarin dose according to INR, aiming for 2.0-3.0.

(3) NOACs: These specifically inhibit a key step in the coagulation cascade, achieving Anti-coagulation while significantly reducing bleeding risk. Examples include the direct thrombin inhibitor dabigatran and the direct factor Xa inhibitors rivaroxaban, apixaban, and edoxaban.

Dabigatran 110 mg twice daily or 150 mg twice daily; rivaroxaban 20 mg once daily; apixaban 5 mg twice daily; edoxaban 60 mg or 30 mg once daily. For elderly (≥75 years), moderate renal impairment (creatinine clearance 0.50-0.85 mL/s), and other high bleeding risk factors, dabigatran dose should be reduced to avoid severe bleeding. All NOACs are contraindicated in end-stage renal disease; warfarin remains the anticoagulant of choice in such cases (Table 3-8).

Table 3-8 Recommended NOAC Dosing for Different Degrees of Renal Impairment

Creatinine Clearance (mL/s)	Dabigatran	Rivaroxaban	Apixaban	Edoxaban
≥0.85	150 mg twice daily	20 mg once daily	5 mg/2.5 mg twice daily	60 mg/30 mg once daily
0.50-0.85	110 mg twice daily	15 mg once daily	5 mg/2.5 mg twice daily	30 mg/15 mg once daily
0.25-0.50	Not recommended	15 mg once daily	Not recommended	Not recommended
<0.25	Not recommended	Not recommended	Not recommended	Not recommended

(iii) Precautions for the Use of Anticoagulant Drugs

1. The value of NOACs in valvular atrial fibrillation patients remains to be explored. Valvular atrial fibrillation refers to atrial fibrillation associated with rheumatic mitral stenosis, mechanical or biological heart valve prostheses, or mitral valve repair. Patients with valvular atrial fibrillation should receive warfarin anti-coagulation therapy.

2. Antithrombotic therapy after percutaneous coronary intervention (PCI) in atrial fibrillation patients. For stable coronary artery disease (SCAD) patients with atrial fibrillation, CHA2DS2-VASc score≥2, and HAS-BLED≤2, it is recommended to administer an oral anticoagulant plus aspirin 100 mg/d and clopidogrel 75 mg/d for at least 1 month after bare-metal stent or new-generation drug-eluting stent implantation, followed by an oral anticoagulant plus aspirin 100 mg/d or clopidogrel 75 mg/d for up to 1 year. For acute coronary syndrome (ACS) patients with atrial fibrillation and HAS-BLED≤2, it is recommended to administer an oral anticoagulant plus aspirin 100 mg/d and clopidogrel 75 mg/d for 6 months, regardless of stent type, followed by an oral anticoagulant plus aspirin 100 mg/d or clopidogrel 75 mg/d for up to 1 year. For coronary artery disease patients (including SCAD and ACS) with HAS-BLED≥3 requiring oral Anti-coagulation, it is recommended to administer an oral anticoagulant plus aspirin 100 mg/d and clopidogrel 75 mg/d for at least 1 month, regardless

of stent type, followed by an oral anticoagulant plus aspirin 100 mg/d or clopidogrel 75 mg/d (duration based on clinical circumstances). During the stable period of coronary artery disease (1 year after myocardial infarction or PCI) without coronary events, long-term oral anti-coagulation (warfarin or NOAC) monotherapy can be considered.

3. Anti-coagulation therapy for thromboembolic patients. Anti-coagulation therapy is not recommended within 2 weeks of an ischemic stroke. If there is no intracranial hemorrhage or hemorrhagic transformation after 2 weeks, anti-coagulation therapy should be initiated, following the same principles as for general atrial fibrillation patients. For atrial fibrillation patients with transient ischemic attack (TIA), anti-coagulation therapy should be initiated as soon as possible after ruling out cerebral infarction or hemorrhage. NOACs are also effective for secondary stroke prevention. If central or peripheral thromboembolic events occur during warfarin anti-coagulation therapy in atrial fibrillation patients, and the anti-coagulation intensity is already within the therapeutic range, increasing the warfarin intensity to achieve an INR of 2.5-3.0 is preferable to adding another antiplatelet drug. If thromboembolic events occur while taking a low-dose NOAC, switching to a higher dose can be considered.

4. Long-term oral warfarin therapy

(1) If the INR has been stable previously, and an occasional INR elevation occurs but does not exceed 3.5, no dose adjustment is necessary immediately. Recheck the INR in 2 days, or reduce the weekly warfarin dose by 10%-15%. If the INR is >4.0 without bleeding, warfarin can be withheld for 1 or several doses, typically for 3 days.

(2) In cases of trauma or minor bleeding, apply pressure to stop the bleeding and observe. If bleeding continues, warfarin can be stopped, and oral vitamin K_1 (10-20 mg) can be administered, which generally terminates the anticoagulant effect of warfarin within 12-24 hours.

(3) For emergency surgery or severe bleeding, intravenous vitamin K_1 (5-10 mg) can be considered. If the effect is inadequate, additional vitamin K_1 can be given, and fresh frozen plasma can be transfused to increase coagulation factors. Prothrombin complex concentrates can more effectively and rapidly reverse excessive anti-coagulation-induced bleeding.

5. After intracranial hemorrhage, Anti-coagulation therapy can be re-initiated 2-4 weeks later. As NOACs significantly reduce the risk of intracranial hemorrhage compared to warfarin, switching to NOACs can be considered for these patients.

(iv) Interruption and Bridging of Antithrombotic Therapy

Bridging therapy refers to the short-term use of unfractionated heparin or low molecular weight heparin as a substitute for Anti-coagulation during warfarin interruption.

1. Classification of Bleeding Risk for Surgical Procedures and Interventions

(1) Procedures and interventions not requiring discontinuation of anticoagulants:

Dental: Extraction of 1-3 teeth, periodontal surgery, abscess drainage, implant positioning.

Ophthalmologic: Cataract or glaucoma surgery, non-surgical endoscopic examinations.

Superficial procedures: Such as abscess drainage, minor skin excisions.

(2) Low bleeding risk procedures and interventions:

Endoscopic biopsy, prostate or bladder biopsy, electrophysiology study and radio-frequency ablation for supra-ventricular tachycardia (including left-sided ablation via transseptal approach), angiography, pacemaker or implantable cardioverter-defibrillator (ICD) implantation (unless anatomically complex, e.g., congenital heart disease).

(3) High bleeding risk procedures and interventions:

Complex left-sided ablation (pulmonary vein isolation, ventricular rate control ablation), spinal or epidural anesthesia, diagnostic lumbar puncture, thoracic surgery, abdominal surgery, major orthopedic surgery, liver biopsy, transurethral resection of the prostate, kidney biopsy.

2. For atrial fibrillation patients receiving warfarin who require non-emergent surgery or procedures with bleeding risk, the following treatment strategies can be adopted.

(1) For patients with a lower thromboembolic risk or who have restored sinus rhythm, bridging therapy may not be necessary. Warfarin can be discontinued for 1 week until the INR returns to the normal range, and warfarin can be re-initiated once hemostasis is adequate.

(2) For patients with a higher thromboembolic risk (mechanical heart valve prosthesis, history of stroke, CHA2DS2-VASc score ≥2), bridging therapy is typically used. For most patients, warfarin is stopped 5 days before surgery, and when the INR is <2.0 (usually 2 days before surgery), full-dose unfractionated heparin or low molecular weight heparin is initiated. Intravenous unfractionated heparin is continued until 6 hours before surgery, or subcutaneous unfractionated heparin or low molecular weight heparin is discontinued 24 hours before surgery. Based on the surgical bleeding risk, heparin anti-coagulation is re-initiated 12-24 hours after surgery; for high bleeding risk procedures, anti-coagulation can be delayed until 48-72 hours after surgery, and warfarin is also restarted.

(3) If the INR is >1.5 but the patient requires early surgery, a low dose of oral vitamin K (1-2 mg) can be given to rapidly normalize the INR.

3. Patients taking non-vitamin K antagonist oral anticoagulants (NOACs) do not require heparin bridging during the perioperative period.

(1) For elective surgery: For low bleeding risk or procedures with easy hemostasis (e.g., dental, cataract, or glaucoma surgery), it is recommended to stop the NOAC 12-24 hours before surgery; for higher bleeding risk surgeries, the NOAC should be stopped at least 24 hours before, with individualized assessment of the stop time based on the patient's renal function; for extremely high bleeding risk procedures (e.g., spinal anesthesia, epidural anesthesia, and lumbar puncture), it is recommended to stop the NOAC more than 48 hours before surgery. After surgery, close monitoring for bleeding is necessary, and typically the NOAC can be restarted 6-8 hours after surgery if hemostasis is adequate; otherwise, the optimal time to resume the NOAC should be determined within 48-72 hours after surgery, based on the patient's bleeding risk and the possibility of further surgery.

(2) For emergency surgical patients, the NOAC should be discontinued; if the surgery can be delayed, it should be performed at least 12 hours (preferably 24 hours) after the last dose; if the surgery cannot be delayed, the bleeding risk should be assessed against the urgency and necessity of the procedure.

(v) Transitioning between Warfarin and NOACs

1. Transitioning from warfarin to NOAC: Discontinue warfarin, check the INR, and immediately initiate the NOAC when the INR is <2.

2. Transitioning from NOAC to warfarin: When transitioning from an NOAC to warfarin, both agents should be administered concomitantly until the INR reaches the target range.

3. Transitioning between NOACs: When transitioning from one NOAC to another, the new NOAC can be started at the next scheduled dose time; patients with impaired renal function may require a delayed dose.

4. Transitioning between NOACs and heparins: When transitioning from a parenteral anticoagulant to an NOAC, the NOAC can be started after discontinuing unfractionated heparin, or at the next scheduled injection for low molecular weight heparin. When transitioning from an NOAC to a parenteral anticoagulant, the parenteral agent should be administered at the next scheduled dose time.

5. Transitioning from antiplatelet agents to NOACs: An NOAC can be started after discontinuing aspirin or clopidogrel.

Ⅱ Control of Ventricular Rate

1. General Principles: Assess the severity of atrial fibrillation symptoms, hemodynamic status, presence of heart failure, and potential precipitating factors comprehensively.

2. Recommended Medications

(1) Oral beta-blockers or non-dihydropyridine calcium channel blockers (verapamil, diltiazem) are recommended for ventricular rate control in paroxysmal, persistent, and permanent atrial fibrillation.

(2) Intravenous beta-blockers (esmolol, metoprolol) or non-dihydropyridine calcium channel blockers (verapamil, diltiazem) are recommended for ventricular rate control in acute atrial fibrillation without pre-excitation syndrome. Intravenous amiodarone is effective for acute atrial fibrillation without pre-excitation syndrome. If hemodynamically unstable, proceed directly to synchronized cardioversion.

(3) For symptomatic atrial fibrillation patients, a ventricular rate control strategy (resting heart rate <80 bpm) is reasonable and feasible.

(4) For patients with rapid ventricular rate, significant symptoms, and inadequate response to medical therapy, while rhythm control is not suitable, atrioventricular node ablation and permanent pacemaker implantation can be performed for ventricular rate control.

Ⅲ Rhythm Control

1. Anti-coagulation before and after cardioversion

(1) For patients with atrial fibrillation or atrial flutter lasting $\geqslant 48$ hours or of unknown duration, regardless of CHA2DS2-VASc score or the method of cardioversion (electrical or pharmacological), anti-coagulation with warfarin or NOACs is recommended for at least 3 weeks before and 4 weeks after cardiover-sion.

(2) For patients with atrial fibrillation or atrial flutter lasting $\geqslant 48$ hours or of unknown duration with hemodynamic instability requiring immediate cardioversion, anti-coagulation should be initiated promptly.

(3) For patients with atrial fibrillation or atrial flutter lasting $\geqslant 48$ hours or of unknown

duration, if anti-coagulation has been less than 3 weeks, trans-esophageal echocardiography can be performed before cardioversion. If no left atrial thrombus is present and anti-coagulation has been therapeutic before the trans-esophageal echocardiogram, cardioversion can proceed, followed by at least 4 weeks of anti-coagulation.

(4) For patients with atrial fibrillation or atrial flutter lasting $<$48 hours and at high risk for stroke, intravenous heparin, low molecular weight heparin, or a NOAC is recommended as soon as possible before or immediately after cardioversion, followed by long-term anti-coagulation. The need for long-term anti-coagulation after cardioversion depends on the assessment of thromboembolic risk.

2. The choice of anti-arrhythmic drugs for cardioversion depends on the underlying heart disease and cardiac function. Flecainide, dofetilide, propafenone, and ibutilide are generally recommended as first-line anti-arrhythmic drugs for atrial fibrillation, with amiodarone as a second-line option.

3. Maintenance of Sinus Rhythm after cardioversion

(1) Based on the patient's underlying heart disease, other conditions, and cardiac function, select an appropriate drug from amiodarone, dofetilide, propafenone, sotalol, or dronedarone for long-term maintenance of sinus rhythm.

(2) Amiodarone is effective for maintaining sinus rhythm, but due to its significant adverse effects, it should only be considered when other drugs are ineffective or contraindicated, and risk assessment is necessary.

(3) For tachycardia-induced cardiomyopathy induced by atrial fibrillation, pharmacological management to sustain sinus rhythm is advisable.

Ⅳ Consultation Process

1. Obtain a detailed medical history: Identify potential precipitating factors for atrial fibrillation episodes, such as infection, electrolyte disturbances, psychological factors, myocardial ischemia, or heart failure exacerbation. Inquire about accompanying symptoms during atrial fibrillation episodes, such as headache, dizziness, chest pain, chest tightness, dyspnea, diarrhea, or abdominal pain. Thoroughly understand the patient's past medical history, especially cardiovascular and cerebrovascular conditions.

2. Perform a comprehensive physical examination, including assessment of lung sounds, heart rhythm, heart murmurs, and peripheral edema.

3. Calculate the CHA2DS2-VASc and HAS-BLED scores for all atrial fibrillation patients.

4. Closely monitor for bleeding events after initiating anticoagulant therapy. For patients on warfarin, regularly monitor coagulation function.

Section 8 Catheter Ablation for Atrial Fibrillation

Ⅰ Indications

1. Symptomatic paroxysmal atrial fibrillation refractory to anti-arrhythmic drugs, or

recurrent paroxysmal atrial fibrillation.

2. For symptomatic persistent atrial fibrillation of relatively short duration, refractory to anti-arrhythmic drugs, and without significant structural heart disease, catheter ablation can be a reasonable choice.

3. For symptomatic atrial fibrillation patients with heart failure and/or reduced left ventricular ejection fraction (LVEF), catheter ablation can be a reasonable choice, but the main symptoms and/or heart failure should be related to atrial fibrillation.

Ⅱ Contraindications for Catheter Ablation

1. Atrial fibrillation patients with contraindications to Anti-coagulation therapy are not suitable for catheter ablation.

2. Presence of thrombus in the left atrium or left atrial appendage.

3. General surgical contraindications: infection, severe hepatic or renal dysfunction, etc.

Ⅲ Perioperative Anti-coagulation Strategy for Atrial Fibrillation

1. The traditional perioperative Anti-coagulation strategy for atrial fibrillation catheter ablation is to discontinue warfarin and use low molecular weight heparin bridging therapy. Alternatively, warfarin can be continued, maintaining an INR at 2-3, which may reduce perioperative thromboembolic events without increasing the risk of severe bleeding.

2. Intravenous heparin is used for anti-coagulation during atrial fibrillation catheter ablation. To reduce the risk of bleeding at the puncture site, the activated clotting time (ACT) should be less than 250 seconds before sheath removal; otherwise, protamine can be used to reverse heparin. Warfarin is started 4-6 hours after sheath removal, in combination with low molecular weight heparin bridging until the INR is therapeutic, or a non-vitamin K antagonist oral anticoagulant (NOAC) is initiated.

3. Anti-coagulation therapy after atrial fibrillation ablation: A consensus has been reached to provide anti-coagulation for the first 2 months after ablation. However, the necessity of anti-coagulation beyond 2 months post-ablation remains unclear.

Ⅳ Follow-up

1. The first 3 months after ablation is considered a "blanking period", during which episodes of atrial fibrillation, atrial flutter, or atrial tachycardia are not considered recurrences.

2. Recurrent atrial fibrillation, atrial flutter, or atrial tachycardia after ablation is recommended for repeat ablation.

3. The use of anti-arrhythmic drugs is reasonable within 1-3 months after ablation.

4. Patients at high risk for stroke (CHADS2 score ⩾2) should receive indefinite anti-coagulation after ablation, especially those aged ⩾75 years or with a history of stroke or transient ischemic attack (TIA).

Ⅴ Inpatient Consultation Process by the Attending Physician

1. Screen for atrial fibrillation patients suitable for catheter ablation and admit for elective

ablation after excluding contraindications.

2. Explain the necessity, risks, surgical costs, and post-procedural follow-up considerations to the patient and family in detail.

3. Calculate the CHA2DS2-VASc and HAS-BLED scores for each atrial fibrillation patient.

Section 9 Temporary Cardiac Pacing

I Definition

Temporary cardiac pacing refers to the use of bipolar endocardial or epicardial electrodes connected to an external pacemaker for diagnostic and therapeutic purposes.

II Principles and Components

A temporary cardiac pacemaker is a battery-powered device that can generate a continuous, stable electrical pulse. The specific waveform of the weak electrical current can stimulate the pacing function or induction function of the heart when dysfunctional, but with preserved excitability, contractility, and myocardial fiber conduction. It acts as a substitute for the normal pacemaker, effectively stimulating the myocardium to contract. The device consists of a pulse generator and electrode leads. Temporary pacing utilizes bipolar catheter electrodes, with stainless steel leads for high resistance to bending, enclosed in a plastic sheath with moderate rigidity and flexibility for easy venous insertion. The tip electrode (distal or cathode) is cylindrical with a flat end for easy removal, while the other electrode (ring or anode) is located 1 cm away, forming a ring shape. The two electrodes are insulated from each other within the catheter (Figure 3-15).

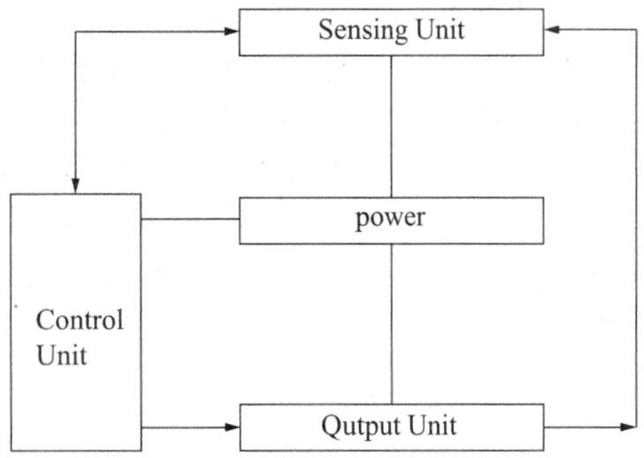

Figure 3-15 Structure diagram of Pulse Generator

III Indications

1. Therapeutic Applications

(1) Slow idioventricular rhythms, symptomatic severe sinus bradycardia, sinus arrest, second-degree or third-degree atrioventricular block.

(2) Reversible factors causing bradyarrhythmias, such as acute myocardial infarction, acute myocarditis, hyperkalemia, drug toxicity, etc.

(3) Recurrent Adams-Stokes syndrome with an indication for permanent pacemaker implantation, but temporary pacing is required due to other reasons precluding immediate permanent pacemaker placement; or for pacemaker-dependent patients requiring replacement of a depleted or malfunctioning permanent pacemaker.

(4) Prior to cardioversion in patients receiving significant doses of anti-arrhythmic drugs that

depress myocardial function, to prevent post-shock asystole.

(5) For patients suspected of sinus node dysfunction, requiring drug therapy or cardioversion.

(6) Prolonged QT interval from various causes, with torsades de pointes ventricular tachycardia.

(7) Paroxysmal supra-ventricular tachycardia, atrial fibrillation, or atrial flutter requiring overdrive suppression.

(8) As a protective measure during major surgical procedures in patients at risk for arrhythmias.

(9) In acute myocardial infarction: Myocardial ischemia can cause sinus node or atrioventricular node dysfunction (sinus arrest, second-degree Type Ⅱ or third-degree atrioventricular block), leading to hemodynamic changes. Temporary pacing can prevent syncope, improve hemodynamics, and avoid further exacerbation of myocardial ischemia. Newly developed intraventricular conduction defects can be an indication for prophylactic pacing. The temporary pacing lead can be removed once sinus node function or atrioventricular conduction recovers; otherwise, permanent pacemaker implantation is required.

(10) Cardiac Surgery:

1) Prophylactic use: In conditions such as Ebstein's anomaly, persistent atrioventricular septal defect, or corrected transposition of the great arteries, surgery near the atrioventricular junction may damage the conduction system, necessitating temporary pacing after thoracotomy.

2) Therapeutic use: For congenital heart disease repairs resulting in atrioventricular block or severe bradycardia, temporary pacing can be used until local edema resolves.

2. Diagnostic Applications: Primarily used for electrophysiological studies.

Ⅳ Pacing Modes and Implantation Methods

1. Pacing Modes

(1) Transvenous endocardial pacing: Currently the most common cardiac pacing method. In emergencies, without fluoroscopy, a bipolar pacing lead or balloon-tipped floating pacing lead can be inserted via the internal jugular or subclavian vein, with positioning guided by intracardiac electrocardiography for rapid bedside pacing (Figure 3-20). For elective endocardial pacing, the femoral vein approach is preferred, followed by the subclavian, internal jugular, or external jugular vein.

(2) Epicardial pacing: Generally used for emergency or prophylactic pacing during open-heart surgery. The electrode is a fine silver wire, with the tip slightly curved into a spiral shape by the surgeon, then sewn into the myocardium, with the tail end exiting the thoracotomy for external temporary pacing. The lead is removed after pacing is terminated.

(3) Transcutaneous pacing: Paddle electrodes are used, with the cathode placed at V_3 and the anode between the left scapular angle and spine. The pacing threshold depends on the patient's chest wall thickness, typically 40-80 mA. This simple, non-invasive method without sterile preparation or fluoroscopy is suitable for emergency resuscitation of cardiac arrest. However, patients may experience discomfort from the strong electrical stimulus, as well as chest muscle contractions, retching, and local skin burning sensation. Most patients can tolerate the procedure

if the pacing threshold is not too high.

(4) Trans-esophageal left atrial pacing: Using a specialized bipolar electrode (5 mm wide, 3-5 cm inter-electrode distance) or a standard bipolar pacing lead, introduced via the nose or mouth into the esophagus at the level of the left atrium. Commonly used for evaluating sinus node function and overdrive suppression of tachyarrhythmias.

(5) Transcutaneous cardiac pacing: This method allows for both artificial ventilation and cardiac pacing during resuscitation.

2. Implantation Method: Transvenous endocardial pacing via the femoral vein is the most commonly used temporary pacing technique.

(1) Venipuncture: The femoral vein lies medial to the femoral artery, which serves as a landmark for indirect localization. The right femoral vein is generally preferred due to the more direct path for lead placement into the right ventricle. Palpate for the most prominent arterial pulsation in the inguinal crease, move 2-3 cm inferiorly, and infiltrate with local anesthetic. Puncture the skin medial to this point, taking care to avoid the artery. Assist localization and artery protection by palpating the femoral artery with the other hand during venipuncture. Advance the needle while applying gentle aspiration; blood return indicates venous entry. Remove the syringe, insert a guidewire through the needle, remove the needle while leaving the guidewire in place, then pass a vessel dilator over the guidewire, followed by the pacing lead, which is advanced under fluoroscopic guidance to the right ventricular apex (Figure 3-16).

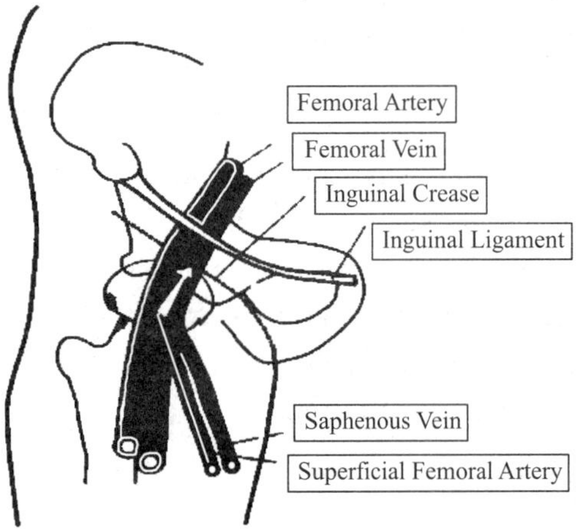

Figure 3-16 Femoral Vein Puncture

(2) Right ventricular lead positioning: Similar to permanent pacemaker implantation, including the following steps: ① Pass the lead across the tricuspid valve; ② Position the lead tip stably in the right ventricle; ③ Acceptable pacing threshold (ideally < 1 mA or 1 V, not exceeding 2 mA); ④ Stable lead position with deep breathing, coughing, or minor body movements; ⑤ The ideal temporary pacing position is the right ventricular apex, with the lead tip pointing inferiorly and leftward on the left anterior oblique view (Figure 3-17).

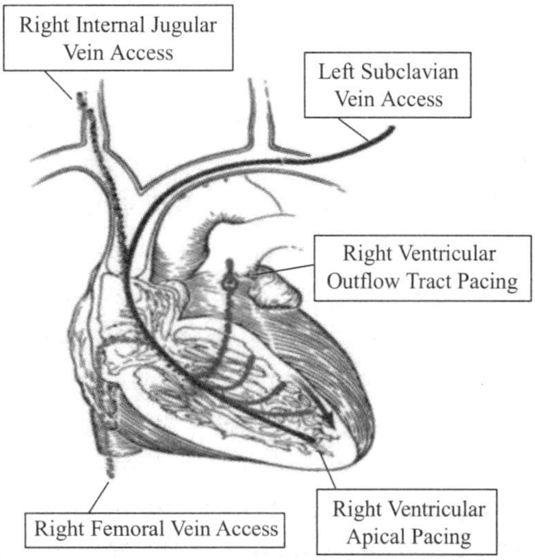

Figure 3-17 Position of the Pacing Electrode Catheter

(3) Lead fixation: After connecting the temporary pacemaker to the lead, pacing

can commence. The pacing output is typically 2-3 times the threshold, with the rate adjusted according to clinical circumstances. A chest X-ray should be obtained immediately after the procedure (during the same session for DSA) to confirm lead position (Figures 3-18, 3-19).

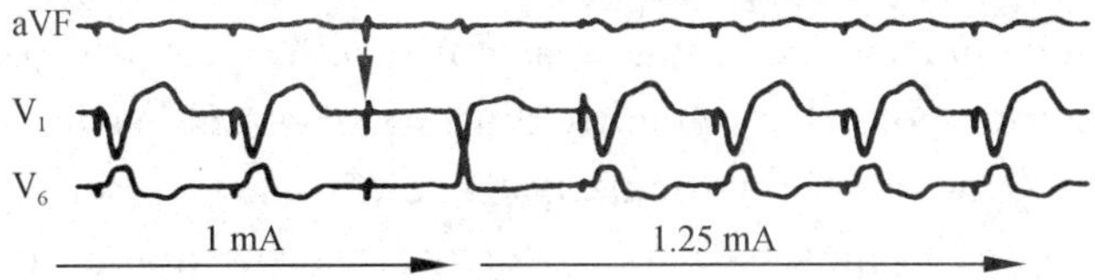

Figure 3-18 Threshold Testing

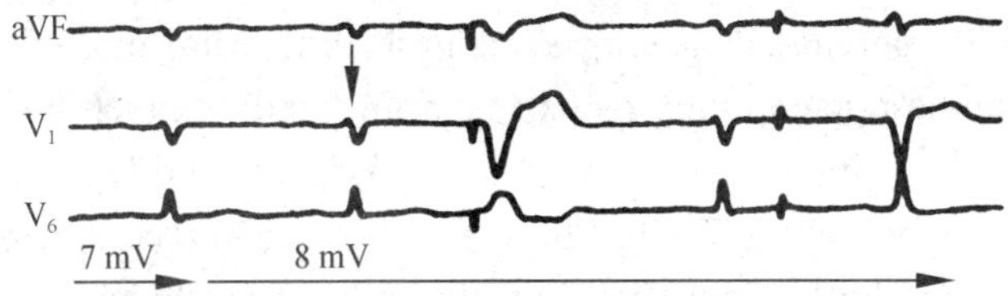

Figure 3-19 Sensitivity Testing

(4) Postoperative care: ① Daily 12-lead electrocardiogram; ② Daily measurement of pacing threshold and sensitivity; ③ Dedicated personnel for monitoring and battery replacement (Figure 3-20).

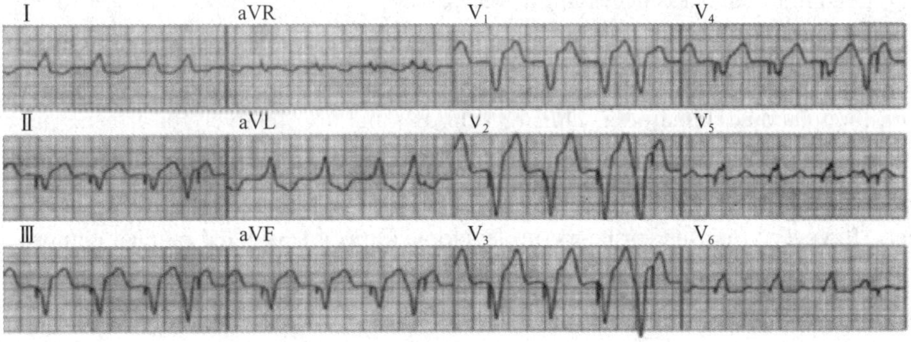

Figure 3-20 ECG of Right Ventricular Apical Pacing

V Procedure-Related Complications and Management

Complications of temporary cardiac pacing are common, with the incidence closely related to the operator's technical proficiency, duration of lead retention, and postoperative care of the pacing system.

1. Lead dislodgement: The most common complication of temporary pacing. Unlike permanent leads, temporary pacing leads have a cylindrical tip without active or passive fixation mechanisms, making dislodgement more likely as the lead does not embed firmly in the trabeculae. Emergency pacing is performed rapidly, without the stringent positioning required for permanent pacemakers, resulting in less stable lead positioning and a higher risk of tip

dislodgement causing pacing failure. Sometimes, pacing can continue, but with an increased threshold or changed QRS morphology. Electrocardiographic signs of dislodgement include intermittent or failure of capture, while fluoroscopy reveals lead tip migration, necessitating repositioning. For minor dislodgement with a slightly increased threshold, increasing the output voltage and pulse width from the external pacemaker may restore adequate pacing.

2. Myocardial Perforation: Due to the rigid nature of plastic pacing leads, patients with enlarged hearts, thin myocardium, particularly those with acute inferior (right ventricular) myocardial infarction, are at increased risk of myocardial perforation if the lead tip exerts excessive pressure, is positioned too high, or if the patient is agitated postoperatively. Clinical manifestations may include precordial pain, diaphragmatic contractions, pacing interruption or intermittent pacing, increase in pacing threshold, precordial or pericardial friction rub, conversion of left bundle branch block pattern to right bundle branch block pattern on paced electrocardiograms, pericardial effusion on echocardiography, and lead tip protruding beyond the cardiac silhouette on the chest X-ray. These findings can serve as evidence of myocardial perforation. Withdrawing the lead tip back into the right ventricle and repositioning typically resolves these symptoms, without leading to cardiac tamponade or severe consequences. However, if cardiac tamponade does occur, immediate pericardiocentesis for decompression is warranted, and surgical pericardial window may be required in some cases.

3. Lead Fracture: The rigid and inflexible nature of plastic leads, coupled with prolonged implantation and patient mobility, can result in partial lead fracture, causing intermittent or loss of pacing. Lead replacement is necessary in such cases.

4. Puncture-related Complications: These complications are closely related to the operator's experience. Common complications include:

(1) Subcutaneous Hematoma: During venous puncture, inadvertent arterial puncture or improper local compression can lead to subcutaneous bleeding, resulting in hematoma formation, pseudo-aneurysm, or arteriovenous fistula. Small hematomas generally require no specific treatment. However, if a pseudo-aneurysm develops, ultrasound-guided manual compression for 20-30 minutes followed by compressive dressing is typically effective in most cases, with only a small proportion requiring vascular surgical intervention.

(2) Infection: As the pacing lead is externalized and connected to an external pacemaker, inadequate local care or prolonged lead implantation can predispose to local or systemic (bacteremia) infections. In general, these infections are mild and can be controlled with antibiotics or lead removal. Therefore, temporary pacing leads should ideally be removed within one week. In the event of bacteremia, prompt lead removal, blood cultures, and targeted antibiotic therapy are warranted. If temporary pacing is still required, a new temporary lead can be inserted through a different venous access while administering antibiotics.

5. Arrhythmias: Placement of any intracardiac lead can potentially induce arrhythmias. The most common arrhythmia observed during temporary pacing lead insertion is ventricular ectopic rhythm, which can often be reduced or eliminated by adjusting the lead tip position and reducing the lead tip pressure. Additionally, electrolyte disturbances, particularly hypokalemia, can increase the risk of ventricular arrhythmias and should be corrected preoperatively.

6. Thrombosis: Temporary pacing via the femoral venous route is associated with an increased risk of deep vein thrombosis, which may be related to postoperative immobilization, prolonged lead implantation, and underlying pro-thrombotic conditions. Therefore, the duration of temporary pacing should be minimized. If prolonged lead retention is necessary, postoperative prophylactic low-molecular-weight heparin should be considered. If thrombosis occurs, immediate anti-coagulation with heparin is warranted, and the pacing lead should be removed only after thrombus resolution to avoid the risk of pulmonary embolism.

Ⅵ Common Clinical Scenarios

1. What Are the Causes of Poor Pacing Function or Sensing Abnormalities After Temporary Pacing?

In most cases, lead dislodgement is the underlying cause. If only the pacing threshold is elevated, increasing the pacing output voltage can be attempted initially. If this is ineffective, prompt bedside chest X-ray should be performed. If minor dislodgement is noted without the lead tip protruding beyond the cardiac silhouette, bedside lead repositioning can be attempted. If this fails, fluoroscopic (DSA) guidance is necessary for lead repositioning. If the chest X-ray reveals the lead tip protruding beyond the cardiac silhouette, immediate DSA-guided lead repositioning is warranted. In facilities with bedside echocardiography and pericardiocentesis capabilities, the original lead can be withdrawn, the lead position readjusted, followed by post-procedural echocardiographic evaluation and close monitoring for cardiac tamponade. If cardiac tamponade occurs, pericardiocentesis can be immediately performed for drainage.

2. Duration of Temporary Pacing Catheter Placement: When Should the Temporary Pacemaker Be Removed?

Temporary pacing is generally recommended for no more than 2 weeks, with a maximum duration of 4 weeks. After reversible factors causing bradyarrhythmias have been addressed and the patient regains an intrinsic rhythm, the pacing rate can be gradually decreased. If monitoring confirms an intrinsic rhythm, the temporary pacemaker can be removed. For patients who received temporary pacing as a bridge to major surgery, the temporary pacemaker should be removed as soon as possible postoperatively. Prior to removal, the patient's rhythm should be closely monitored. If an intrinsic rhythm is present, immediate removal can be performed. However, if the patient remains pacing-dependent, the pacing rate should be gradually decreased until an intrinsic rhythm emerges, and removal can proceed once a stable intrinsic rhythm is observed.

3. How to Manage Difficulties in Passing the Pacing Catheter Through the Tricuspid Valve?

The pacing lead can be formed into a curve within the right atrium or withdrawn into the inferior vena cava, allowing the lead tip to enter the hepatic veins and create a curve before advancing into the right ventricular apex.

4. Is Routine Anti-coagulation Therapy Required After Temporary Pace-maker Insertion?

Temporary pacing via the femoral venous route is associated with a relatively higher risk of venous thrombosis. Currently, there is no accurate data on the incidence of thrombosis during temporary pacing lead implantation. However, studies on permanent pacemaker implantation suggest a venous thrombosis rate exceeding 30%, indicating the need for Anti-coagulation during lead implantation and awareness of potential thromboembolic events during lead removal.

5. Miscellaneous Details

(1) Exercise caution when moving patients and secure the temporary pacemaker appropriately. Conscious patients should maintain bedrest and limit activity after pacemaker placement, while unconscious patients should be minimally disturbed to prevent lead dislodgement or right ventricular perforation.

(2) For patients undergoing surgery requiring protective pacing, continuous electrocautery should be avoided to prevent pacemaker over-sensing. Alternatively, the pacemaker can be programmed to VOO mode.

(3) Hyperkalemia and metabolic acidosis can increase the pacing threshold, leading to loss of capture, while hypoxemia and hypokalemia can decrease the pacing threshold, potentially inducing ventricular fibrillation.

(4) Diaphragmatic stimulation is primarily caused by deep lead positioning, with the electrode in close proximity to the phrenic nerve. Patients may experience abdominal pulsations or intractable hiccups, which can be alleviated by gently withdrawing the lead.

Ⅶ Consultation Process

1. For patients meeting the indications for temporary cardiac pacing and without contraindications, temporary pacing should be performed promptly to prevent Stokes-Adams attacks or sudden cardiac death.

2. During the procedure, be vigilant for potential complications such as subcutaneous hematoma, pneumothorax, myocardial perforation, cardiac tamponade, inadvertent subclavian or femoral artery puncture.

3. Postoperatively, closely monitor pacemaker function, including pacing and sensing parameters.

4. For patients meeting the indications for permanent pacemaker implantation, arrange for early permanent pacemaker placement.

Section 10 Clinical Significance and Management of Various Premature Contractions

Ⅰ Definition

Premature beats, also known as premature contractions, refer to the premature occurrence of impulses from an ectopic focus (such as the atria, ventricles, or atrioventricular junction) other than the sinus node, leading to early heart contractions. On an electrocardiogram (ECG), this manifests as premature P-QRS complexes.

Premature contractions are the most common form of ectopic rhythms and can be classified into three types based on their origin: atrial, atrioventricular junctional, and ventricular.

Ventricular premature contractions (VPCs) are the most prevalent, followed by atrial premature contractions (APCs), while atrioventricular junctional premature contractions are relatively uncommon. Premature contractions can occur sporadically or frequently, irregularly or regularly after each one or several normal beats, forming bigeminal or trigeminal rhythms. They commonly occur in conditions such as coronary artery disease, rheumatic heart disease, hypertensive heart disease, cardiomyopathies, and can also be observed in healthy individuals or in association with quinidine, procainamide, digoxin, or antimony toxicity, hypokalemia, cardiac surgery, or mechanical stimulation during cardiac catheterization procedures.

Ⅱ Etiologies

1. Structural Heart Disease: Any structural heart disease can lead to premature contractions, commonly observed in coronary artery disease, advanced valvular heart disease, cardiomyopathies, myocarditis, thyrotoxic heart disease, mitral valve prolapse, and heart failure.

2. Drugs and Electrolyte Disturbances: Digoxin, antimony compounds, quinidine, sympathomimetic agents, chloroform, cyclopropane anesthetics, acid-base imbalances, and electrolyte disturbances can precipitate premature contractions.

3. Neurological Abnormalities: Premature contractions can be triggered by emotional stress, anxiety, fatigue, indigestion, excessive smoking, alcohol consumption, strong tea, insomnia, or sudden positional changes.

4. Endocrine Disorders: Conditions such as hyperthyroidism, adrenal disorders, and anemia can precipitate premature contractions.

5. Healthy Individuals: Premature contractions can occur in healthy individuals across all age groups, although less common in children and more prevalent in middle-aged and older adults. This may be related to autonomic nervous system dysfunction.

Ⅲ Diagnosis

1. History and Symptoms: Premature contractions can be asymptomatic or present with palpitations or a skipped beat sensation. Frequent premature contractions can cause fatigue, dizziness, or exacerbate angina or heart failure in patients with pre-existing heart disease. Some patients may experience severe anxiety, insomnia, and a vicious cycle due to frequent premature contractions. The medical history should be carefully reviewed for conditions such as hypertension, coronary artery disease, cardiomyopathy, rheumatic heart disease, and recent illnesses, fever, diarrhea, or use of digoxin, anti-arrhythmic drugs, or diuretics, which can precipitate premature contractions.

2. Physical Examination: Auscultation may reveal an irregular rhythm with a compensatory pause following premature contractions. The first heart sound is often accentuated, while the second heart sound may be diminished or absent with premature contractions. In bigeminal or trigeminal rhythms, longer pauses can be audible after every two or three heartbeats, respectively. Premature contractions occurring between two normal beats may present as three consecutive beats. Palpation may reveal intermittent pulse deficits.

3. Diagnostic Tests: The ECG is diagnostic for premature contractions, which are

characterized by one or more premature P-QRS complexes compared to the underlying rhythm (Figures 3-21 to 3-23).

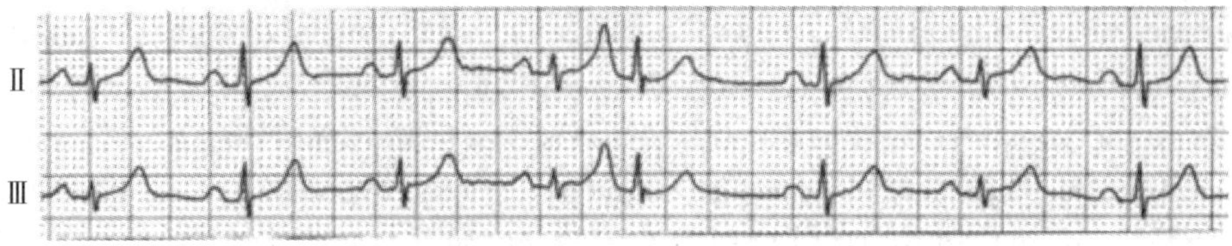

Figure 3-21 Atrial Premature Contraction

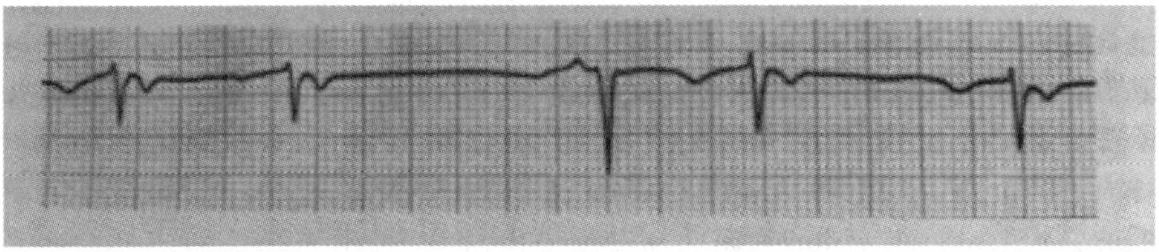

Figure 3-22 Atrioventricular Junctional Premature Contraction

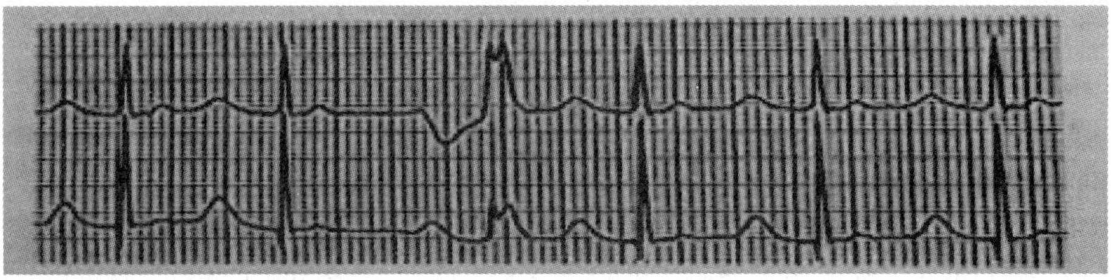

Figure 3-23 Ventricular Premature Contraction

Ⅳ Clinical Significance

In healthy individuals and patients without structural heart disease, premature contractions of various types are generally clinically insignificant. However, frequent and complex ventricular premature contractions (such as ventricular premature contraction runs, multi-focal ventricular premature contractions, or R-on-T ventricular premature contractions) can potentially degenerate into life-threatening ventricular tachyarrhythmias, but the occurrence of the latter mainly depends on the presence, type, and severity of structural heart disease. Ventricular premature contractions associated with acute myocardial infarction, coronary ischemia, cardiomyopathies, hypokalemia, digoxin or anti-arrhythmic drug toxicity, and congenital or acquired long QT syndromes are more prone to progressing to ventricular tachycardia or ventricular fibrillation. Additionally, long-term frequent ventricular premature contractions can lead to a cardiomyopathy known as tachycardia-induced cardiomyopathy, with clinical manifestations and cardiac findings similar to dilated cardiomyopathy. For individuals with ventricular premature contractions $\geqslant 5\%$, even in the absence of symptoms, follow-up is recommended to prevent the development of tachycardia-induced cardiomyopathy. If left ventricular function is already impaired without other causes of heart failure, tachycardia-induced cardiomyopathy secondary to ventricular premature contractions should be considered.

V Treatment

1. Treatment Principles: Treatment principles should be guided by the presence or absence of structural heart disease, the impact on cardiac output, and the potential for progression to severe arrhythmias. In healthy individuals or those without significant symptoms, specific treatment is generally not required. For patients without structural heart disease but with prominent symptoms, treatment aims to alleviate symptoms and eliminate precipitating factors. In patients with structural heart disease and premature contractions, the primary focus should be on treating the underlying condition, potentially combined with anti-arrhythmic drugs.

2. Anti-arrhythmic Drugs for Premature Contractions

(1) Class Ⅰa anti-arrhythmic drugs (e.g., quinidine): These moderate sodium channel blockers are broad-spectrum antiarrhythmics effective against atrial, atrioventricular junctional, and ventricular premature contractions. They are contraindicated in digoxin toxicity, pregnancy, severe hepatic or renal impairment, and hypokalemia.

(2) Class Ⅰb anti-arrhythmic drugs (e.g., phenytoin sodium): These mild sodium channel blockers are primarily used for ventricular arrhythmias, but phenytoin sodium is also effective against atrial and ventricular premature contractions associated with digoxin toxicity.

(3) Class Ⅰc anti-arrhythmic drugs (e.g., propafenone): These potent sodium channel blockers are broad-spectrum antiarrhythmics effective against ventricular premature contractions but can also induce pro-arrhythmic effects, limiting their clinical use.

(4) Class Ⅱ anti-arrhythmic drugs (beta-blockers, e.g., atenolol, metoprolol): These are often the first-line agents, blocking cardiac beta receptors and counteracting the effects of sympathetic stimulation and catecholamines. Control of atrial premature contractions or a heart rate reduction to 50-55 beats/min or lack of significant heart rate acceleration with exercise indicates an adequate dose. Metoprolol should be avoided in acute left ventricular failure, pulmonary edema, atrioventricular conduction block, chronic bronchitis, and asthma. Beta-blockers should be tapered gradually and not abruptly discontinued.

(5) Class Ⅲ anti-arrhythmic drugs (amiodarone): By reducing potassium efflux and prolonging the action potential duration and effective refractory period, amiodarone is effective but has a slow onset of action and potential adverse effects. Regular monitoring of thyroid function and chest CT is recommended to detect potential complications like drug-induced hyperthyroidism or pulmonary fibrosis. Amiodarone is reserved for cases refractory to other agents or with significant symptoms.

(6) Class Ⅳ anti-arrhythmic drugs (calcium channel blockers, e.g., verapamil, diltiazem): By blocking extracellular calcium influx, slowing atrioventricular nodal conduction, and prolonging the effective refractory period, these agents are effective against atrial premature contractions by preventing impulse transmission to the ventricles and eliminating atrioventricular nodal re-entry circuits. However, they are contraindicated in heart failure, shock, atrioventricular conduction block, and sick sinus syndrome. Concomitant use with digoxin should be avoided due to the risk of increased digoxin levels and toxicity.

For patients with premature contractions, the risks and benefits of long-term anti-arrhythmic drug therapy should be carefully considered. Class Ⅰ anti-arrhythmic drugs are contraindicated in patients with heart failure and myocardial infarction. Potentially life-threatening ventricular premature contractions often require urgent intravenous therapy. In the early phase of acute myocardial infarction, intravenous amiodarone or lidocaine can be considered. Post-myocardial infarction, in the absence of contraindications, beta-blockers or amiodarone are commonly used. In long QT syndrome, Class Ⅰ drugs are contraindicated; beta-blockers, phenytoin, or mexiletine can be used in congenital cases, while acquired cases may benefit from addressing the underlying cause and considering isoproterenol or atrial / ventricular pacing.

3. Interventional Arrhythmia Treatment: Radio-frequency catheter ablation is an effective treatment option for ventricular premature contractions in addition to anti-arrhythmic drugs. Current guidelines recommend catheter ablation for frequent ventricular premature contractions with clinical symptoms, recurrent non-sustained ventricular tachycardia, or ventricular fibrillation triggered by similar monomorphic ventricular premature contractions, as well as tachycardia-induced cardiomyopathy secondary to frequent ventricular premature contractions.

Ⅵ Common Questions in Consultation

1. Diagnostic Evaluation for Patients with Premature Contractions

(1) 12-lead or 18-lead ECG: Routine tests for diagnosis and localization of the origin of premature contractions.

(2) 24-hour Holter monitoring: Provides valuable information on the type and frequency of premature contractions, guiding treatment selection.

(3) Cardiac imaging: Primarily echocardiography, chest X-ray, and cardiac magnetic resonance imaging. Routine echocardiography can assess cardiac structure and function, while further imaging with MRI or nuclear studies may be required in some cases.

(4) Thyroid function and electrolyte tests: To rule out reversible precipitating factors.

(5) Evaluation for associated conditions: Screening for underlying conditions like coronary artery disease or hypertension.

2. Ventricular Premature Contractions Requiring Treatment: In general, infrequent ventricular premature contractions without structural heart disease do not require intervention, and lifestyle modifications to eliminate precipitating factors may be sufficient.

Intervention is typically recommended for frequent and symptomatic ventricular premature contractions, based on the "10% rule"—specifically, >10,000 ventricular premature contractions in 24 hours or >10% of total heart beats. Significant symptoms should be carefully evaluated to determine their relationship to ventricular premature contractions. Particular attention should be given to ventricular premature contractions in patients with structural heart disease, where treatment of the underlying condition and potential adjunctive anti-arrhythmic therapy is warranted. Ventricular premature contractions requiring urgent attention include those associated with dizziness, syncope, structural heart disease (e.g., coronary artery disease, acute myocardial infarction, cardiomyopathy, valvular disease), genetic arrhythmia syndromes or family history, evidence of cardiac structural / functional impairment (e.g., cardiomegaly, left ventricular ejection fraction <40%, heart failure), multi-focal or repetitive ventricular premature contractions, R-on-T ventricular premature contractions in the setting of acute myocardial infarction or QT prolongation, ventricular premature contractions sharing the same mechanism as ventricular tachycardia, and ventricular premature contractions triggering hemodynamically unstable ventricular tachycardia.

3. Risk Stratification of Ventricular Premature Contractions: The Lown grading system is commonly used for risk stratification of ventricular premature contractions, with higher grades indicating increased risk of sudden cardiac death, particularly in acute myocardial infarction patients. The Lown grading system is as follows: Grade 0—no ventricular premature contractions; Grade Ⅰ—<30 ventricular premature contractions / hour; Grade Ⅱ—>30 ventricular premature contractions / hour; Grade Ⅲ—multiform ventricular premature contractions; Grade Ⅳa—bigeminal or trigeminal ventricular premature contractions; Grade Ⅳb—ventricular tachycardia; Grade Ⅴ—R-on-T ventricular premature contractions.

Most experts currently agree that the Lown grading system is only applicable to ventricular arrhythmias in myocardial infarction patients, mainly because R-on-T ventricular premature contractions can be observed in healthy individuals and pacemaker recipients without necessarily progressing to ventricular tachycardia or fibrillation.

4. How to Assess the Risk of Ventricular Premature Contractions (VPCs). Clin-ically, the risk of VPCs is primarily assessed based on the following factors: ① Underlying cardiac conditions, such as severe myocardial infarction, severe ischemia, myocarditis, or ventricular aneurysm; ② Cardiac functional status; ③ Presence of electrolyte imbalances. In patients with good cardiac function and no structural heart disease, VPCs are generally considered benign arrhythmias. However, in patients with severe structural heart disease and significantly impaired cardiac function, such as VPCs ≥ Grade Ⅲ, the arrhythmia is considered high-risk with a possibility of sudden cardiac death.

5. Management Principles for Perioperative VPCs. Perioperative arrhythmias are relatively common and can be related to the patient's preexisting conditions or comorbidities, intraoperative anesthetic agents, electrolyte imbalances, hypoxia and carbon dioxide retention, changes in body temperature, anesthetic procedures, and surgical stimulation. The severity depends on the type of arrhythmia and the resulting hemodynamic changes. For perioperative patients with VPCs, if preoperative evaluation suggests a high likelihood of functional VPCs and there are clear indications for surgery, Holter monitoring may not be required, and surgery can proceed with close intraoperative and postoperative monitoring and management of any changes. Intraoperatively, if VPCs occur, the patient should be evaluated for potential internal environment disturbances and treated accordingly. Generally, atrial premature contractions are benign and do not require special treatment. For ventricular premature contractions, a distinction should be made between monomorphic and polymorphic forms. If monomorphic VPCs are infrequent, especially if present before anesthesia, no further treatment is needed. However, if the frequency increases significantly, treatment is required. On the other hand, if polymorphic VPCs, R-on-T phenomenon, or significant hemodynamic compromise occurs, immediate treatment is necessary, particularly if the VPCs are new-onset or associated with myocardial ischemia.

6. Indications for Catheter Ablation in Patients with VPCs. Catheter ablation for VPCs is primarily indicated in the following situations: ① VPCs associated with structural heart disease or potential for polymorphic ventricular tachycardia or ventricular fibrillation, such as those with R-on-T phenomenon or triggering ventricular fibrillation; ② Frequent (>20% of total heartbeats) and symptomatic VPCs, especially those originating from the right ventricular outflow tract, which can lead to left ventricular enlargement and dysfunction; ③ VPCs that persist despite anti-arrhythmic drug therapy or are associated with intolerable side effects; ④ Patients with frequent VPCs who are unaware of the condition, but echocardiography shows significant impairment of cardiac function. In such cases, catheter ablation may significantly improve cardiac function.

Ⅶ Consultation Process

1. Obtain a detailed medical history, focusing on cardiovascular and cerebrovascular disease history.

2. Perform routine electrocardiography, 24-hour Holter monitoring, and echocardiography to evaluate the severity of VPCs.

3. Identify the underlying cause of VPCs and rule out thyroid disorders and electrolyte imbalances. Treat the primary condition accordingly.

4. Determine the treatment approach based on the presence of structural heart disease, impact on cardiac output, and the potential for developing severe arrhythmias. In healthy individuals or those without significant symptoms, no special treatment may be required. In patients without structural heart disease but with significant symptoms, treatment aims to relieve symptoms and eliminate triggers. For patients with structural heart disease and VPCs, treatment should focus on managing the underlying condition while considering anti-arrhythmic drugs.

5. Indications for radio-frequency catheter ablation: Catheter ablation may be considered for frequent and symptomatic VPCs, recurrent ventricular tachycardia triggered by similar monomorphic VPCs, ventricular fibrillation, or tachycardia-induced cardiomyopathy due to frequent VPCs.

Chapter 4

Hypertension

Section 1 Hypertensive Emergencies

I Definition and Classification

Hypertensive emergencies include hypertensive crises and hypertensive urgencies. A hypertensive crisis refers to a sudden and significant elevation of blood pressure (generally above 180/120 mmHg) in patients with primary or secondary hypertension, often triggered by certain factors, accompanied by progressive impairment of vital target organs, such as the brain, heart, and kidneys. This includes hypertensive encephalopathy, intracranial hemorrhage (cerebral hemorrhage and subarachnoid hemorrhage), cerebral infarction, acute heart failure, pulmonary edema, acute coronary syndromes (unstable angina, non-ST-segment elevation myocardial infarction, and ST-segment elevation myocardial infarction), aortic dissection, and eclampsia. These patients require immediate blood pressure lowering (not necessarily to normal levels) to prevent or minimize target organ damage, usually necessitating hospitalization for parenteral anti-hypertensive therapy. A hypertensive urgency refers to a significant elevation in blood pressure without acute target organ damage, where patients may experience symptoms related to the elevated blood pressure, such as headache, chest discomfort, nosebleeds, and restlessness. A considerable number of patients exhibit poor medication adherence or inadequate treatment. The degree of blood pressure elevation is not the standard for distinguishing between hypertensive crises and urgencies; the sole criterion is the presence or absence of newly developed, progressive, severe target organ damage.

The prevalence of hypertensive emergencies varies considerably across studies. Multiple factors can precipitate hypertensive emergencies, including heart failure, cerebrovascular events, kidney damage, poly-pharmacy, poor adherence, and socioeconomic factors like lack of access to basic healthcare, medical insurance, and smoking. Research also suggests that most patients with hypertensive emergencies had previously known hypertension but failed to adhere to their medication regimen.

Currently, there is a lack of evidence-based studies examining the incidence and mortality of hypertensive emergencies to guide clinical practice. Relevant research has primarily focused on comparing the efficacy of anti-hypertensive drugs, blood pressure control, or treatment adherence. Although hypertensive emergencies account for only a small proportion of hypertensive patients, they carry significant clinical importance. Without timely and effective treatment, these conditions can severely impact prognosis and even threaten life, making them one of the most common consultations encountered by cardiologists.

Ⅱ Clinical Manifestations

The clinical manifestations of hypertensive emergencies are complex and varied, primarily reflecting the target organ damage caused by the acute blood pressure elevation. Neurological symptoms are the most common, including aphasia, dilated pupils, projectile vomiting, hemiplegia, impaired consciousness, and seizure-like episodes. The presence of severe headache, nausea, vomiting, nuchal rigidity, altered mental status, and meningeal signs should raise suspicion for a potential subarachnoid hemorrhage.

Respiratory distress, chest pain, cyanosis, lung crackles, tachycardia, cardiomegaly, and frothy pink sputum suggest acute heart failure. If the electrocardiogram shows significant ischemic changes and cardiac biomarkers are positive, acute coronary syndrome should be considered. The presence of tearing chest or abdominal pain may indicate acute aortic dissection. Oliguria, anuria, proteinuria, and elevated serum creatinine and blood urea nitrogen indicate acute kidney injury. Blurred vision, and fundoscopic findings of optic disc edema, retinal hemorrhages, and exudates suggest retinal artery involvement.

In hypertensive urgencies, patients do not exhibit clear clinical manifestations of target organ damage. Their symptoms often reflect autonomic dysfunction, such as pallor, restlessness, diaphoresis, palpitations, tremors, frequent urination, and tachycardia (possibly >110 bpm). Other symptoms may include nosebleeds, dizziness, and headaches, which could be attributed to the elevated blood pressure alone without acute or permanent organ damage.

Ⅲ Clinical Assessment

Clinical assessment is crucial in hypertensive emergencies. By obtaining a thorough history, evaluating symptoms and signs, and reviewing available diagnostic tests, clinicians can rapidly determine whether the acute blood pressure elevation is accompanied by target organ damage or life-threatening conditions, allowing for appropriate emergent management.

When taking the medical history, several aspects should be addressed: the patient's history of hypertension, previous treatment regimens and blood pressure control, potential triggers for the current elevation, and any specific medication use. Evaluation of specific symptoms can help identify potential target organ involvement.

Ancillary tests should focus on the following: laboratory tests to assess for electrolyte disturbances (hypokalemia and hypomagnesemia) that may precipitate arrhythmias, as well as liver and kidney function, complete blood count, and urinalysis to evaluate target organ function; electrocardiogram to assess for coronary ischemia or left ventricular hypertrophy; chest X-ray for patients with chest pain or dyspnea to evaluate for pulmonary edema; and head CT or MRI for patients with neurological deficits or altered mental status.

Ⅳ Treatment

When a hypertensive emergency is suspected, initial treatment should not be delayed due to the ongoing process of overall patient evaluation. Patients with hypertensive emergencies should be admitted to the emergency department or an intensive care unit for continuous blood pressure monitoring. Appropriate anti-hypertensive agents should be administered promptly, and effective sedatives may be considered to alleviate patient anxiety. Additionally, specific management should be provided based on the target organ damage present.

Immediate blood pressure lowering is required in hypertensive emergencies to prevent further target organ damage. Prior to the treatment, the route of administration, choice of medication, target blood pressure level, and rate of blood pressure reduction should be determined. Clinical application should consider the pharmacological and pharmacokinetic properties of the drugs, as well as their effects on cardiac output, systemic vascular resistance, target organ perfusion, and potential adverse reactions. The ideal agent should have a predictable anti-hypertensive potency and speed of action, with the ability to titrate the intensity as needed. Generally, short-acting intravenous anti-hypertensive agents are commonly used, depending on the clinical scenario. During the blood pressure lowering process, close monitoring of target organ function is essential, including changes in neurological symptoms and signs, as well as worsening chest pain. Since target organ damage is already present, excessively rapid or excessive blood pressure reduction can compromise tissue perfusion pressure, potentially precipitating ischemic events. Therefore, the initial target is not to normalize blood pressure but to gradually lower it to a moderately elevated level, maximally preventing or minimizing damage to vital organs such as the heart, brain, and kidneys.

For patients with hypertensive urgencies, oral anti-hypertensive agents can generally be used for blood pressure control. Initial treatment can be initiated in the outpatient or emergency department setting, with monitoring for 5-6 hours after medication administration. Dosage adjustments can be made within 2-3 days in the outpatient clinic, followed by the use of long-acting formulations to achieve the ultimate target blood pressure. Patients with hypertensive urgencies and high-risk factors, such as cardiovascular disease, may require inpatient treatment. Conversely, over-treatment should be avoided in patients without complications but with relatively high blood pressure levels. In these cases, intravenous or large oral loading doses of anti-hypertensive agents can potentially induce adverse effects or hypotension, leading to subsequent harm, and should be avoided.

V Common Questions in Consultation

1. Is the severity of the condition directly proportional to the degree of blood pressure elevation?

A common clinical question is whether higher blood pressure levels correlate with more severe disease in patients with hypertensive emergencies. In reality, this is not necessarily the case, as the degree of acute target organ damage is not directly proportional to the blood pressure level. Some hypertensive emergencies may not present with exceptionally high blood pressure values, such as those occurring during pregnancy or in certain cases of acute glomerulonephritis. However, if blood pressure is not promptly controlled to a reasonable range, serious organ damage or life-threatening consequences can ensue, necessitating urgent attention. Conversely, patients with acute pulmonary edema, aortic dissection, or myocardial infarction should be managed as hypertensive emergencies even if their blood pressure is only moderately elevated.

Additionally, some patients may present with relatively high blood pressure levels without clear evidence of target organ damage, requiring a differentiated treatment approach.

2. Pace and target for blood pressure control in hypertensive emergencies. The first goal of anti-hypertensive treatment in hypertensive emergencies is to lower blood pressure to a safe level within 30-60 minutes. As patients have varying baseline blood pressure levels and concomitant target organ damage, this safe level must be determined based on individual circumstances. *The 2010 Chinese Guidelines for the Management of Hypertension* recommend that within the first hour of treatment, the target should be a reduction in mean arterial pressure not exceeding 25% of the pre-treatment level. However, most experts suggest lowering blood pressure by approximately 10% in the first hour, followed by a further 10%-15% reduction over the next 2-4 hours, with the exception of aortic dissection cases. During emergency blood pressure lowering, it is crucial to recognize the importance of intrinsic blood pressure regulatory mechanisms. If blood pressure is abruptly reduced through treatment, the auto-regulatory capacity of the vascular bed is compromised, potentially leading to inadequate tissue perfusion, ischemia, and infarction.

The second goal of anti-hypertensive treatment is to gradually lower blood pressure to a second target level after achieving the first goal. This involves slowing the rate of intravenous administration and introducing oral medications. *The 2010 Chinese Guidelines for the Management of Hypertension* recommend reducing blood pressure to a relatively safe level of around 160/100 mmHg within the subsequent 2-6 hours, with appropriate adjustments based on the patient's baseline blood pressure and specific clinical condition.

The third goal is to gradually lower blood pressure to normal levels over the following 24-48 hours if the patient can tolerate the second target blood pressure level and their clinical condition remains stable. During this phase, the specific treatment plan should be individualized, taking into consideration factors such as the patient's age, duration of hypertension, degree of blood pressure elevation, target organ damage, and concomitant clinical conditions. The aim is to maximize target organ protection and provide appropriate management for any existing target organ damage.

3. Considerations during anti-hypertensive treatment in hypertensive emergencies. Hypertensive emergencies are life-threatening conditions, and anti-hypertensive treatment is crucial. However, the following aspects should be considered: First, the clinical pathophysiology of hypertensive emergencies is complex, and the application of treatment guidelines should be combined with principles of individualized therapy. Second, short-acting intravenous anti-hypertensive agents are preferable for the clinical management of hypertensive emergencies, avoiding oral or sublingual administration of rapid-acting agents (e.g., nifedipine). Third, pharmacological treatment should be complemented by general supportive measures, such as rest, oxygen supplementation, maintenance of vital signs, and appropriate sedation. Fourth, if the patient presents with focal neurological deficits, emergency blood pressure lowering is not recommended before brain imaging, unless there is a critically elevated intracranial pressure.

4. Considerations in the treatment of hypertensive urgencies. For patients with hypertensive

urgencies, blood pressure can be slowly lowered to 160/100 mmHg within 24-48 hours. There is no evidence that emergency anti-hypertensive treatment improves outcomes in these situations. After the initial blood pressure control in the emergency department, patients with hypertensive urgencies should be advised on adjustments to their oral anti-hypertensive regimen and recommended for regular follow-up in a hypertension clinic. Many patients may continue with their previous sub-optimal treatment plan after the emergency department visit due to a lack of understanding, leading to recurrent hypertensive urgencies and potentially severe consequences.

Ⅵ Consultation Process

1. Assess the patient's vital signs and general condition. If signs of instability such as decreased oxygen saturation, hypotension, oliguria, cold and clammy skin, or altered mental status are present, immediately initiate emergency interventions like mechanical ventilation, fluid resuscitation, and vasopressor support.

2. Obtain crucial history, including family history of hypertension, chronic hypertension history, baseline anti-hypertensive medication use and blood pressure control, presence of underlying heart disease or chronic kidney disease, history of renal impairment, acute or chronic onset, presence of altered mental status, oliguria, cold and clammy skin suggestive of shock, or associated neurological manifestations like blurred vision, hemiparesis, hemianopsia, dysarthria, dizziness, projectile vomiting, or headache.

3. Pay attention to important physical examination findings, such as level of consciousness, presence of cyanosis, presence of dry or moist crackles, jugular venous distension, cardiomegaly on percussion, lower extremity edema, or focal neurological deficits.

4. Promptly obtain relevant investigations like complete blood count, renal function tests, electrolytes, BNP or NT-proBNP, cardiac enzymes, cardiac biomarkers, arterial blood gas analysis, electrocardiogram, chest X-ray, and head CT scan. If initial findings suggest acute coronary syndrome, proceed with emergency coronary angiography. If acute heart failure is suspected, expedite an echocardiogram. If renal impairment is considered, expedite a renal ultrasound. If aortic dissection is suspected, urgently obtain a CT angiogram of the entire aorta.

5. After diagnosis, initiate targeted treatment. For example, if head CT suggests acute stroke, consult the relevant specialty for further management. If electrocardiogram and cardiac biomarkers indicate acute coronary syndrome, proceed with timely revascularization therapy. For heart failure, initiate diuretics, vasodilators, and, if necessary, inotropic support or mechanical interventions; once symptoms improve, investigate the underlying etiology. If laboratory tests reveal renal impairment with electrolyte and acid-base disturbances, consider dialysis or hemofiltration if necessary. For aortic dissection, aggressively control blood pressure and consult cardio-thoracic surgery for potential emergency surgical intervention.

6. After ruling out life-threatening emergencies, proceed with further investigations for dynamic blood pressure monitoring and assessment of hypertensive target organ damage.

Section 2 Hypertensive Encephalopathy

I Definition and Pathogenesis

Hypertensive encephalopathy is a clinical syndrome characterized by a temporary disturbance in cerebral circulatory function, resulting from a sudden elevation in blood pressure exceeding the auto-regulatory threshold (mean arterial pressure >140 mmHg), leading to cerebral hyper-perfusion, increased capillary pressure, enhanced osmotic pressure, brain edema, elevated intracranial pressure, and potentially brain herniation. Any type of hypertension or acute severe blood pressure elevation from any cause can precipitate hypertensive encephalopathy. Clinically, it most commonly results from accelerated malignant hypertension, particularly in patients with concomitant renal failure or cerebrovascular atherosclerosis, accounting for approximately 12% of cases. Secondary causes like acute or chronic glomerulonephritis, eclampsia, pheochromocytoma, etc., can also lead to hypertensive encephalopathy, although it is less common in primary aldosteronism and renovascular hypertension.

The exact pathogenesis of hypertensive encephalopathy remains unclear, with two main proposed mechanisms: the over-auto-regulation (small artery spasm) theory and the auto-regulatory breakthrough theory. The latter is more widely accepted, suggesting that a rapid rise in blood pressure overwhelms the cerebral auto-regulatory mechanisms, leading to passive vasodilation, increased cerebral blood flow, and extravasation of fluid from the vascular bed into the brain interstitium due to increased capillary pressure exceeding the interstitial pressure. This rapid development of brain edema and elevated intracranial pressure is further exacerbated by small artery spasm induced by the abrupt blood pressure elevation.

II Clinical Presentation

Hypertensive encephalopathy has an acute onset and severe clinical course, characterized primarily by central nervous system dysfunction. It is one of the critical conditions frequently encountered in cardiology consultations. In addition to a sudden rise in blood pressure, patients typically present with severe headache and altered mental status. Other manifestations may include blindness, loss of vision, numbness, motor deficits, localized or diffuse retinal arteriolar spasm, though hemorrhages, exudates, or papilledema are not necessarily present. Prompt and appropriate blood pressure lowering can rapidly improve the clinical symptoms. If left untreated, hypertensive encephalopathy can progress to brain herniation, although cerebral thrombosis or hemorrhage is relatively rare but carries grave consequences if present.

III Clinical Assessment and Diagnosis

A significant elevation in blood pressure, along with brain edema and increased intracranial pressure, should raise suspicion for hypertensive encephalopathy. Patients typically have a history of primary or secondary hypertension and develop an acute blood pressure spike after precipitating factors like excessive exertion, alcohol consumption, discontinuation of anti-hypertensive medications, or mental stress. Within 12-48 hours of the marked blood pressure elevation, they manifest neurological and psychiatric abnormalities, predominantly due to increased intracranial pressure and focal brain tissue injury. Neuroimaging (CT or MRI) excludes intracranial hemorrhage or subarachnoid hemorrhage but may reveal characteristic parieto-occipital edema. The diagnosis of hypertensive encephalopathy should integrate clinical symptoms, signs, and neuroimaging findings, with neuroimaging playing a crucial role.

Ⅳ Management of Hypertensive Encephalopathy

The key to managing hypertensive encephalopathy is lowering blood pressure while maintaining cerebral perfusion and minimizing the impact on intracranial pressure. Treatment should aim to reduce brain edema, lower intracranial pressure, and avoid medications that decrease cerebral blood flow. The management encompasses three main aspects: ① General measures, including blood pressure monitoring, electrocardiographic monitoring, establishing intravenous access, and controlling psychiatric symptoms; ② Anti-hypertensive therapy, typically with intravenous agents. The rate of blood pressure reduction should be individualized, not too rapid or excessive, to prevent compromised perfusion to vital organs like the heart, kidneys, and brain; ③ Reduction of intracranial pressure and brain edema, usually achieved through dehydration and diuresis to alleviate brain edema, stabilize intracranial pressure, and relieve symptoms.

Ⅴ Common Questions in Consultation

1. Considerations in blood pressure management for hypertensive ence-phalopathy. The treatment of hypertensive encephalopathy primarily involves intravenous anti-hypertensive agents. *The 2010 Chinese Guidelines for the Management of Hypertension* recommend lowering systolic blood pressure by 20%-25% within 1 hour, with the reduction not exceeding 50%, and maintaining diastolic blood pressure generally above 110 mmHg. Commonly used agents include nicardipine, labetalol, and urapidil. Sodium nitroprusside should be used cautiously as it may increase intracranial pressure, impair cerebral perfusion, and potentially cause accumulation toxicity. For patients with coronary artery disease or heart failure, nitroglycerin can be considered. Mannitol and diuretics should be added if intracranial pressure is significantly elevated. The use of pure beta-blockers, clonidine, and methyldopa is generally avoided. For pheochromocytoma patients with hypertensive encephalopathy, α-adrenergic receptor blockers like phenoxybenzamine should be selected. Pregnant women with hypertension should receive intravenous magnesium sulfate. Once the target blood pressure is achieved, oral calcium channel blockers, angiotensin-converting enzyme inhibitors, or other agents can be initiated.

2. Management of prominent psychiatric symptoms in hypertensive ence-phalopathy. Patients with hypertensive encephalopathy often exhibit psychiatric abnormalities, including agitation, delirium, and even recurrent seizures. Controlling these symptoms can aid in blood pressure control. When psychiatric symptoms arise, patients should be kept at bed rest, with fluid restriction and head elevation at 15°-20°. Diazepam can be administered as a slow intravenous infusion, or a chloral hydrate retention enema can be given. For agitated patients, intramuscular phenobarbital may be considered. In the presence of symptoms and signs of elevated intracranial

pressure, rapid intravenous infusion of 250 mL of 20% mannitol or intravenous furosemide 40-60 mg can effectively reduce intracranial pressure and improve symptoms. Generally, psychiatric symptoms tend to resolve with appropriate blood pressure lowering and intracranial pressure control.

3. Prognosis of hypertensive encephalopathy. Early diagnosis, prompt treatment, and timely blood pressure reduction are crucial in hypertensive encephalopathy. Most patients can recover within 3-48 hours with effective pharmacological treatment, showing complete resolution of abnormal lesions on imaging without any residual deficits, indicating a favorable prognosis. However, if treatment is delayed, irreversible brain damage, paralysis, or life-threatening consequences may ensue. Therefore, early diagnosis and treatment have a significant impact on the prognosis.

VI Consultation Process

1. Assess the patient's vital signs and general condition. If signs of instability such as decreased oxygen saturation, hypotension, oliguria, cold and clammy skin, or altered mental status are present, immediately initiate emergency interventions like mechanical ventilation, fluid resuscitation, and vasopressor support.

2. Obtain crucial history, including family history of hypertension, chronic hypertension history, baseline anti-hypertensive medication use and blood pressure control, presence of underlying heart disease or chronic kidney disease, history of renal impairment, acute onset, sudden or paroxysmal elevation in blood pressure, presence of altered mental status or psychiatric changes, or associated symptoms like blurred vision, hemiparesis, hemianopsia, dysarthria, projectile vomiting, headache suggestive of elevated intracranial pressure or neurological involvement.

3. Pay attention to important physical examination findings, such as level of consciousness, cardiomegaly on percussion, or focal neurological deficits.

4. Promptly obtain relevant investigations like complete blood count, renal function tests, electrolytes, BNP or NT-proBNP, cardiac enzymes, cardiac biomarkers, electrocardiogram, and head CT scan. If renal impairment is present, expedite renal ultrasound and renal artery imaging. If heart failure is suspected, expedite an echocardiogram.

5. After diagnosis, initiate targeted treatment. For example, if head CT suggests acute stroke, consult the relevant specialty for further management; promptly initiate blood pressure lowering; if intracranial pressure is elevated, consider intracranial pressure-lowering measures.

6. After ruling out life-threatening emergencies and common causes, proceed with further investigations for secondary causes of hypertension.

Section 3 Management of Hypertensive Aortic Dissection

I Overview

Aortic dissection (AD) is a severe, emergent cardiovascular condition characterized by the separation of the aortic wall layers due to an intimal tear, allowing blood to enter the media and propagate along the length of the aorta, forming a dissecting hematoma.

Aortic dissection is a rare disease, with an annual incidence of approximately 6/100,000 based on data from the Oxford Vascular Study. It has an acute onset and rapid progression, with relatively high rates of misdiagnosis and missed diagnosis, posing significant risks and grave consequences. Among hypertensive emergencies, acute aortic dissection represents the most urgent clinical situation.

Ⅱ Classification

There are several classification systems for aortic dissection, with the DeBakey and Stanford classifications being the most widely used clinically. Introduced in 1965, the DeBakey classification divides aortic dissections into three types based on the location of the originating intimal tear and the extent of dissection propagation: Type Ⅰ involves an originating tear in the ascending aorta, extending distally into the aortic arch and descending aorta; Type Ⅱ refers to a tear originating in the ascending aorta but confined to the ascending aorta; Type Ⅲ involves a tear originating distal to the left subclavian artery in the descending aorta, extending distally and potentially involving the thoracic and abdominal aorta, with Type Ⅲa limited to the descending thoracic aorta and Type Ⅲb extending into the abdominal aorta.

The Stanford classification is another commonly used system, dividing aortic dissections into two types based on the involvement of the ascending aorta, which is more practical in clinical practice. Stanford Type A dissections involve the ascending aorta, corresponding to DeBakey Types Ⅰ and Ⅱ, while Stanford Type B dissections involve the descending aorta distal to the left subclavian artery, corresponding to DeBakey Type Ⅲ.

Based on the time of onset, aortic dissections can also be classified as acute (within 14 days), sub-acute (15-90 days), or chronic (more than 90 days).

Ⅲ Clinical Presentation

Approximately 80% of patients experience a typical sudden, severe, tearing chest pain in the acute phase, with 40% reporting back pain and 25% reporting abdominal pain. Type A dissections more commonly present with chest pain, while Type B dissections are more likely to manifest as back or abdominal pain. Patients typically experience an immediate, rapidly peaking, severe, tearing or ripping pain that is unbearable, often exacerbated by each heartbeat, accompanied by a sense of suffocation and an extreme fear of impending death. The migratory nature of the pain is a characteristic feature, with less than 15% of Type A dissections and nearly 20% of Type B dissections exhibiting this pattern. Nearly 50% of the patients may present with shock, anxiety, diaphoresis, pallor, cold and clammy skin, and tachycardia due to the excruciating pain. Unlike typical shock, the blood pressure may not correlate with the shock presentation and may not be significantly reduced, or even elevated, possibly due to renal ischemia from renal artery involvement or obstruction of the aortic arch and descending aorta. A significant drop in blood pressure often indicates impending external rupture of the dissection.

Aortic dissection can extend into the pericardial sac or left pleural space, causing cardiac tamponade or hemothorax, or rupture into the esophagus, trachea, or abdominal cavity, leading to shock, chest pain, syncope, dyspnea, palpitations, hematemesis, and hemoptysis. Involvement of the coronary artery ostia can result in myocardial ischemia and angina, with severe cases potentially leading to myocardial infarction. Dissection into the pericardial sac can cause cardiac tamponade, rapidly deteriorating the patient's condition and potentially resulting in death. If the dissection involves the upper or lower extremity arteries, symptoms such as absent pulse, pain, pallor, coolness, numbness, and sensory disturbances may occur in the affected areas. Involvement of the carotid arteries can lead to cerebral hypo-perfusion, causing dizziness, syncope, or even coma. Insufficient collateral circulation to the vertebrobasilar system can result in contra-lateral hemiplegia, ipsilateral visual disturbances, or blindness. Dissection involving the intercostal or vertebral arteries can cause paraplegia, with sensory deficits below the level of the lesion, often accompanied by urinary retention. Compression of the recurrent laryngeal nerve can cause hoarseness, while involvement of the sympathetic ganglia can lead to Horner's syndrome. Extension to the iliac arteries can result in peripheral nerve ischemia and necrosis, manifesting as numbness, paresthesias, decreased muscle tone, or complete paralysis of the extremities. In approximately one-third to one-half of patients, the aortic dissection can involve the abdominal aorta and its branches, presenting as severe abdominal pain, predominantly in the upper abdomen, often accompanied by nausea and vomiting, mimicking various acute abdominal conditions. Compression of the esophagus, mediastinum, or vagus nerve can cause dysphagia, while rupture into the esophagus can lead to hematemesis. Dissection involving the mesenteric or abdominal aortic branches can cause intestinal necrosis and hematochezia. Rupture into the peritoneal cavity can result in peritoneal signs. Involvement of the renal arteries can cause flank or costovertebral angle pain, with a palpable mass in the renal area, and some patients may present with gross hematuria. Bronchial compression by the dissecting hematoma can lead to bronchospasm, causing dyspnea and respiratory distress. Rupture into the pleural space, typically on the left side, can cause chest pain, dyspnea, cough, or hemoptysis, potentially leading to hemorrhagic shock and life-threatening consequences. Renal artery dissection can result in acute renal ischemia or acute renovascular hypertension.

Ⅳ Diagnosis

If severe chest pain is accompanied by a difference in blood pressure between the two upper limbs of more than 20 mmHg, aortic dissection should be considered, and emergency electrocardiography (ECG) and chest X-ray examinations should be performed promptly. Emergency ECG can differentiate between aortic dissection and acute myocardial infarction, but myocardial infarction may coexist when the dissection involves the ostia of the coronary arteries; 20% of acute Stanford type A aortic dissections may exhibit signs of myocardial ischemia or infarction on ECG. In 60% of the patients, emergency chest X-ray may reveal widening of the aortic shadow and can rule out the presence of pleural effusion or pneumothorax. If the emergency ECG and chest X-ray findings highly suggest aortic dissection and preliminarily exclude other conditions, computed tomographic angiography (CTA) of the aorta and echocardiography should be performed immediately. If the emergency CTA reveals a double-lumen sign in the aorta, aortic dissection can be preliminarily diagnosed, and echocardiography can determine whether the dissection involves the ascending aorta and aortic valve, and whether there is cardiac tamponade. Aortic angiography may also be necessary.

V Anti-hypertensive Treatment

Hypertension complicated by acute aortic dissection is considered a hypertensive emergency, and compared to other types of hypertensive emergencies, acute aortic dissection has a higher short-term mortality and disability rate, requiring more urgent and rapid blood pressure reduction. Once acute aortic dissection is suspected, the patient's blood pressure must be rapidly lowered to a normal-to-low level, with a systolic pressure of 100-120 mmHg. Since acute aortic dissection involving the ascending aorta or aortic arch is a surgical emergency, the anti-hypertensive treatment for these patients should consider surgical requirements.

The shear stress on the aortic wall depends on the force and rate of ventricular contraction and the stroke volume. The chosen medication must help reduce these three factors, and reflex tachycardia should be particularly well controlled during blood pressure lowering.

The principle of anti-hypertensive treatment is to rapidly reduce and maintain blood pressure at the lowest possible level while ensuring adequate organ perfusion, with a systolic pressure of at least 120 mmHg and ideally around 100 mmHg if organ perfusion is maintained, and a heart rate of 60-80 beats/min. The European Society of Cardiology recommends using a combination of anesthetic analgesics, intravenous beta-blockers, and vasodilators. If morphine is used for analgesia, beta-blockers such as esmolol, labetalol, metoprolol, or propranolol can be combined with vasodilators like nitroprusside or nicardipine. Verapamil and diltiazem can be alternatives if beta-blockers are not tolerated.

Since the vasodilating effect of nitroprusside can lead to a compensatory increase in heart rate, it should be used in combination with a beta-blocker and is not the first choice. Nicardipine has a similar efficacy to nitroprusside but a higher safety profile, making it more widely applicable and generally able to replace the traditional vasodilator nitroprusside in most cases. Urapidil has a rapid onset, moderate duration, and easy control of the rate and extent of blood pressure reduction, without compromising target organ perfusion during the perioperative period or causing coronary steal phenomena or other adverse reactions. It can also be a preferred option, particularly suitable for aortic dissection patients with impaired renal function.

Rapid blood pressure reduction can trigger sympathetic nervous system excitation, reflexively increasing myocardial contractility. Abrupt changes in blood pressure and increased left ventricular contractility can exacerbate the risk of aortic rupture. Therefore, the concomitant use of beta-blockers (such as esmolol) can reduce myocardial contractility and slow the heart rate. Beta-blockers should be administered before anti-hypertensive medications but should be avoided if aortic valve regurgitation or suspected cardiac tamponade is present. Additionally, labetalol, which has both alpha and beta-blocking effects, can effectively lower dp / dt and arterial pressure, exhibiting a good therapeutic effect on aortic dissection, and can be used as a single agent without the need for combination therapy. If necessary, oral ACEIs, ARBs, or low-dose diuretics can be added, but caution should be taken as ACEIs may cause cough as a side effect, potentially exacerbating the condition. Diazoxide and hydralazine can reflexively excite the sympathetic nervous system, increasing the shear stress on the aortic wall, and are therefore contraindicated. In patients with obstruction of major aortic branches, excessive blood pressure lowering should be avoided as it may worsen ischemia. During medication administration, vital signs, especially blood pressure, should be closely monitored, with invasive blood pressure monitoring being preferable, or at least non-invasive blood pressure measurements repeated every 5 minutes.

Ⅵ Common Questions in Consultation

1. Use of commonly administered intravenous anti-hypertensive agents. Nitro-prusside: Diluted in 5% glucose solution, initial dose is typically 0.3-0.5 μg/(kg·min), increased by 0.5 μg/(kg·min) every 15-20 minutes based on blood pressure, maximum dose 10 μg/(kg·min).

Urapidil: Initial dose of 12.5-25 mg diluted and administered intravenously, maintenance dose of 100-400 μg/min by continuous intravenous infusion.

Nicardipine: Diluted and administered by continuous intravenous infusion at 0.5-10 μg/(kg·min), with the rate adjusted based on blood pressure.

Esmolol: Initial dose of 250-500 μg/kg administered directly intravenously (without dilution), maintenance dose of 50-300 μg/(kg·min) by continuous intravenous infusion.

Labetalol: Initial dose of 20-100 mg diluted and administered intravenously, maintenance dose of 0.5-2.0 mg/min by continuous intravenous infusion, not exceeding 300 mg in 24 hours.

2. Management of hypotension in acute aortic dissection patients. If a suspected aortic dissection patient presents with severe hypotension, cardiac tamponade or aortic rupture should be considered, requiring prompt volume expansion. Before initiating aggressive treatment, the possibility of false hypotension must be carefully ruled out, which may result from measuring the blood pressure of an extremity affected by the dissection. If urgent vasopressor therapy is required for refractory hypotension, norepinephrine (8-12 μg/min initial, 2-4 μg/min maintenance) or epinephrine (0.1-0.5 mg diluted in saline and administered intravenously) is preferred over dopamine, as dopamine can increase dp/dt. Dopamine should be used in low doses only when improving renal perfusion is necessary.

3. Caution with "inferior wall myocardial infarction". Acute myocardial infarction induced by aortic dissection is generally seen more often in DeBakey Type Ⅰ or Ⅱ (Stanford Type A) dissections. A retrospective study indicated that approximately 5% of Stanford type A dissections are complicated by acute myocardial infarction, with an extremely high mortality rate of around 36%. The mechanisms by which aortic dissection induces myocardial infarction include intimal tear involving the coronary ostia, compression of the coronary artery by the dissection, obstruction of the coronary artery by floating intimal debris, and coronary artery spasm caused by the dissection. The dissection tends to affect the right coronary artery more than the left, resulting in a predominance of inferior wall myocardial infarctions. Therefore, in patients diagnosed with inferior wall myocardial infarction, it is necessary to rule out the possibility of aortic dissection before proceeding with thrombolysis or anti-coagulation. If conditions permit, emergency

coronary angiography plus aortic angiography can establish the diagnosis; if angiography is not available, echocardiography can help differentiate between the two conditions, primarily by directly visualizing the flapping intimal flap and detecting aortic regurgitation. Patients with aortic dissection complicated by acute myocardial infarction may exhibit certain suggestive features, such as severe pain refractory to analgesics, signs of aortic insufficiency or absent pulses, ST-T wave changes on ECG that deviate from the usual pattern, presentations unexplained by acute myocardial infarction alone (e.g., stroke, leg pain), and findings on echocardiography.

To sum up, the clinical relationship between aortic dissection and acute myocardial infarction is complex, and making an accurate early diagnosis directly impacts prognosis. By considering factors such as the nature of chest pain, aortic valve insufficiency, absent pulse, ECG changes, and bedside echocardiography, clinicians can differentiate between the two conditions in most patients without significant difficulty. In patients presenting several days after symptom onset, analysis of ECG evolution, cardiac biomarkers, and echocardiographic findings can provide important diagnostic clues, while further investigations such as CT, MRI, and aortic angiography can establish the diagnosis. The key is for clinicians to maintain a high index of suspicion for aortic dissection, carefully considering and ruling it out to avoid misdiagnosis or missed diagnosis.

Ⅶ Consultation Procedure

1. Assess the patient's vital signs. If there is evidence of life-threatening instability, such as decreased oxygen saturation, shallow and rapid breathing, hypotension, or malignant arrhythmias, immediately initiate emergency management, including mechanical ventilation, cardioversion, temporary pacing, anti-arrhythmic therapy, and vasopressor support to maintain blood pressure.

2. Obtain critical medical history, including family history of hypertension, personal history of chronic hypertension, current anti-hypertensive medication use and degree of blood pressure control, presence of underlying cardiac disease, diabetes, coronary artery disease, or renal impairment. Determine if the current episode is acute in onset, characterized by tearing chest pain, associated with symptoms such as dizziness, amaurosis fugax, hoarseness, paresthesias, paraplegia, or oliguria, and whether the patient exhibits altered mental status, angina, acute abdomen, acute renal failure, or shock.

3. Perform a thorough physical examination, paying particular attention to signs of ischemia in the upper or lower extremities, such as absent pulses or pallor. Note any significant discrepancies in blood pressure between arms or between arms and legs, inability to obtain blood pressure in one extremity, markedly diminished femoral pulse on one side, and the presence of valvular murmurs. Carefully exclude the possibility of false hypotension.

4. Rapidly obtain relevant diagnostic studies, including arterial blood gas analysis, complete blood count, renal function tests, electrolytes, cardiac enzymes, biomarkers, electrocardiogram, chest radiography, B-type natriuretic peptide (BNP) or N-terminal pro-BNP, and D-dimer. Proceed with comprehensive computed tomographic angiography (CTA) of the aorta as soon as possible to establish the diagnosis and classify the dissection. Determine promptly whether acute renal failure is present. In patients diagnosed with inferior wall myocardial infarction who are

suspected of concomitant aortic dissection, perform emergency coronary angiography plus aortic angiography if feasible; if angiography is unavailable, echocardiography can help differentiate between the two conditions.

5. Once the diagnosis is confirmed, initiate treatment promptly: rapidly lower the blood pressure to a normal-to-low range, with a systolic pressure of 100-120 mmHg; provide analgesia if pain is significant; if refractory hypotension occurs, administer norepinephrine or epinephrine as vasopressor therapy. Consult cardio-thoracic surgery to evaluate the need for emergency surgical intervention.

Section 4 Characteristics of Hypertension in the Elderly

I Increased Systolic Blood Pressure and Widened Pulse Pressure

Isolated systolic hypertension accounts for over 60% of hypertension cases in the elderly population, with an increasing prevalence as age advances. Concurrently, the incidence of stroke also rises. In the elderly, wider pulse pressure correlates positively with overall mortality and cardiovascular events. The underlying pathophysiology involves decreased aortic elasticity due to arteriosclerosis, leading to inadequate diastolic aortic recoil and increased peripheral resistance during systole, resulting in elevated systolic blood pressure and reduced diastolic blood pressure, thereby widening the pulse pressure.

II Increased Blood Pressure Variability: Manifested as a Higher Prevalence of Morning Hypertension, Orthostatic Hypotension, and Postprandial Hypotension

Morning hypertension in the elderly refers to home self-measured blood pressure readings≥135/85 mmHg within 1 hour of awakening, or ambulatory blood pressure monitoring readings≥135/85 mmHg within 2 hours of arising, or office blood pressure readings≥140/90 mmHg between 6:00 am and 10:00 am. The prevalence of morning hypertension is 19.4% in individuals aged 40-79 years and 21.8% in those aged 80 years or older. In the morning, increased sympathetic activity and elevated levels of vasoconstrictive catecholamines, activation of the renin-angiotensin-aldosterone system, and increased cortisol secretion collectively contribute to the observed rise in blood pressure and increased risk. The morning hours represent a peak period for cerebrovascular and cardiovascular events, with elevated blood pressure being a significant precipitating factor.

Orthostatic blood pressure variability encompasses both orthostatic hypotension and orthostatic hypertension. Orthostatic hypotension is defined as a decrease in systolic blood pressure of≥20 mmHg or a decrease in diastolic blood pressure of≥10 mmHg within 3 minutes of changing from a supine to an upright position, accompanied by symptoms of reduced perfusion such as dizziness, lightheadedness, weakness, nausea, blurred vision, pallor, or diaphoresis. The occurrence of orthostatic hypotension often leads to adverse events and necessitates prompt identification and management of the underlying cause (e.g., volume depletion) and adjustment of therapeutic regimens, with appropriate additional diagnostic evaluation. Conversely, orthostatic hypertension, characterized by an increase in systolic blood pressure exceeding 20 mmHg upon assuming an upright posture from a supine position, is another manifestation of impaired blood pressure regulation in the elderly. Patients with orthostatic hypertension tend to be older and have a higher prevalence of left ventricular hypertrophy, coronary artery disease, and asymptomatic cerebrovascular disease compared to those with hypertension complicated by orthostatic hypotension. The overall prevalence of orthostatic hypotension in individuals aged 65 years and older ranges from 20% to 50%, while the prevalence in the elderly hypertensive population with orthostatic hypotension is even higher, with a 2- to 3-fold increase in cerebrovascular and cardiovascular events. The causes of orthostatic blood pressure variability include: ①age-related degenerative changes in the cardiovascular system, such as decreased sensitivity of baroreceptors, reduced vascular compliance due to arteriosclerosis, and attenuated heart rate responses; ②medication effects, such as those associated with commonly prescribed anti-hypertensives, anti-psychotics, tricyclic antidepressants, and anti-neoplastic agents; and ③underlying medical conditions leading to volume depletion, autonomic dysfunction, or peripheral neuropathy.

Postprandial hypotension is defined as a decrease in systolic blood pressure of more than 20 mmHg within 2 hours after a meal, a postprandial systolic blood pressure below 90 mmHg in individuals with a pre-meal systolic blood pressure of 100 mmHg or higher, or the development of symptoms suggestive of cerebral or myocardial ischemia, even if the blood pressure decrease does not meet the aforementioned criteria. The prevalence of postprandial hypotension is 24%-36% among elderly individuals receiving home care and 74.7% among hospitalized elderly patients in China. The underlying mechanism primarily involves an increase in splanchnic blood flow after meals, resulting in decreased venous return and cardiac output. The sensitivity of pressure sensors decreases, and the compensatory function of the sympathetic nervous system is impaired. Additionally, the secretion of vasoactive peptides with vasodilatory effects increases after meals.

Ⅲ Common Abnormalities in Blood Pressure Circadian Rhythm

Abnormalities in blood pressure circadian rhythm are prevalent, manifesting as a nocturnal blood pressure decline of less than 10% (non-dipper pattern), greater than 20% (extreme-dipper pattern), or the absence of a circadian rhythm (reverse-dipper pattern). These abnormalities increase the risk of target organ damage to the heart, brain, and kidneys, which is associated with arterial stiffening, increased vascular wall rigidity, and reduced function of the central blood pressure regulatory mechanisms in the elderly.

Ⅳ Increased Prevalence of White-Coat Hypertension

The prevalence of white-coat hypertension is approximately 13%. The underlying causes and mechanisms may involve increased psychological stress and enhanced sympathetic activity in medical environments, as well as metabolic disorders such as dyslipidemia and dysglycemia.

Ⅴ Increased Incidence of Pseudo-Hypertension

Pseudo-hypertension is more common in elderly individuals with severe arterial stiffening and is also frequently observed in patients with diabetes mellitus and uremic syndrome. The prevalence ranges from 1.7% to 50.0%, with a tendency to increase with age. Pseudo-hypertension results from decreased arterial compliance and increased arterial stiffness. Due to the progression of atherosclerosis in peripheral muscular arteries, a higher cuff pressure is required to compress the artery, leading to a discrepancy between cuff-measured blood pressure and direct blood pressure measurements, causing apparent elevated blood pressure readings. The Osler's maneuver using the cuff method can aid in the differential diagnosis. If the radial or brachial artery can be palpated clearly when the cuff pressure exceeds the patient's systolic pressure, the Osler's maneuver is positive; otherwise, it is negative.

Ⅵ Presence of Secondary Hypertension

Secondary hypertension, such as renovascular hypertension, renal hypertension, primary aldosteronism, and sleep apnea syndrome, is not uncommon. In some cases, secondary hypertension may be caused by atherosclerotic vascular lesions. For elderly patients with difficult-to-control hypertension, in addition to assessing the accuracy of diagnostics, the appropriateness of treatment, adherence, and potential factors affecting blood pressure control (e.g., poor sleep, concomitant use of blood pressure-altering medications), further examinations should be conducted to rule out contributing factors for secondary hypertension.

Ⅶ Consultation Process

1. Definition of hypertension in the elderly: Age ≥65, with a systolic blood pressure≥140 mmHg and/or diastolic blood pressure≥90 mmHg on at least three separate measurements without the use of antihypertensive medications.

2. Characteristics of hypertension in the elderly: Elevated systolic pressure, increased pulse pressure, greater blood pressure variability, increased prevalence of morning hypertension, tendency for orthostatic hypotension and postprandial hypotension, and common occurrence of abnormal circadian rhythms.

3. Elderly hypertensive patients are prone to pseudo-hypertension and white-coat hypertension, necessitating the evaluation of both clinic and ambulatory blood pressure measurements. The Osler's cuff method may be required in some cases.

4. Careful assessment of risk factors, target organ damage, and clinical complications is essential in elderly hypertensive patients.

5. Secondary hypertension should not be overlooked in elderly hypertensive patients.

Section 5 Treatment Strategies for Hypertension in the Elderly

Ⅰ Diagnosis of Hypertension in the Elderly

1. Hypertension in the elderly: Age ≥65, with sustained or ≥3 separate measurements of seated systolic blood pressure (SBP) ≥140 mmHg and/or diastolic blood pressure (DBP) ≥90 mmHg on different days.

2. Isolated systolic hypertension in the elderly: SBP ≥140 mmHg and DBP <90 mmHg (Table 4-1).

Table 4-1 Measurement Methods and Significance

Measurement Method	Device	Blood Pressure (mmHg)	Clinical Significance
Clinic Blood Pressure	Mercury Sphygmomanometer, Electronic Blood Pressure Mon-itor	≥140/90	Standard method for diagnosing hypertension and grading severity; primary basis for management decisions
Ambulatory Blood Pressure	Monitoring | Ambulatory Blood Pressure Monitor	24 h ≥130/80 Daytime≥135/85, Nighttime	① Assess hypertension; ② Diagnose whitecoat hypertension; ③ Identify masked hypertension; ④ Investigate causes of treatment-resistant hyper-tension; ⑤ Evaluate the degree of blood pressure elevation, short-term variability, and circadian rhythm
Home Blood Pressure Monitoring	Upper Arm Electronic Blood Pressure Monitor	≥ 135/85	① Long-term monitoring of daily blood pressure; ② Avoid white-coat effect; ③ Assist in evalua-ting treatment effectiveness; ④ Not recommen-ded for patients with high anxiety

Ⅱ Initial Management of Elderly Hypertensive Patients

Risk stratification assessment: Other cardiovascular risk factors, subclinical target organ damage, and clinical diseases.

Ⅲ Treatment Goals for Elderly Hypertensive Patients

The treatment goal for elderly hypertension is to maximally reduce the risk of cardiovascular complications and mortality. All reversible cardiovascular risk factors, subclinical target organ damage, and coexisting clinical diseases should be treated.

1. Initial Treatment Thresholds

(1) Age ≥65 and <80: ≥150/90 mmHg.

(2) Age ≥80: ≥160/90 mmHg.

2. Blood Pressure Target Values

(1) For patients aged ≥65, blood pressure should be lowered to <150/90 mmHg, and further to <140/90 mmHg if tolerated.

(2) For patients aged ≥80, blood pressure generally should not be lowered below 130/60 mmHg.

1) For very elderly patients without coexisting clinical diseases (e.g., chronic cerebrovascular disease, coronary artery disease, heart failure, diabetes mellitus, chronic kidney disease), the target blood pressure is <145-150/90 mmHg.

2) For patients with coexisting cardiovascular, cerebrovascular, or renal diseases, first lower blood pressure to <150/90 mmHg, and if well-tolerated, further lower to <140/90 mmHg.

Ⅳ Examination Selection for Elderly Hypertensive Patients

A comprehensive physical examination is emphasized in elderly hypertensive patients to assess the functional status of various organs. The following aspects should be particularly emphasized:

(1) Renal function assessment: Elderly individuals often have decreased renal function, but serum creatinine and blood urea nitrogen levels may still be within the normal range, leading to potential oversight. In such cases, creatinine clearance should be calculated and adjusted for age. Patients with proteinuria require special attention. Renal and renal artery ultrasound examinations can be performed to assess renal and renal vascular resistance. If necessary, adrenal CT scan can be conducted, and if serum creatinine changes are observed, renal scintigraphy can be performed to evaluate the glomerular filtration rate of both kidneys.

(2) Echocardiography should be performed for all elderly hypertensive patients.

(3) Carotid and vertebral artery ultrasound examinations should be performed for all elderly hypertensive patients.

(4) Brain CT scan should be conducted to assess cerebral conditions, including the degree of brain atrophy and lacunar infarcts.

(5) All patients should undergo blood lipid, blood glucose, and blood uric acid tests.

(6) If feasible, vascular function tests, such as pulse wave velocity (PWV) and ankle-brachial index (ABI), can be performed to assess vascular stiffness.

(7) If possible, blood pressure should be measured in all four limbs for comparison in elderly patients.

Ⅴ Choice of Pharmacological Treatment

The ideal medication for hypertension in the elderly should meet the following conditions: smooth and effective; safe with minimal side effects; simple to administer with good compliance. Commonly used antihypertensive drugs include five classes: calcium channel blockers (CCBs), angiotensin-converting enzyme inhibitors (ACEIs), angiotensin receptor blockers (ARBs), diuretics, and beta-receptor blockers, as well as fixed-dose combination preparations composed of the above drugs. In addition, α-receptor blockers can also be used as adjuvant therapy for patients with benign prostatic hyperplasia and refractory hypertension.

Initial monotherapy is suitable for the following patients: ① Blood pressure < 160/100 mmHg; ② Systolic blood pressure 150-179 mmHg/diastolic blood pressure < 60 mmHg; ③ Risk stratification is moderate risk.

Initial combination drug therapy is suitable for the following patients: ① Blood pressure ≥ 160/100 mmHg; ② Systolic blood pressure > 180 mmHg/diastolic blood pressure < 60 mmHg; ③ Blood pressure higher than the target value by 20/10 mmHg; ④ Risk stratification is high risk.

Ⅵ Blood Pressure Lowering Strategies for Coexisting Cardiovascular and Cerebrovascular Diseases

Blood pressure lowering strategies for coexisting cardiovascular and cerebrovascular diseases are presented in Table 4-2.

Table 4-2 Blood Pressure Lowering Strategies for Coexisting Cardiovascular and Cerebrovascular Diseases

Coexisting Disease	Blood Pressure Treatment Goals	Recommended Medications
Stroke	In the acute phase, if blood pressure remains elevated ≥200/110 mmHg, gradually lower blood pressure (24-hour reduction <25%); In the chronic phase, target blood pressure <140/90 mmHg	In the chronic phase, ACEIs / ARBs, diuretics, long-acting CCBs
Coronary Artery Disease	Target blood pressure <140/90 mmHg	β-blockers and ACEIs / ARBs; Add CCBs if blood pressure is difficult to control or if vasospastic angina is present
Chronic Heart Failure	Target blood pressure <140/90 mmHg	If no contraindications, use diuretics / beta-blockers / ACEIs / ARBs and aldosterone receptor antagonists; Add amlodipine or nifedipine if blood pressure is not controlled
Atrial Fibrillation		First choice: ACEIs / ARBs; For sust ained rapid atrial fibrillation, use beta-blockers or nondihydropyridine CCBs to control ventricular rate
Renal Impairment	Target blood pressure <140/90 mmHg; If proteinuria is present and tolerated, further lower blood pressure	If no contraindications, first choice: ACEIs or ARBs; If blood pressure is not controlled, add dihydropyridine CCBs; If fluid retention is present, add loop diuretics
Diabetes Mellitus	Target blood pressure <140/90 mmHg; If tolerated, further lower blood pressure	First choice: ARBs or ACEIs; Can be combined with long-acting dihydropyridine CCBs or thiazide diuretics

1. Blood Pressure Lowering Strategies for Hypertensive Emergencies. Blood pressure lowering strategies for hypertensive emergencies are presented in Table 4-3.

Table 4-3 Blood Pressure Lowering Strategies for Hypertensive Emergencies

Hypertensive Emergencies in the Nervous System			
Disease Conditions	Blood Pressure Treatment Goals	Commonly Used Medications	Precautions
Hypertensive Encephalopathy	For BP>160-180/100-110 mmHg, reduce DBP by 20%-25% within 1 hour	Nicardipine, labetalol, sodium nitroprusside, etc.	Avoid drugs that reduce cerebral blood flow; consider alleviation of brain edema / reduction of intracranial pres-sure; monitor intra-cranial pressure when using sodium nitro-prusside; add mannitol / diuretics for marked intracranial hypertension

(Continued)

<table>
<tr><th colspan="4">Hypertensive Emergencies in the Nervous System</th></tr>
<tr><th>Disease Conditions</th><th>Blood Pressure Treatment Goals</th><th>Commonly Used Medications</th><th>Precautions</th></tr>
<tr><td>Ischemic Stroke</td><td>When SBP>220 mmHg or DBP > 120-140 mmHg, reduce BP by 10%-15%, closely monitoring associated neurolog-ical symptoms</td><td>Nicardipine, labetalol, urapidil, sodium nitroprusside, etc.; oral options: captopril or nicardipine</td><td rowspan="4">Sublingual nitroglycerin causing abrupt BP reduction significantly increases cardiovascular risk and should be avoided; betablockers may reduce cerebral blood flow and are not recommended in the acute phase</td></tr>
<tr><td>Brain Infarction</td><td>When SBP>200/130 mmHg, reduce by<10%-15% within 24 hours, maintain DBP<120 mmHg</td><td></td></tr>
<tr><td>Hemorrhagic Stroke</td><td>For primary spontaneous intracerebral hemorrhage, there is no clear blood pressure target. It is recommended to maintain systolic blood pressure≤180 mmHg or mean arterial pressure (MAP) <130 mmHg, with individualized determination</td><td>Labetalol, urapidil, nicardipine, angiotensin-converting enzyme inhibitors (ACEIs), diuretics, etc.</td></tr>
<tr><td>Subarachnoid Hemorrhage</td><td>The initial blood pressure reduction target should be within 25%. For patients with normal blood pressure, maintain systolic blood pressure between 130-160 mmHg to prevent worsening of bleeding and excessive blood pressure dec-rease</td><td>Nimodipine, nicardipine, betareceptor bl-ockers, ACEIs, etc.</td></tr>
<tr><th colspan="4">Cardiovascular Emergencies</th></tr>
<tr><td>Acute Heart Failure</td><td>Reduce BP to normal range within 1 hour, maintain SBP≥90 mmHg or 10%-15% reduction</td><td>Vasodilators (nitroglycerin or isosorbide dinitrate / sodium nitroprusside), diuretics (furosemide), ACEIs, urapidil, morphine, digoxin, etc.</td><td>Use labetalol / non-dihydropyridine CCBs cautiously; do not abruptly stop Ⅳ antihypertensives after symptom relief to avoid BP rebound; if condition fluctuates, add oral antihypertensives and gradually taper Ⅳ drugs; avoid excessive BP reduction</td></tr>
<tr><td>Acute Coronary Syndrome</td><td>For non-ST-elevation non-diabetic patients, target BP <140/90 mmHg; for non-ST-elevation diabetic or chronic kidney disease patients, target BP 130/80 mmHg</td><td>Nitroglycerin plus esmolol or labetalol / nic-ardipine</td><td>Monitor ischemic chest pain, ECG, and cardiac biomarkers dynamically, and observe vital signs and hemo-dynamics</td></tr>
</table>

(Continued)

Hypertensive Emergencies in the Nervous System			
Disease Conditions	Blood Pressure Treatment Goals	Commonly Used Medications	Precautions
Cardiovascular Emergencies			
Acute Aortic Dissection	If tolerated, reduce BP to 90-110/60-70 mmHg within 30 minutes, and heart rate to 60-75 bpm, maintaining BP in lower range	Sodium nitroprusside or nicardipine combined with labetalol / urapidil / esmolol or metoprolol	Avoid hydralazine; in cases of major aortic branch obstruction, excessive BP reduc-tion may exacerbate ischemia
Acute Kidney Injury			
Renal insufficiency / Renal failure	Strict BP control, lower to 130/80 mmHg or below	Loop diuretics, urapi-dil, nicardipine, nifedipine, nitroglycerin	For diabetic nephropathy with GFR>20 mL/min, ACEIs can be first choice; when SCr>3 mg/dL, ACEIs generally not used
Other Conditions			
Pheochromocytoma	Reduce DBP to around 110 mmHg or by 10%-15% within 30-60 minutes. If tolerated, further lower BP to 160/100 mmHg within 2-6 hours, and gradually to baseline over 24-48 hours	Labetalol, urapidil, and nicardipine	After beta-blocker-induced vasodilation, α-adrenergic vasoconstrictor activity may predominate, leading to further BP elevation
Perioperative Hypertension	Reduce DBP to around 110 mmHg or by 10%-15% within 30-60 minutes. If tolerated, lower BP to 160/100 mmHg within 2-6 hours, and gradually to baseline over 24-48 hours	Sodium nitroprusside, nitroglycerin or nicardipine combined with labetalol / urapidil /esmolol or diltiazem	Avoid ACEIs or diure-tics
Eclampsia and Pre-eclampsia	Reduce DBP to 90-100 mmHg	For pre-eclampsia, Ⅳ labetalol or sodium nitroprusside / nitroglycerin drip, then switch to oral methyldopa / labetalol when BP is stable	Avoid ACEIs, use beta-blockers (risk of fetal growth retardation) and diuretics cauti-ously

2. Chronic Blood Pressure Lowering Strategies for Elderly Hypertension. The chronic blood pressure lowering strategies for elderly hypertension are presented in Figures 4-1 to 4-9.

Ⅶ Consultation Process

1. Definition of hypertension in the elderly: Age≥65, with sustained or≥3 separate measurements of seated systolic blood pressure (SBP) ≥140 mmHg and/or diastolic blood pressure (DBP) ≥90 mmHg on different days. Isolated systolic hypertension in the elderly is defined as SBP≥140 mmHg and DBP<90 mmHg.

2. Initial risk stratification assessment for elderly hypertensive patients includes evaluation of cardiovascular risk factors, target organ damage, and coexisting clinical conditions.

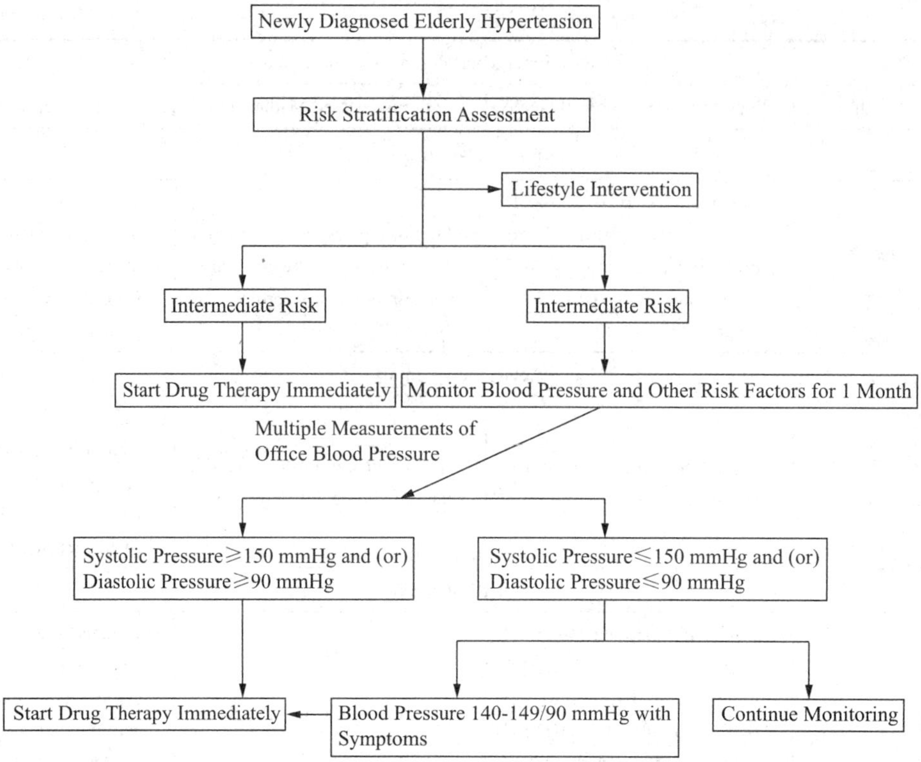

Figure 4-1 Assessment and Monitoring Procedure for Newly Diagnosed Elderly Hypertensive Patients

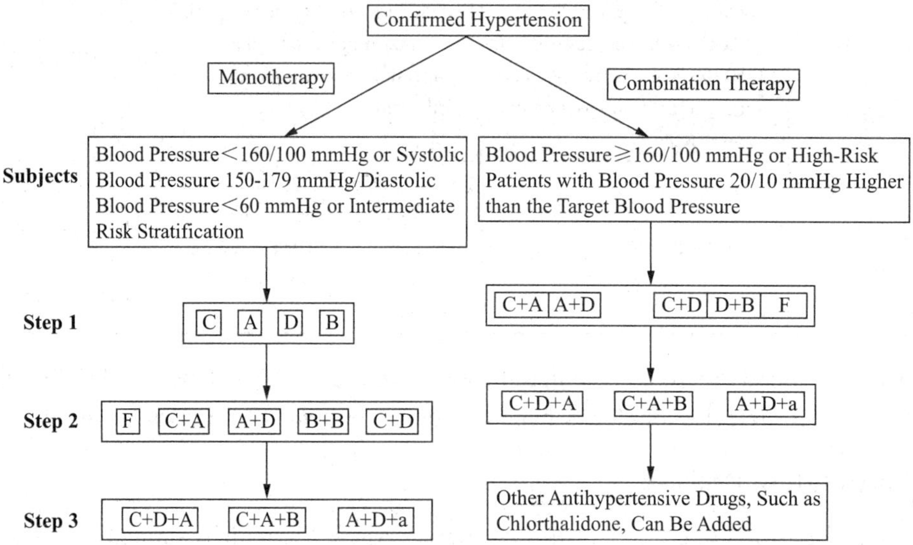

Figure 4-2 Drug Selection Process for Elderly Hypertensive Patients

3. For elderly hypertensive patients:

(1) Initial treatment thresholds: ① Age≥65 and<80: ≥150/90 mmHg; ② Age≥80: ≥160/90 mmHg.

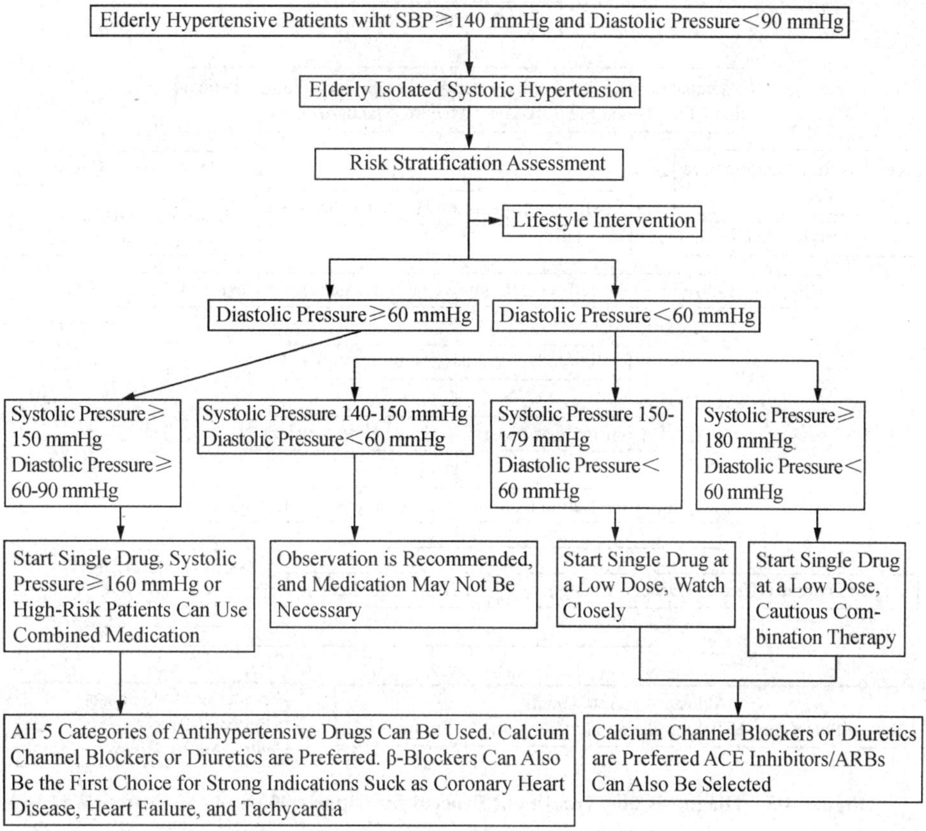

Figure 4-3 Diagnosis and Treatment Process for Elderly Isolated Systolic Hypertension

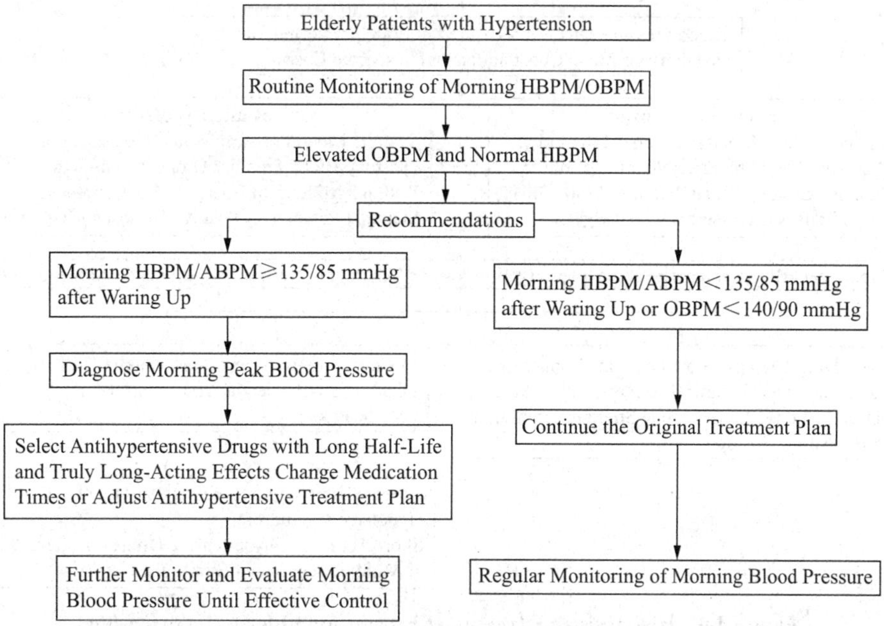

Figure 4-4 Diagnosis and Treatment Process for Elderly Morning Hypertension

Note: ABPM, Ambulatory Blood Pressure Monitoring; HBPM, Home Blood Pressure Monitoring; OBPM, Office Blood Pressure

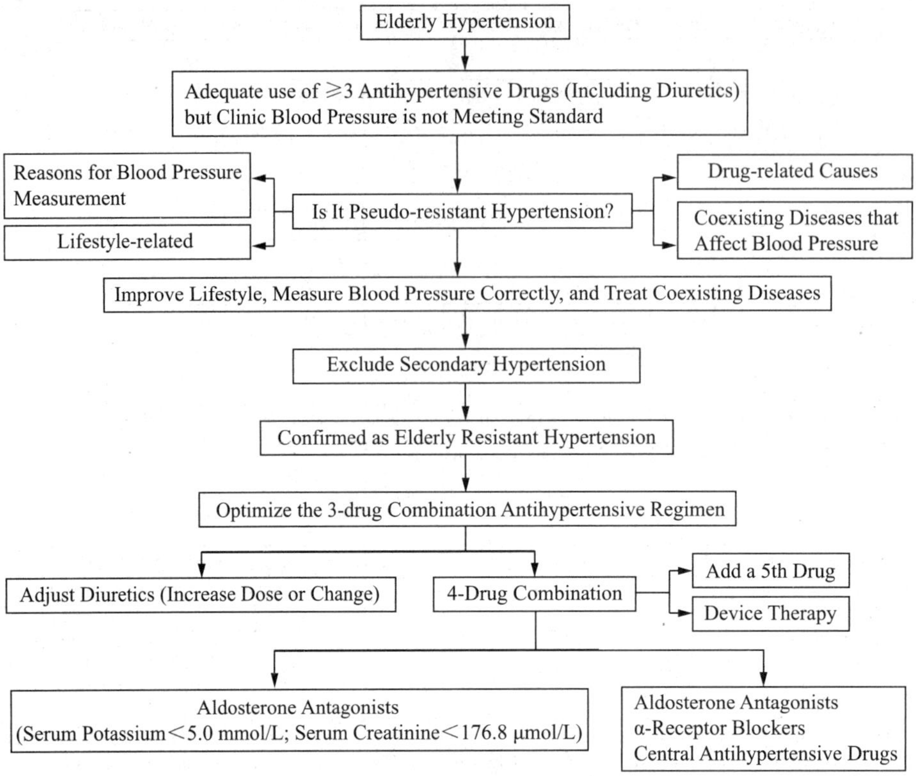
Elderly Hypertension
Adequate use of ≥3 Antihypertensive Drugs (Including Diuretics) but Clinic Blood Pressure is not Meeting Standard
Reasons for Blood Pressure Measurement
Lifestyle-related
Is It Pseudo-resistant Hypertension?
Drug-related Causes
Coexisting Diseases that Affect Blood Pressure
Improve Lifestyle, Measure Blood Pressure Correctly, and Treat Coexisting Diseases
Exclude Secondary Hypertension
Confirmed as Elderly Resistant Hypertension
Optimize the 3-drug Combination Antihypertensive Regimen
Adjust Diuretics (Increase Dose or Change)
4-Drug Combination
Add a 5th Drug
Device Therapy
Aldosterone Antagonists (Serum Potassium<5.0 mmol/L; Serum Creatinine<176.8 μmol/L)
Aldosterone Antagonists
α-Receptor Blockers
Central Antihypertensive Drugs

Figure 4-5 Diagnosis and Treatment Process for Elderly Morning Hypertension

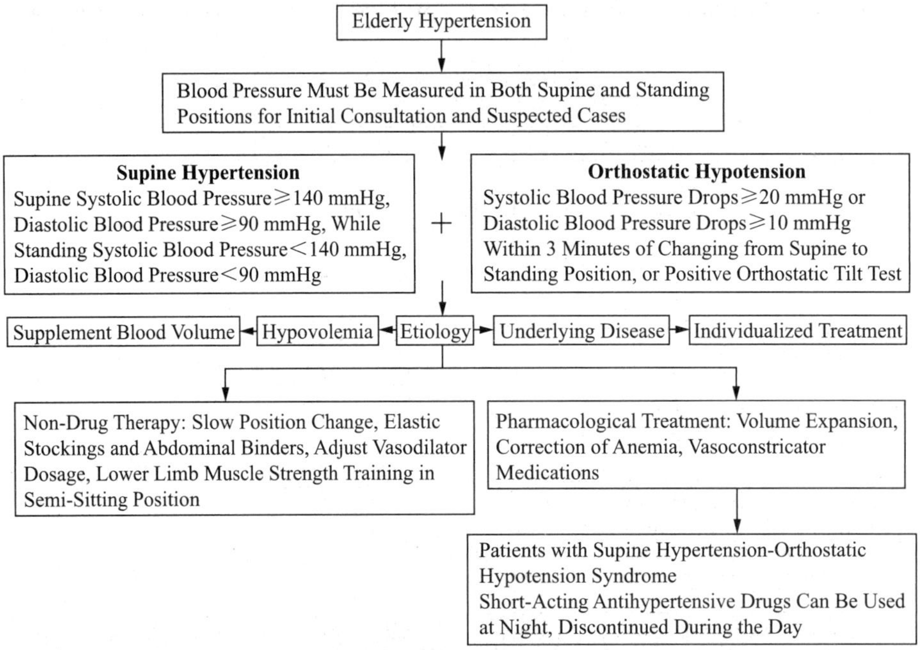
Elderly Hypertension
Blood Pressure Must Be Measured in Both Supine and Standing Positions for Initial Consultation and Suspected Cases
Supine Hypertension
Supine Systolic Blood Pressure≥140 mmHg, Diastolic Blood Pressure≥90 mmHg, While Standing Systolic Blood Pressure<140 mmHg, Diastolic Blood Pressure<90 mmHg
+
Orthostatic Hypotension
Systolic Blood Pressure Drops≥20 mmHg or Diastolic Blood Pressure Drops≥10 mmHg Within 3 Minutes of Changing from Supine to Standing Position, or Positive Orthostatic Tilt Test
Supplement Blood Volume
Hypovolemia
Etiology
Underlying Disease
Individualized Treatment
Non-Drug Therapy: Slow Position Change, Elastic Stockings and Abdominal Binders, Adjust Vasodilator Dosage, Lower Limb Muscle Strength Training in Semi-Sitting Position
Pharmacological Treatment: Volume Expansion, Correction of Anemia, Vasoconstricator Medications
Patients with Supine Hypertension-Orthostatic Hypotension Syndrome
Short-Acting Antihypertensive Drugs Can Be Used at Night, Discontinued During the Day

Figure 4-6 Diagnosis and Treatment Process for Elderly Hypertension with Orthostatic Blood Pressure Variation

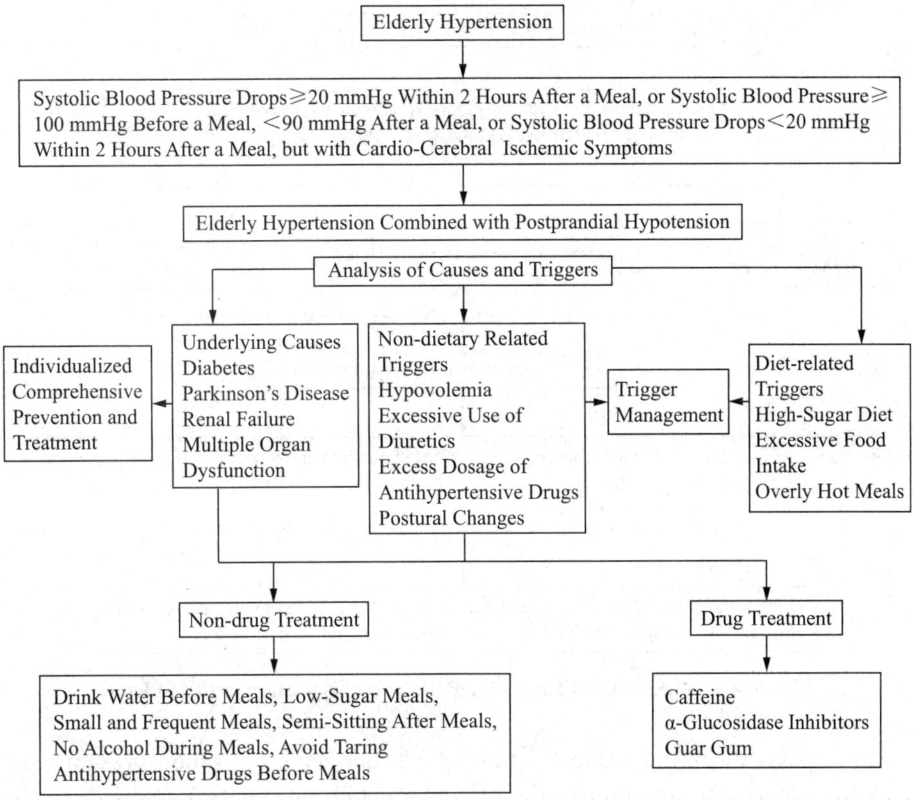

Figure 4-7 Diagnosis and Treatment Process for Elderly Hypertension with Postprandial Hypotension

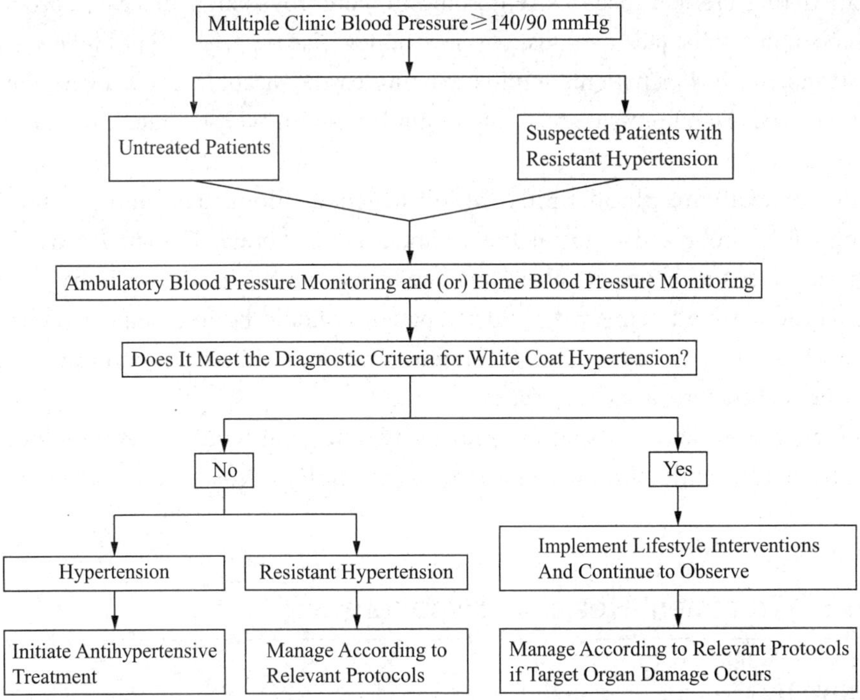

Figure 4-8 Diagnosis and Treatment Process for White Coat Hypertension

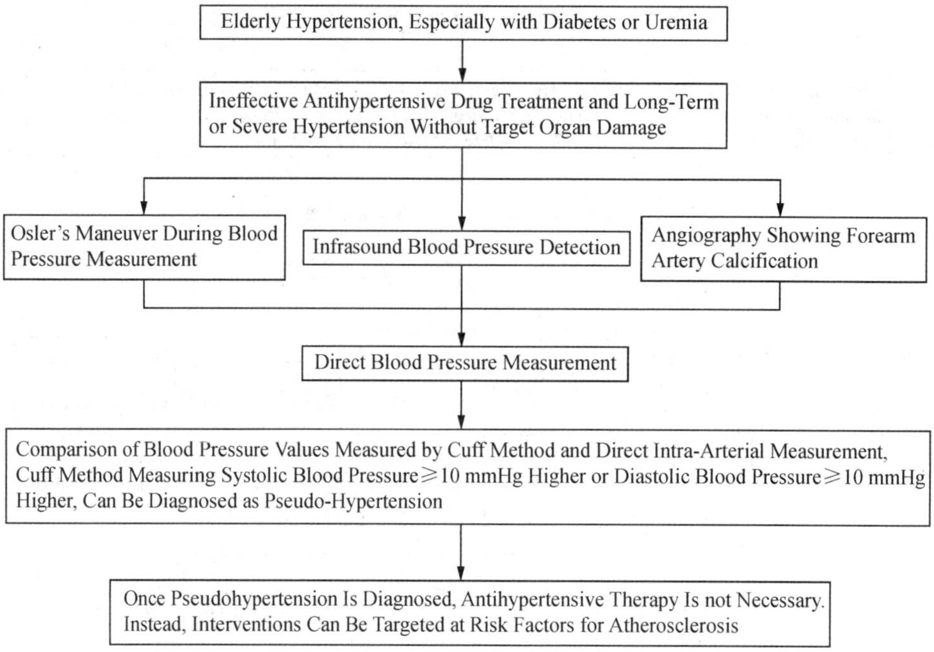
Elderly Hypertension, Especially with Diabetes or Uremia
Ineffective Antihypertensive Drug Treatment and Long-Term or Severe Hypertension Without Target Organ Damage
Osler's Maneuver During Blood Pressure Measurement
Infrasound Blood Pressure Detection
Angiography Showing Forearm Artery Calcification
Direct Blood Pressure Measurement
Comparison of Blood Pressure Values Measured by Cuff Method and Direct Intra-Arterial Measurement, Cuff Method Measuring Systolic Blood Pressure≥10 mmHg Higher or Diastolic Blood Pressure≥10 mmHg Higher, Can Be Diagnosed as Pseudo-Hypertension
Once Pseudohypertension Is Diagnosed, Antihypertensive Therapy Is not Necessary. Instead, Interventions Can Be Targeted at Risk Factors for Atherosclerosis

Figure 4-9　Diagnostic Process for Pseudo-Hypertension in the Elderly

(2) Blood pressure target values: ① For patients aged≥65, blood pressure should be lowered to<150/90 mmHg, and further to<140/90 mmHg if tolerated; ② For patients aged≥80, blood pressure generally should not be lowered below 130/60 mmHg. a. For very elderly patients without coexisting clinical diseases (e.g., chronic cerebrovascular disease, coronary artery disease, heart failure, diabetes mellitus, chronic kidney disease), the target blood pressure is<145-150/90 mmHg. b. For patients with coexisting cardiovascular, cerebrovascular, or renal diseases, first lower blood pressure to<150/90 mmHg, and if well-tolerated, further lower to<140/90 mmHg.

4. Further evaluate blood lipids, blood glucose, blood uric acid, renal function, echocardiography, carotid and vertebral artery ultrasound, and brain CT scan. If feasible, perform vascular function tests and compare blood pressure measurements in all four limbs.

5. Antihypertensive treatment for elderly patients should be individualized based on age and staged blood pressure lowering. Treatment strategies should be tailored to coexisting cardiovascular and cerebrovascular diseases.

6. Acute hypertension and special types of hypertension require specific blood pressure lowering strategies, while chronic hypertension primarily involves gradual blood pressure reduction.

Section 6　Treatment-Resistant Hypertension

I　Definition

The Chinese Guidelines for the Management of Hypertension (2010) defined treatment-resistant hypertension as blood pressure remaining above the target level despite lifestyle modifications and the concomitant use of an appropriate combination of at least three antihypertensive agents (including a diuretic) at optimal doses, or the requirement of four or more medications to achieve blood pressure control. Treatment-resistant hypertension (RH) accounts for 15%-20% of hypertensive patients.

The 2013 Chinese Expert Consensus on the Diagnosis and Treatment of Treatment-Resistant Hypertension redefined treatment-resistant hypertension as blood pressure remaining uncontrolled for at least one month despite lifestyle modifications and the concomitant use of a tolerable combination of at least three antihypertensive agents (including a diuretic) at optimal doses, or the requirement of four or more medications to effectively control blood pressure. Compared to the guidelines, the consensus added a one-month time frame to minimize the probability of misdiagnosis.

Ⅱ Evaluation and Diagnostic Approach for Treatment-Resistant Hypertension

In the clinical evaluation of treatment-resistant hypertension, the diagnostic criteria should first be met, followed by the identification of the underlying causes, which is the most critical issue in the diagnosis of treatment-resistant hypertension. The common factors contributing to difficult-to-control hypertension include the following:

1. Factors related to clinicians or patients

(1) Inaccurate blood pressure measurement: The diagnosis of hypertension currently relies on clinic blood pressure measurements. Clinicians are required to follow proper measurement protocols, such as ensuring appropriate cuff tightness, with the cuff covering two-thirds of the arm length and the bladder encircling more than two-thirds of the arm circumference. At least two measurements should be taken, with a 1-minute interval between them. If the difference between two consecutive readings is <5 mmHg, the lower value is considered accurate. The higher value should be recorded if there is a discrepancy between the arms.

Patients should avoid consuming stimulants like coffee or strong tea before the examination, empty their bladder, rest quietly for at least 5 minutes in a comfortable position and temperature before blood pressure measurement.

(2) White-coat hypertension: This phenomenon manifests as higher blood pressure readings when measured by a physician, especially by senior physicians, while self-measured or community-measured readings are lower. The prevalence is not low, reaching 20%-30%, particularly among the elderly. To rule out white-coat hypertension, home blood pressure monitoring or 24-hour ambulatory blood pressure monitoring can be employed. For home monitoring, blood pressure is typically measured twice daily (morning before medication and evening at least 12 hours after the morning dose or before bedtime), with three readings each time, and the average of the two closest values is calculated. A home blood pressure reading ≥135/85 mmHg can be diagnostic for hypertension. For 24-hour ambulatory monitoring, the diagnostic criteria are ≥130/80 mmHg over 24 hours, ≥135/85 mmHg during the day, and ≥120/70 mmHg at night.

(3) Pseudo-hypertension: In clinical practice, elderly patients with atherosclerosis often

have cuff-measured blood pressure readings that are higher than the actual intra-arterial pressure, a condition known as pseudo-hypertension. The more severe the atherosclerosis, the more pronounced the pseudo-hypertension. Pseudo-hypertension should be suspected in the following situations: ① Blood pressure remains elevated after antihypertensive treatment, but the patient exhibits symptoms of hypotension (e.g., dizziness, fatigue); ② Evidence of severe brachial artery atherosclerosis, such as severe calcification on X-ray examination; ③ High blood pressure without target organ damage; ④ Significantly higher brachial artery blood pressure compared to lower extremity artery blood pressure; ⑤ Severe isolated systolic hypertension. Clinically, if the brachial artery pulse remains palpable despite cuff inflation above the measured systolic pressure, pseudo-hypertension should be considered.

(4) Poor patient adherence: Intermittent changing or self-discontinuation of medications are the main manifestations of poor treatment adherence. Possible reasons can be analyzed from the following aspects:

① Physician-related issues: At each visit, physicians frequently change treatment plans solely based on the current blood pressure reading without thorough history-taking; lack of experience leading to suboptimal dosing, irrational combination therapy, or failure to include a diuretic when more than three antihypertensive agents are prescribed. ② Patient-related issues: Some patients cannot afford the medications; some find it inconvenient to adhere to regular medication schedules, especially when multiple drugs or multiple daily doses are required; some discontinue medications due to fear of adverse effects. ③ Drug-related issues: Intolerable adverse effects from the medications themselves force patients to discontinue or switch therapies.

(5) Unhealthy lifestyles: Such as excessive dietary salt intake (>18 g/day), high-fat diets, severe obesity, heavy smoking, alcohol abuse, excessive anxiety, chronic stressful work environments, and chronic pain.

2. Drug-Related Factors

(1) Suboptimal dosing or irrational combination of antihypertensive medications themselves.

(2) Concomitant use of drugs that can interfere with blood pressure control while taking oral antihypertensives. Clinically, common drugs that affect blood pressure include non-steroidal anti-inflammatory drugs, corticosteroids, sympathomimetics, cyclosporine, tacrolimus, erythropoietin, cocaine, amphetamines, and other addictive substances. Common herbal medicines implicated include ephedra, ginseng, astragalus, asarum, licorice, and aconite. Women of childbearing age should also be asked about oral contraceptive use.

3. Secondary Hypertension: In cases of secondary hypertension, blood pressure is often elevated and less responsive to conventional antihypertensive medications if the underlying condition is not treated. Common causes of secondary hypertension include sleep apnea, primary aldosteronism, renal parenchymal disease, renovascular hypertension, chronic kidney disease, pheochromocytoma, chronic steroid therapy and Cushing's syndrome, aortic stenosis, thyroid and parathyroid disorders, and intracranial tumors. Psychological factors leading to refractory hypertension should also be considered.

To sum up, the recommended diagnostic and therapeutic approach for refractory hypertension involves detailed history-taking and physical examination to identify pseudoresistance, assess the accuracy of blood pressure measurement, rule out white-coat and pseudo-hypertension, evaluate adherence, optimize medication dosing and combination therapy, address lifestyle factors, and identify any concomitant medications that may interfere with blood pressure control. The next step is to actively investigate for secondary causes of hypertension, involving relevant specialties when necessary. Once true treatment resistance is confirmed after excluding the above factors, the focus shifts to identifying the underlying reasons for drug resistance and assessing target organ damage.

Ⅲ Treatment of Refractory Hypertension

1. Basic Therapy

(1) Maximizing Patient Adherence: Physicians should thoroughly consider adherence issues before prescribing antihypertensive medications. This includes simplifying regimens, preferring long-acting formulations, selecting cost-effective options based on the patient's financial situation, increasing follow-up frequency, encouraging self-monitoring of blood pressure, enhancing patient education, and establishing multidisciplinary teams (physicians, nurses, pharmacists, dietitians) where feasible to support adherence.

(2) Lifestyle Modifications: Key interventions include weight reduction (targeting a body mass index below 24 kg/m^2), alcohol restriction (<30 g/day for men, half for women or low body weight), dietary sodium restriction (<6 g/day), adoption of a high-fiber, low-fat diet with controlled caloric intake, increased physical activity (30 minutes, 3-5 times per week), and stress management techniques to maintain psychological well-being.

(3) Treatment of Underlying Secondary Causes.

(4) Discontinuation of Interfering Medications: Drugs that impair blood pressure control, especially non-steroidal anti-inflammatory drugs, should be discontinued if possible. If discontinuation is challenging, dose reduction is recommended. Close blood pressure monitoring is necessary when initiating such medications.

2. Pharmacological Treatment

(1) Basic Principles: An individualized approach is essential, selecting antihypertensive agents based on the patient's specific conditions and tolerability. Long-acting formulations should be preferred to effectively control nocturnal, morning, and 24-hour blood pressure. Rational combination therapy should be employed to maximize efficacy while minimizing adverse effects. Proper diuretic use is crucial.

(2) Drug Selection: For patients with high renin and sympathetic activity, renin-angiotensin-aldosterone system inhibitors (RASIs) [angiotensin Ⅱ receptor blockers (ARBs) or angiotensin-converting enzyme inhibitors (ACEIs)] and beta-blockers are the mainstay. For volume overload and low circulating renin-angiotensin system activity, calcium channel blockers (CCBs) and diuretics are preferred. In cases of high dietary salt intake, thiazide diuretic doses should be appropriately increased, emphasizing strict sodium restriction. For severe renal impairment, loop diuretics are indicated. In non-dialysis chronic kidney disease, CCB doses should be increased, potentially combining dihydropyridine and non-dihydropyridine CCBs, due to limitations in RASI use or dosing. For obese patients, RASI doses should be escalated. In isolated systolic

hypertension or the elderly, higher CCB doses are recommended.

The typical triple therapy regimen consists of a RASI + CCB + thiazide diuretic at standard or maximally tolerated doses. If the blood pressure remains uncontrolled, the addition of a mineralocorticoid receptor antagonist or a beta-blocker, alpha-blocker, or central sympatholytic agent (e.g., clonidine, methyldopa) as a fifth drug can be considered after carefully evaluating renal function and the risk of hyperkalemia.

3. For a subset of patients with true treatment-resistant hypertension despite optimal lifestyle modifications and intensive pharmacological treatment, renal denervation (RDN) represents an emerging interventional approach. Excessive renal sympathetic nerve activity plays a crucial role in the pathogenesis and maintenance of hypertension. The anatomical localization of renal nerve fibers predominantly along the renal artery adventitia allows for selective ablation by RDN. The Symplicity HTN-1 and HTN-2 trials demonstrated the efficacy of RDN in treating resistant hypertension, and this approach offers advantages of minimal invasiveness and high procedural success rates. However, RDN remains in its early stages, with initiation in 2007 internationally and the first reports in China in 2011. Many issues require further investigation, such as the lack of robust evidence on the long-term impact of RDN on cardiovascular events and mortality, as well as potential procedural complications like renal artery dissection, aneurysm formation, and stenosis. Therefore, clinicians are advised to conduct thorough pre-procedural evaluations, strictly adhere to procedural indications, and implement RDN judiciously and systematically.

Ⅳ Common Questions in Consultation

1. How to interpret the results of 24-hour ambulatory blood pressure monitoring (ABPM) in patients with resistant hypertension?

ABPM reflects the specific situation of a patient's blood pressure fluctuations within a day. The results generally include: ① Blood pressure (BP) status, including the average BP over 24 hours, the highest and lowest values and their occurrence times; the average BP, highest and lowest values, and their occurrence times during the daytime (8:00-23:00) and nighttime (23:00-8:00). The diagnostic criteria for hypertension based on ABPM are: 24-hour average BP ≥130/80 mmHg, daytime BP ≥135/85 mmHg, and nighttime BP ≥120/70 mmHg. ② BP rhythm: In normal individuals, the BP fluctuation follows a long-spoon shape, with the lowest trough occurring at 2:00-3:00 at night, known as the nocturnal dip. The BP rises sharply in the early morning and remains at a relatively high level during the day, often with two peaks (8:00-9:00 and 16:00-18:00). After 18:00, it shows a slow downward trend. Hypertensive patients often exhibit a reverse-spoon pattern, with a shallow nocturnal dip, a nighttime BP reduction of <10% compared to daytime, or no obvious nocturnal dip, and sometimes even higher nighttime BP than daytime.

When using antihypertensive drugs for resistant hypertension, attention should be paid to chronotherapy. Based on ABPM, the timing of morning, midday, and evening BP peaks should be determined, and different antihypertensive drugs with varying durations of action should be selected and administered at appropriate times according to the BP peak and trough periods, to maximize the effects of the medications.

2. What should be done if the patient's BP remains uncontrolled despite the combination of four antihypertensive drugs?

When resistant hypertension occurs, a 24-hour ABPM should be performed first to exclude "white coat" hypertension and clarify the specific situation of the patient's BP elevation. It can also help assess patient compliance, confirm and improve relevant lifestyles, discontinue or reduce drugs that affect BP, and most importantly, screen for secondary hypertension. If the BP remains high after the above measures, oral medications should be adjusted, with attention to increasing the dose of diuretics, including mineralocorticoid receptor antagonists, combining drugs with different mechanisms of action, and individualizing the timing of antihypertensive drug administration according to the time of BP elevation. If all methods fail, it is advisable to temporarily discontinue drug therapy, closely monitor BP, and initiate a new treatment plan, which may help break the vicious cycle of BP elevation.

3. What are the considerations for antihypertensive treatment in isolated systolic hypertension?

Isolated systolic hypertension is common in the elderly. The first-line antihypertensive drugs are diuretics or long-acting calcium channel blockers (CCBs). In the presence of heart failure and kidney disease, angiotensin-converting enzyme inhibitors (ACEIs) are preferred. For patients with myocardial infarction, beta-blockers and ACEIs can be used. Combination therapy is often required, with common regimens including CCB + ACEI, diuretic + angiotensin receptor blocker (ARB)/ACEI, CCB + diuretic, and CCB + beta-blocker. During BP reduction, attention should be paid to the decrease in diastolic BP. The HOT trial showed that when diastolic BP drops below 70 mmHg, cardiovascular mortality increases significantly, and if it falls below 55 mmHg, cardiovascular disease increases by 99%. Therefore, when treating isolated systolic hypertension in the elderly, it is necessary to maintain a certain level of diastolic BP and avoid excessive lowering.

V Consultation Process

1. First, clarify whether the patient meets the diagnostic criteria for resistant hypertension.

2. Conduct a detailed medical history inquiry and physical examination to identify pseudo-resistant hypertension.

3. Further investigate the causes of resistant hypertension, including factors related to clinicians or patients, drug factors, and secondary hypertension, and identify reversible factors.

4. Complete examinations including renal function, electrolytes, endocrine tests related to secondary hypertension, echocardiography, renal ultrasound, renal artery CTA, enhanced CT scan of the adrenal glands, and ABPM.

5. Treatment plan: basic treatment, drug therapy, and invasive interventional surgery.

Section 7 Secondary Hypertension

Secondary hypertension accounts for 5%-10% of all hypertension cases. Due to the large base of hypertensive patients in China, secondary hypertension is not uncommon. Moreover, some cases of secondary hypertension can be cured through etiological treatment, making early diagnosis of secondary hypertension crucial. According to statistics, there are more than 50 causes of secondary hypertension, with renal parenchymal hypertension being the most common, followed by renovascular hypertension and endocrine hypertension. Obstructive sleep apnea syndrome is also frequently encountered. The following sections will discuss these conditions in detail.

I Renal Parenchymal Hypertension

1. Etiology. Renal parenchymal hypertension can be primary or secondary. There are many causes, with primary causes including acute and chronic glomerulonephritis, chronic pyelonephritis, polycystic kidney disease, IgA nephropathy, etc. Secondary causes include diabetic nephropathy, lupus nephritis, multiple myeloma, hepatitis B-related kidney disease, and others. According to epidemiological statistics, the incidence of hypertension in chronic nephritis is 60%-80%, reaching 90% in sclerosing nephritis and over 95% in end-stage renal failure.

2. Clinical Clues. Renal parenchymal diseases can lead to hypertension, and conversely, hypertension can cause kidney damage, accelerating the progression of renal parenchymal diseases and forming a vicious cycle. Therefore, renal parenchymal hypertension generally presents as grade 2 or higher hypertension, predominantly with elevated systolic blood pressure and a large pulse pressure. In some critical cases, diastolic blood pressure may also be significantly elevated. Patients are often insensitive to antihypertensive drugs, frequently requiring a combination of three or more medications. Compared to primary hypertension of the same level, renal parenchymal hypertension is associated with more severe target organ damage, such as more severe fundus lesions and more cardiovascular complications. It is also more likely to progress to malignant hypertension, resulting in a worse prognosis than primary hypertension.

3. Diagnosis

(1) Blood pressure ≥140/90 mmHg.

(2) History of renal parenchymal diseases such as acute or chronic nephritis, pyelonephritis, or polycystic kidney disease. Clinical manifestations of oliguria, edema (mainly facial edema), hematuria, and proteinuria often suggest the presence of renal parenchymal lesions.

(3) Laboratory tests: Urine routine examination may reveal hematuria, proteinuria, or granular casts. In chronic kidney disease, complete blood count may show anemia. Renal function tests may indicate elevated blood urea nitrogen and serum creatinine levels. Electrolyte disturbances such as hyperkalemia, hyponatremia, hypocalcemia, and hyperphosphatemia may be present. Blood gas analysis may suggest metabolic acidosis. Ultrasound and CT can demonstrate various renal parenchymal lesions. Definitive diagnosis relies on renal biopsy.

4. Treatment

(1) Non-pharmacological treatment: As with primary hypertension, smoking cessation, alcohol abstinence, moderate exercise, and maintaining a good mental state are recommended. A low-salt diet is advised, but renal parenchymal hypertension patients require stricter sodium

control, generally recommended at <3 g/day. Dietary protein intake should also be restricted.

(2) Pharmacological treatment: ACEIs, ARBs, CCBs, diuretics, beta-blockers, and vasodilators can all be used, with ACEIs, ARBs, and CCBs being the most widely applied. ACEIs or ARBs can delay the deterioration of renal function in the early and middle stages. However, caution should be exercised in cases of low blood volume or late-stage disease (creatinine clearance <30 mL/min or serum creatinine>265 μmol/L), as they may worsen renal function. Therefore, dynamic monitoring of renal function is necessary when using ACEIs or ARBs. Generally, if the increase from baseline exceeds 30%, discontinuation of the drug is recommended. Additionally, due to their potassium-elevating effect, serum potassium levels should be monitored during treatment.

Ⅱ Renovascular Hypertension

1. Etiology. Renovascular hypertension is caused by stenosis of the main trunk or branches of the unilateral or bilateral renal arteries, leading to renal ischemia and activation of the renin-angiotensin-aldosterone system, resulting in hypertension. Common causes include polyarteritis nodosa, congenital fibromuscular dysplasia of the renal artery, and atherosclerosis. The first two are more common in young people, while the latter is more common in the elderly.

2. Clinical Clues

① Blood pressure is often grade 2 or higher, and blood pressure in the four limbs is often asymmetric. ② Sudden worsening of previously well-controlled hypertension. ③ Hypokalemia occurring without the use of diuretics. ④ Unilateral renal atrophy found on examination. ⑤ Coexistence of other severe obstructive vascular diseases (coronary heart disease, cervical vascular murmurs, peripheral vascular lesions). ⑥ Periumbilical vascular murmurs. ⑦ Significant blood pressure reduction or easily induced acute renal insufficiency with ACEIs or ARBs. ⑧ Elevated serum creatinine that cannot be explained by other causes. ⑨ Paroxysmal pulmonary edema disproportionate to left ventricular function.

3. Diagnosis

(1) Blood pressure ≥140/90 mmHg, age of onset under 35 or over 50 years, short disease course, rapid progression, and insensitivity to antihypertensive drugs. Patients with polyarteritis nodosa may also have low-grade fever.

(2) Vascular murmurs heard in the periumbilical region, transmitted unilaterally.

(3) Laboratory tests: Significantly elevated renin activity, weakly positive urine protein, slightly elevated serum creatinine, and slightly decreased serum potassium. In cases caused by polyarteritis nodosa, erythrocyte sedimentation rate and C-reactive protein may also be elevated.

(4) Auxiliary examinations: Ultrasound may reveal unilateral renal atrophy. Color Doppler ultrasound can detect stenosis at the origin of the renal artery. Enhanced CT or MRA of the renal arteries can clarify the location of renal artery stenosis. Renal function tests, such as renal scintigraphy or split renal glomerular filtration rate, may show decreased function of one kidney. Definitive diagnosis relies on renal arteriography.

4. Treatment

(1) Conservative drug therapy: ACEIs and ARBs are effective in the antihypertensive

treatment of renovascular hypertension patients. However, caution should be exercised as they are a double-edged sword. On one hand, they can exert a strong antihypertensive effect by inhibiting the renin-angiotensin-aldosterone system. On the other hand, they block the contraction of efferent arterioles, leading to a decrease in glomerular filtration rate of the affected kidney, renal function damage, and even acute renal insufficiency. Therefore, for these patients, treatment should start with a low dose and gradually increase, with close monitoring of renal function. If serum creatinine rises >30% from baseline, the drug should be discontinued, especially in patients with bilateral or single functional kidney renal artery stenosis. For patients with contraindications to ACEIs or ARBs, CCBs are a safe and effective choice. Other drugs such as beta-blockers, α-blockers, non-specific vasodilators, and centrally acting antihypertensive agents can also be considered.

(2) Renal artery revascularization: Treatment options include percutaneous transluminal angioplasty (PTA), percutaneous renal artery stent implantation, and vascular bypass surgery. In recent years, with the maturity of interventional surgery, it has basically replaced surgical treatment. For renal artery stenosis caused by fibromuscular dysplasia and polyarteritis nodosa, PTA is recommended, and stent implantation is not advised. Patients with polyarteritis nodosa should not undergo surgery during the active inflammatory period. Generally, glucocorticoid treatment should be administered to reduce the erythrocyte sedimentation rate to the normal range for 3-6 months before considering PTA. For renal artery stenosis caused by atherosclerosis, stent implantation is recommended, but there is a possibility of in-stent restenosis after the procedure.

Ⅲ Endocrine Hypertension

Endocrine hypertension includes endocrine diseases with hypertension as the main manifestation, such as primary aldosteronism and pheochromocytoma, as well as endocrine diseases with hypertensive manifestations, such as acromegaly and hyperthyroidism. Endocrine hypertension is mainly concentrated in the young and middle-aged population. If diagnosed early and given correct treatment, most cases can be completely cured, or at least the damage caused by hypertension to the related target organs (mainly the heart, brain, and kidneys) can be alleviated.

1. Primary Aldosteronism (PA)

(1) Etiology: PA is mainly caused by adrenal cortical lesions leading to increased aldosterone secretion. It belongs to mineralocorticoid excess syndrome independent of the renin-angiotensin system. The common types are adrenal adenoma and hyperplasia, with adenoma mostly being aldosteronoma and hyperplasia mostly being idiopathic aldosteronism. Aldosterone carcinoma is rare. Some patients have familial genetic diseases, known as glucocorticoid-remediable aldosteronism.

(2) Clinical clues:

1) Hypertension with hypokalemia.

2) Moderate to severe hypertension, resistant to conventional antihypertensive drugs.

3) Adrenal incidentaloma and hypertension.

4) Early-onset hypertension (<20 years old).

5) Severe hypokalemia induced by conventional doses of potassium-sparing diuretics.

6) Family history of PA.

(3) Diagnosis

1) Screening is performed for patients with a high suspicion of PA. The commonly used tool is the measurement of the plasma aldosterone to renin ratio (ARR), with units in ng. Due to different laboratory conditions, the diagnostic criteria, sensitivity, and specificity of ARR vary. If ARR >20, the sensitivity is 78% and the specificity is 83%; if ARR >50, the sensitivity is 10%. If ARR is normal, PA is excluded. Patients with abnormal ARR should undergo further confirmatory tests.

2) Confirmatory tests: Options include captopril suppression test, oral sodium loading test, intravenous saline infusion test, posture test, and fludrocortisone suppression test. Currently, the captopril suppression test is commonly used in clinical practice. If suppressed, PA is excluded; if not suppressed, PA is confirmed.

3) For patients diagnosed with PA, adrenal CT should be performed to further differentiate between hyperplasia and adenoma. It should be emphasized that before conducting the above tests, drugs that may affect the renin-angiotensin-aldosterone system, such as β-blockers, ACEIs, ARBs, dihydropyridine calcium channel blockers, and spironolactone, must be discontinued for at least 2 weeks, and diuretics for more than 4 weeks. Hypokalemia needs to be corrected first. Drugs with less influence include non-dihydropyridine calcium channel blockers and α-blockers.

(4) Treatment: For aldosteronoma, surgical resection is the first choice, which can achieve a radical cure. Patients with idiopathic hyperaldosteronism have poor surgical outcomes and should receive drug therapy. Sometimes, when it is difficult to determine hyperplasia or adenoma, drug therapy can be initiated first, with continued observation and regular CT reexaminations. Small adenomas that were not detected initially may sometimes become apparent during follow-up. For drug therapy, oral mineralocorticoid receptor antagonist spironolactone is recommended. Usually, a small dose can improve hypokalemia, but a large dose is required to achieve an antihypertensive effect. For patients who cannot tolerate spironolactone, dihydropyridine calcium channel blockers can be selected, as they can directly inhibit aldosterone and block mineralocorticoid receptors. For patients with glucocorticoid-remediable aldosteronism, glucocorticoid therapy is the first choice. Aldosterone carcinoma has a poor prognosis, and the opportunity for surgical cure is often lost at the time of discovery. Chemotherapeutic drugs such as mitotane and aminoglutethimide can temporarily alleviate the clinical symptoms brought about by increased aldosterone but have no significant improvement on the course of the disease.

2. Pheochromocytoma

(1) Etiology: 80%-90% of pheochromocytomas are located in the adrenal medulla, mostly unilateral and rarely bilateral. Extra-adrenal pheochromocytomas are called paragangliomas, mainly located in the abdomen, mostly near the abdominal aorta (10%-15%), and rarely outside the abdomen. The tumor continuously or intermittently releases large amounts of catecholamines, causing sustained or paroxysmal hypertension and dysfunction and metabolic disorders of multiple organs. 90% of pheochromocytomas are benign.

(2) Clinical clues: The typical manifestation is paroxysmal hypertension accompanied by sympathetic excitation, such as tachycardia, sweating, headache, and pallor. Hypertension can

also be persistent, and some patients may experience paroxysmal hypotension or even shock.

(3) Diagnosis

1) Blood and urine catecholamine and metabolite measurements: These include vanillyl mandelic acid (VMA), metanephrine (MN), and normetanephrine (NMN). In patients with persistent hypertension, these indicators are significantly elevated. In patients with paroxysmal hypertension, they may not be elevated during normal periods but will be higher than normal after an attack.

2) Pharmacological tests: In patients with persistent hypertension, if urine catecholamines and their metabolites are significantly elevated, pharmacological tests may not be necessary. For paroxysmal cases, if symptoms do not occur for a long time, a glucagon stimulation test can be performed.

3) Localization diagnosis: It is advisable to perform this after blood pressure is controlled with α-blockers. Tumors located in the adrenal glands can generally be clearly identified in terms of specific location and size through ultrasound, CT, or MRI. Localization of extra-adrenal tumors is more difficult. Octreotide scintigraphy and I-MIBG can help locate the tumor. If the location still cannot be determined, segmental blood samples from the vena cava can be taken to measure catecholamine concentrations. Based on the concentration differences, the approximate location of the tumor can be determined, followed by further judgment with CT and MRI.

4) Treatment: Surgical resection is the fundamental treatment. However, surgery has certain risks. Especially when manipulating the tumor, a sudden release of large amounts of catecholamines may cause a sharp increase in blood pressure and/or arrhythmia. Therefore, α-blockers should be used for at least 2 weeks before surgery to reduce blood pressure, reduce cardiac load, and expand the previously reduced blood volume.

Ⅳ Obstructive Sleep Apnea Syndrome (OSAS)

1. Etiology. OSAS is a common but easily overlooked disease. It is a chronic sleep-disordered breathing disease characterized by upper airway obstruction due to certain factors, resulting in sleep apnea accompanied by hypoxia, snoring, daytime sleepiness, and other symptoms. It mainly causes hypertension through multiple mechanisms such as activating the renin-angiotensin-aldosterone system, autonomic dysfunction, damaging vascular endothelial function, and activating inflammatory responses. Epidemiological surveys show that the prevalence of OSAS in hypertensive patients is 30%-50%, while the detection rate of hypertension in OSAS patients is as high as 50%-92%.

2. Clinical Clues

(1) Patients are mostly obese or have abnormal upper airway anatomical structures, with a higher prevalence in males than females.

(2) Blood pressure is characterized by nighttime blood pressure elevation, significant morning blood pressure elevation, and blood pressure rhythm disturbances, presenting as non-dipper or reverse-dipper patterns. Along with apnea, blood pressure periodically rises. The effect of drug treatment alone is poor, and resistant hypertension is common.

(3) Snoring during sleep is irregular, with disturbed breathing and sleep structure. Repeated

apnea and awakenings occur, or patients feel suffocated. Nocturia is increased, and patients experience headache and dry mouth upon waking in the morning. Daytime sleepiness is significant, and memory is impaired.

3. Diagnosis

(1) OSAS diagnostic criteria: Mainly based on medical history, physical signs, and polysomnography monitoring results. Diagnostic criteria: ① Clinically typical nighttime snoring accompanied by apnea, daytime sleepiness, and physical examination revealing narrowing and obstruction of any part of the upper airway, with an apnea-hypopnea index (AHI) ≥5 times/h. ② For patients with no obvious daytime sleepiness, AHI≥10 times/h or AHI≥5 times/h, along with one or more comorbidities such as cognitive dysfunction, coronary heart disease, cerebrovascular disease, diabetes, and insomnia, the diagnosis can also be confirmed.

(2) Diagnosis of OSAS-related hypertension: Patients have both hypertension and OSAS, with a clear correlation between the two.

4. Treatment

(1) General treatment: Weight loss; changing sleep position: sleeping on the side, raising the head of the bed; quitting smoking and drinking alcohol; avoiding sedatives.

(2) Drug therapy: The efficacy is uncertain. Acetazolamide, medroxyprogesterone, and protriptyline can be used for treatment. Modafinil has the effect of improving daytime sleepiness and is suitable for patients whose sleepiness symptoms do not significantly improve after continuous positive airway pressure (CPAP) treatment, with a certain degree of efficacy.

(3) CPAP: Currently, it is an effective and most commonly used method for treating OSAS.

(4) Oral appliance therapy and surgical treatments such as septoplasty, nasal polypectomy, and uvulopalatopharyngoplasty also have certain efficacy.

V Common Questions in Consultation

1. For patients with hypertension combined with hypokalemia, what examinations should be performed to further clarify whether there is secondary hypertension?

Several types of secondary hypertension are more likely to be associated with hypokalemia, such as renal artery stenosis, primary aldosteronism, hyperthyroidism, and Cushing's syndrome. In clinical practice, screening for these diseases is mainly performed. First, check whether the patient is taking potassium-sparing diuretics. If so, it is recommended to discontinue them and correct hypokalemia with oral or intravenous potassium supplementation. Second, check the current oral antihypertensive drugs. If the blood pressure is not particularly high, it is recommended to discontinue all antihypertensive drugs first. If antihypertensive drugs must be used, it is recommended to discontinue drugs that affect the RAS system, such as ACEIs and ARBs, and choose antihypertensive drugs that have less impact on the RAS system. Then, measure the plasma aldosterone / renin ratio (ARR), perform a posture test or captopril test, check 24-hour urinary potassium and sodium, thyroid function, serum cortisol, and perform renal and renal artery ultrasound and adrenal enhanced CT. Generally, the cause can be found through the above examinations.

2. If potassium is normal, can primary aldosteronism be excluded?

The answer is no. In the early stage of primary aldosteronism, there may be no hypokalemia, and only hypertension is present. However, aldosterone is increased, and the renin system is suppressed, resulting in an elevated plasma aldosterone / renin ratio. Therefore, it is not possible to determine whether it is primary aldosteronism based solely on whether potassium is decreased.

3. How to deal with a hypertensive crisis caused by pheochromocytoma?

Immediately administer a slow intravenous injection of phentolamine 1-5 mg, while closely monitoring blood pressure. When the blood pressure drops to around 160/100 mmHg, immediately stop the injection and switch to a slow intravenous drip of 10-15 mg dissolved in 500 mL of 5% glucose saline. Alternatively, sublingual nifedipine 10 mg can be used to lower blood pressure.

Ⅵ Consultation Process

1. Renal Parenchymal Hypertension

(1) Carefully inquire about the medical history to understand whether there is a history of various chronic kidney diseases and clarify the chronological relationship between kidney disease and hypertension.

(2) Pay attention to whether there are clinical symptoms and signs of renal parenchymal damage, such as oliguria, edema (mainly facial edema), hematuria, and proteinuria. Check renal function, electrolytes, urine routine, blood gas analysis, ultrasound, and CT to further clarify the evidence of renal parenchymal damage.

(3) Treatment: Treatment of underlying renal disease, general treatment, and drug therapy.

2. Renovascular Hypertension

(1) Carefully inquire about the medical history for the following clues: blood pressure is mostly grade 2 or above, and blood pressure in the four limbs is often asymmetric; sudden worsening of previously well-controlled hypertension; hypokalemia occurring without the use of diuretics; unilateral renal atrophy found on examination; coexistence of other severe obstructive vascular diseases (coronary heart disease, cervical vascular murmurs, peripheral vascular lesions); periumbilical vascular murmurs; significant blood pressure reduction or easily induced acute renal insufficiency with ACEIs or ARBs; elevated serum creatinine that cannot be explained by other causes; paroxysmal pulmonary edema disproportionate to left ventricular function.

(2) Complete bilateral renal and renal artery color Doppler ultrasound, renal artery CTA, and glomerular filtration rate examinations. If necessary, further perform renal arteriography for definitive diagnosis.

(3) Conservative drug therapy and interventional treatment.

3. Endocrine Hypertension

(1) Primary Aldosteronism

1) Carefully inquire about the medical history for the following clues: hypertension with hypokalemia; moderate to severe hypertension, resistant to conventional antihypertensive drugs; adrenal incidentaloma and hypertension; early-onset hypertension (<20 years old); severe hypokalemia induced by conventional doses of potassium-sparing diuretics; family history of

primary aldosteronism; suspicious patients screened out.

2) Further screen patients with a high suspicion of primary aldosteronism. The commonly used method is the measurement of the plasma aldosterone / renin ratio (ARR). Patients with abnormal ARR need further confirmatory tests to clarify the diagnosis.

3) Treatment: For aldosteronoma, surgical resection is the first choice. For idiopathic aldosteronism, drug therapy should be used. Sometimes, when it is difficult to determine hyperplasia or adenoma, drug therapy can be initiated first, with continued observation and regular CT reexaminations.

(2) Pheochromocytoma

1) Inquire about the medical history for the following clues: paroxysmal hypertension accompanied by sympathetic excitation or even shock.

2) For patients with suspected pheochromocytoma, measure blood and urine catecholamines and their metabolites. For patients with paroxysmal hypertension, if symptoms do not occur for a long time, a glucagon stimulation test can be performed.

3) Use color Doppler ultrasound, CT, MRI, and radionuclide scanning for localization diagnosis.

4) Treatment: Surgical resection is the fundamental treatment. α-blockers should be used for at least 2 weeks before surgery.

4. Obstructive Sleep Apnea Syndrome

(1) Inquire about the medical history for the following clues: obesity, abnormal upper airway anatomical structures, blood pressure characterized by nighttime blood pressure elevation, significant morning blood pressure elevation, blood pressure rhythm disturbances presenting as non-dipper or reverse-dipper patterns, periodic blood pressure elevation accompanying apnea, poor effect of drug treatment alone, and common resistant hypertension. Snoring during sleep is irregular, with disturbed breathing and sleep structure. Repeated apnea and awakenings occur, or patients feel suffocated. Nocturia is increased, and patients experience headache and dry mouth upon waking in the morning. Daytime sleepiness is significant, and memory is impaired.

(2) Combine medical history, physical signs, and polysomnography (PSG) monitoring results to clarify the diagnosis.

(3) Treatment: General treatment, drug therapy, CPAP treatment; oral appliance therapy and surgical treatments such as uvulopalatopharyngoplasty.

Chapter 5

Pericardial and Valvular Heart Diseases

Section 1 Pericardial Effusion

I Definition

Pericardial effusion (hydropericardium) refers to the excess of fluid between the visceral and parietal layers of the pericardium, which is seen in exudative pericarditis and other non-inflammatory pericardial diseases.

II Etiology

Pericardial effusion is classified into two major categories: infectious and non-infectious.

1. Infectious causes include viruses, bacteria, fungi, protozoa, rickettsia, etc.

2. Non-infectious causes include tumors, autoimmune diseases, endocrine and metabolic diseases, trauma, radiation, post-myocardial infarction, etc.

III Clinical Manifestations

The patient's symptoms depend on the degree of cardiac compression by the effusion. Mild cases may have no obvious symptoms, while the most prominent symptom is dyspnea. In severe cases, patients may experience orthopnea. Acute cardiac tamponade can lead to shock and acute circulatory failure, while subacute or chronic cardiac tamponade manifests as systemic venous congestion and paradoxical pulse. Physical signs also depend on the amount of effusion, including enlarged cardiac dullness, weakened apex beat, distant and muffled heart sounds, dullness below the left scapula, and bronchial breathing sounds caused by left lung compression, known as the pericardial effusion sign (Ewart's sign). Other signs include jugular venous distension, hepatomegaly, ascites, and lower extremity edema.

IV Diagnosis

1. Chest X-ray: An enlarged cardiac silhouette on both sides suggests pericardial effusion, generally exceeding 300 mL. A flask-shaped cardiac silhouette indicates pericardial effusion exceeding 1, 000 mL. In adults, X-ray may not detect effusion volumes <250 mL, and in children, <150 mL.

2. Electrocardiogram (ECG): Low voltage, tachycardia, and electrical alternans may be observed.

3. Echocardiography: It can confirm the diagnosis of pericardial effusion and assess its

severity, as well as guide pericardiocentesis. A maximum diastolic dark space <10 mm between the pericardium and epicardium indicates a small amount of pericardial effusion, 10-19 mm indicates a moderate amount, and >20 mm indicates a large amount.

4. Magnetic resonance imaging (MRI): It can clearly show the volume and distribution of pericardial effusion and distinguish the nature of the effusion. Low signal intensity generally indicates non-hemorrhagic exudate, such as that caused by viral infections.

5. Pericardiocentesis: It can confirm the presence of pericardial effusion, examine the effusion to clarify the etiology, drain the effusion to relieve symptoms of cardiac tamponade, and allow intrapericardial administration of drugs for treatment.

6. Pericardial biopsy: It helps to clarify the etiology.

V Treatment

1. If emergency treatment is needed, pericardiocentesis should be performed promptly. If necessary, a drainage tube can be placed for 4-5 days. In cases of late-stage tumor metastasis with uncontrollable tumor growth, continuous drainage may be required.

2. Etiological treatment: Infectious pericardial effusion: Anti-infective treatment is effective for different types of infections, and different anti-infective drugs are selected according to the specific infection. Tuberculous pericardial effusion: Anti-tuberculosis treatment is administered, generally using a triple therapy of isoniazid, ethambutol, and streptomycin. Glucocorticoids can promote the absorption of pericardial effusion. For large amounts of pericardial effusion, pericardiocentesis and drainage are preferred. Bacterial pericardial effusion: Antibiotics can be selected based on drug sensitivity. If purulent effusion is present without identified bacteria, the first choice is a combination of semi-synthetic anti-staphylococcal antibiotics and aminoglycosides. Fungal pericardial effusion: Appropriate antifungal drugs are used for treatment. If constrictive pericarditis with symptoms of cardiac tamponade develops, pericardiectomy is also required. Other infections, such as those caused by mycoplasma, amoeba, schistosoma, filaria, toxoplasma, etc., are treated with corresponding anti-infective therapies. Pericardial effusion occurring a few days after acute myocardial infarction is generally transient and does not require treatment. If there is significant chest pain, high-dose aspirin can be given. Other non-steroidal anti-inflammatory drugs and corticosteroids should be avoided as much as possible, as they may increase the risk of cardiac rupture. If it is post-myocardial infarction syndrome, it is generally self-limiting. For patients with severe fever and chest pain, aspirin or non-steroidal anti-inflammatory drugs can be given. If recurrent, anticoagulants should be discontinued to avoid pericardial hemorrhage, and corticosteroid therapy should be administered. For corticosteroid-dependent recurrent pericarditis, colchicine can be given.

Uremic pericardial effusion generally resolves after dialysis treatment. If chest pain is significant, non-steroidal anti-inflammatory drugs can be given. If recurrent pericardial effusion persists after dialysis, intrapericardial injection of triamcinolone after pericardiocentesis may be effective. For neoplastic pericardial effusion, the main goal is to relieve symptoms of dyspnea, generally by pericardiocentesis and continuous pericardial drainage. If tumor treatment is effective, pericardial effusion may decrease or disappear. For rheumatic autoimmune pericardial effusion, corresponding treatments are given. For rheumatic fever, penicillin is used. For systemic lupus erythematosus, rheumatoid arthritis, and systemic sclerosis, immunosuppressants and/or glucocorticoids are administered. Pericardial effusion caused by hypothyroidism is treated with thyroid hormone replacement therapy.

3. Surgical treatment: This includes subxiphoid pericardial window drainage, partial or complete pericardial resection via thoracotomy, and thoracoscopic pericardial resection. The purpose of surgical treatment is to relieve existing or potential pericardial obstruction, remove pericardial effusion, reduce the possibility of pericardial effusion recurrence, and prevent late pericardial constriction. For tuberculous pericardial effusion, if recurrent large amounts of pericardial effusion persist after drug treatment or if compressive symptoms occur due to exudative-constrictive lesions or early constrictive pericarditis, pericardiectomy should be performed 4-6 weeks after anti-tuberculosis treatment. For uremic pericardial effusion with cardiac tamponade, surgical pericardial window or pericardiectomy can be performed. For pericardial effusion caused by other etiologies, if constrictive pericarditis develops with symptoms of cardiac tamponade, pericardiectomy is required.

Ⅵ Common Questions Encountered in Consultation

1. Consultation type: An urgent consultation suggests that the patient is in a relatively critical state due to large amounts of pericardial effusion leading to hemodynamic instability, and emergency pericardiocentesis may be needed to alleviate symptoms. If it is a routine consultation, it is generally to clarify the etiology and determine the next diagnostic and treatment plan.

2. Consulting department: The consulting department can provide an initial consideration of the etiology of pericardial effusion. For example, in the oncology department, tumor metastasis and hypoproteinemia are more likely. In the radiotherapy department, in addition to tumors, radiation injury should also be considered. In the endocrinology department, hypothyroidism is a likely cause. In the respiratory department, infectious pericardial effusion is more likely. An initial judgment is made, and then a corresponding diagnosis is made based on medical history, physical examination, and auxiliary examinations. If pericardiotomy is required, the possibility of post-pericardiotomy syndrome should be considered. After cardiothoracic or cardiac surgery, pacemaker implantation, cardiac catheterization, atrial tachycardia or atrial fibrillation ablation, or coronary intervention, pericardial hemorrhage should be considered.

3. Determining the etiology of pericardial effusion: The etiological diagnosis of pericardial effusion can generally be made based on medical history, physical examination, and corresponding tests. For example, thyroid function tests can diagnose pericardial effusion caused by hypothyroidism. If there is a history of uremia or long-term hemodialysis, uremic pericardial effusion can be diagnosed. If there is a history of surgery or cardiac trauma, it may be post-cardiac injury syndrome. If it occurs a few days after acute myocardial infarction, post-myocardial infarction pericarditis should be considered. If it occurs 2-3 weeks after acute myocardial infarction, the diagnosis of post-myocardial infarction syndrome should be considered, which is generally related to autoimmunity. If the onset is acute, with a history of upper respiratory tract infection, persistent fever, chest pain, pericardial friction rub, and a small

amount of pericardial effusion that is prone to recurrence, acute specific pericardial effusion should be considered. If there is a history of primary tuberculosis, with symptoms such as fever, fatigue, and night sweats, and a gradual onset with a large amount of pericardial effusion, tuberculous pericardial effusion should be considered. If the onset is acute, with high fever, chills, night sweats, dyspnea, transient significant chest pain, and a marked increase in white blood cell count, the possibility of purulent pericardial effusion is high. If there is a history of tumor, with no symptoms or progressive dyspnea as the main manifestation, neoplastic pericardial effusion should be considered. If there is a history of tumor radiotherapy, especially with a high radiation dose, radiation-induced pericardial effusion should be considered. If the patient has a history of rheumatic diseases, combined with systemic manifestations such as joint pain, fever, kidney damage, and rash, pericardial effusion caused by rheumatic autoimmune diseases should be considered. If echocardiography shows that the amount of pericardial effusion reaches a certain level, pericardiocentesis can be performed to clarify the etiology.

When common etiologies of pericardial effusion cannot explain the condition, rare causes should be considered, such as fungal infections (generally seen in congenital immunodeficiency, use of immunosuppressants, AIDS, or long-term use of broad-spectrum antibiotics in burn patients), amebic infections (with hepatic or pleural amebiasis, characteristic chocolate-colored pericardial pus, and cultivation of amebic trophozoites), filariasis (with characteristic chylous pericardial effusion and detection of microfilariae), non-infectious causes such as cholesterol pericardial effusion (golden yellow effusion with cholesterol content exceeding 700 mg/L), drug-induced pericardial effusion (such as phenytoin sodium, isoniazid, doxorubicin, penicillin, and amlodipine), and other conditions such as hypoproteinemia, nephrotic syndrome, acute and chronic heart failure, beriberi, and pericardial effusion caused by compression of pericardial venous drainage by adjacent mediastinal tumors.

4. Prognosis of pericardial effusion: The prognosis is determined by the etiology of the effusion. For malignant tumors, the overall prognosis is poor, depending on whether it is primary or metastatic, the pathological type of the tumor, and the treatment effect. Additionally, it is related to the patient's underlying disease and the rate of effusion accumulation. Mild cases may have no impact, while severe cases can lead to death. Some patients with pericardial effusion may eventually develop constrictive pericarditis, and the prognosis then depends on whether pericardiectomy is performed.

Ⅶ Consultation Process

1. Assess the patient's vital signs. If hemodynamic instability occurs, immediately perform pericardiocentesis and drainage. Stabilizing vital signs is a prerequisite.

2. Collect medical history: Pericardial effusion is commonly seen in tumors, tuberculosis, hypothyroidism, trauma, maintenance dialysis, postoperative complications, etc. Inquire about weight loss or even cachexia, history of trauma, long-term dialysis, surgical history, fever, apathy, etc.

3. Key points of physical examination: Patients often present with dyspnea, and in severe cases, orthopnea. Pay attention to the presence of jugular venous distension, hepatomegaly,

ascites, and lower extremity edema. Note whether the heart rate is fast, blood pressure is low, and whether there is enlarged cardiac dullness, weakened apex beat, and distant and muffled heart sounds on cardiac examination.

4. Auxiliary examinations: To confirm the presence of pericardial effusion, perform examinations such as ECG, chest X-ray, and echocardiography. To clarify the etiology of pericardial effusion, perform effusion analysis, cardiac MRI, and pericardial biopsy.

5. Etiological treatment after diagnosis: If caused by tuberculosis, administer anti-tuberculosis treatment. If caused by hypothyroidism, supplement thyroid hormone. If caused by rheumatic autoimmune diseases, administer glucocorticoid-related treatment. Some patients require surgical treatment to remove part or all of the pericardium to reduce pericardial effusion recurrence and prevent pericardial constriction.

Section 2 Viral Myocarditis

I Definition

Viral myocarditis refers to the inflammatory lesions of the myocardium caused by viral infection, which can be focal or diffuse, and can also be classified as acute, subacute, or chronic. The inflammation can involve myocardial cells, interstitial tissue, vascular components, and the pericardium.

II Etiology and Pathogenesis

Currently, the viruses that have been proven to cause myocarditis include: small ribonucleic acid viruses, such as coxsackievirus, echovirus, and poliovirus; arthropod-borne viruses, such as dengue virus, epidemic hemorrhagic fever virus, yellow fever virus, etc.; adenovirus; influenza virus; paramyxoviruses, such as mumps virus, measles virus, respiratory syncytial virus, etc.; herpesviruses; rubella virus; rabies virus; hepatitis virus; respiratory and enteric viruses; meningitis viruses, etc. Among them, coxsackievirus, echovirus, influenza virus, mumps virus, and poliovirus are the most common.

Various viruses primarily cause myocardial damage through three mechanisms: ① Direct invasion of the myocardium; ② Myocardial damage and microvascular injury mediated by multiple cytokines and nitric oxide; ③ Virus-mediated immune damage, mainly T-cell immunity.

III Clinical Manifestations

The clinical manifestations of viral myocarditis vary greatly. Mild cases, such as focal infections, may have no symptoms, or may present with chest tightness, palpitations, shortness of breath, fatigue, etc. Severe cases may manifest as severe arrhythmia, heart failure, cardiogenic shock, etc. Pericardial involvement can lead to severe chest pain, and even sudden death. Half of the patients have a history of respiratory or gastrointestinal prodromal infections 1-3 weeks before the onset of the disease. Physical signs include enlarged heart borders, tachycardia, various arrhythmias (premature contractions are common), systolic murmurs at the apex, and in severe cases, gallop rhythm, alternating pulse, pulmonary rales, hepatomegaly, as well as other signs of heart failure and cardiogenic shock.

Serological tests may show a slight increase or normal white blood cell count, increased erythrocyte sedimentation rate, and elevated myocardial enzymes. The electrocardiogram is non-specific and may show various arrhythmias, with premature contractions being the most common. Chest X-rays and echocardiography may show cardiac enlargement or reduced cardiac function. Virological tests, such as isolating viruses from throat swabs, feces, blood, or pericardial fluid, can help with the diagnosis. A 4-fold increase in viral neutralizing antibody titers or complement fixation titers is of diagnostic significance. Detection of viruses, viral gene fragments, or viral protein antigens in endomyocardial or myocardial biopsies can confirm the diagnosis of viral myocarditis, but negative results do not exclude the diagnosis.

Ⅳ Diagnosis

The diagnostic criteria for viral myocarditis in Chinese adults are as follows.

1. History and physical signs: Within 3 weeks after viral infections such as upper respiratory tract infections or diarrhea, cardiac manifestations appear, such as unexplained severe post-infection fatigue, chest tightness, dizziness (due to reduced cardiac output), significantly weakened first heart sound at the apex, diastolic gallop rhythm, pericardial friction rub, enlarged heart borders, congestive heart failure, or Ards syndrome, etc.

2. New-onset arrhythmias or electrocardiographic changes within 3 weeks after the above infections:

(1) Sinus tachycardia, atrioventricular conduction block, sinoatrial block, or bundle branch block.

(2) Multifocal, paired ventricular premature contractions, ectopic atrial or junctional tachycardia, paroxysmal or non-paroxysmal ventricular tachycardia, atrial or ventricular flutter or fibrillation.

(3) ST-segment depression ⩾0.01 mV in two or more leads, or abnormal ST-segment elevation, or appearance of abnormal Q waves.

3. Reference indicators of myocardial injury: During the course of the disease, serum cardiac troponin I or troponin T (emphasizing quantitative measurement), creatine kinase isoenzyme significantly elevated. Echocardiography suggests cardiac chamber enlargement or abnormal ventricular wall motion, and/or radionuclide cardiac function examination confirms reduced left ventricular systolic or diastolic function.

4. Etiological evidence:

(1) Detection of viruses, viral gene fragments, or viral protein antigens from the endocardium, myocardium, pericardium, or pericardial puncture fluid during the acute phase.

(2) Viral antibodies: The titer of the same type of viral antibody in the second serum sample is 4 times higher than that in the first serum sample (the two serum samples should be taken more than 2 weeks apart), or a single antibody titer ⩾640 is positive, and 320 is suspicious (if based on 1 : 32, it is better to use ⩾256 as positive and 128 as suspicious).

(3) Virus specificity: IgM ⩾1 : 320 is positive. If there is also positive enterovirus nucleic

acid in the blood, it further supports a recent viral infection.

If the patient simultaneously meets any two items in "1", "2" [(1), (2), (3) any one item], and "3", after excluding other causes of myocardial diseases, acute viral myocarditis can be clinically diagnosed. If the patient also meets item (1) in "4", viral myocarditis can be etiologically confirmed. If only items (2) and (3) in "4" are met, it can only be etiologically diagnosed as acute viral myocarditis.

If the patient has one or more manifestations including Ards syndrome, congestive heart failure with or without myocardial infarction-like electrocardiographic changes, cardiogenic shock, acute renal failure, sustained ventricular tachycardia with hypotension, or myopericarditis, it can be diagnosed as severe viral myocarditis.

V Treatment

1. Rest in bed, physical activity should generally be restricted for 6 months during the acute phase.

2. Integrated traditional Chinese and Western medicine treatment: Astragalus, taurine, and coenzyme Q10 in combination have antiviral, immunomodulatory, and cardiac function improvement effects.

3. Treatment of complications: If heart failure occurs, diuretics, ACEIs, vasodilators, digitalis, and other positive inotropic drugs are needed. If severe conduction block occurs, temporary pacing treatment should be considered. For patients with atrioventricular conduction block, refractory heart failure, severe conditions, or autoimmune situations, the use of glucocorticoids can be considered.

If severe heart failure occurs, endotracheal intubation and assisted ventilation are required. If combined with cardiogenic shock, cardiac assist devices (such as extracorporeal membrane oxygenation) can be used.

4. Antiviral therapy: If the viral type is identified, specific antiviral therapy can be considered, especially for enteroviruses, which can improve the 10-year prognosis.

5. High-dose intravenous immunoglobulin: It can improve heart failure by regulating immune and inflammatory responses, but the evidence is insufficient.

VI Common Questions and Precautions in Consultation

1. Need to be differentiated from other myocarditis:

(1) Beta-receptor hyperactivity syndrome: Mainly seen in young and middle-aged women, with symptoms such as palpitations, chest tightness, dizziness, and tachycardia. The electrocardiogram may show premature contractions and ST-T changes. Patients have manifestations of sympathetic excitation such as irritability, insomnia, and sweating. The heart is not enlarged. Symptoms can be improved after treatment with beta-receptor blockers, and the electrocardiogram can also return to normal.

(2) Rheumatic myocarditis: There are abnormalities such as increased anti-O and increased erythrocyte sedimentation rate.

(3) Allergic or toxic myocarditis: There is a history of drug use, such as cocaine,

chemotherapy drug doxorubicin, penicillin, sulfonamides, etc.

(4) Syphilitic myocarditis: There is a history of syphilis infection, and the serological Kahn and Wassermann reactions are positive.

(5) Other infectious myocarditis: Diseases such as typhoid fever, toxoplasmosis, and Legionnaires' disease all have corresponding other clinical manifestations.

(6) Isolated myocarditis: Idiopathic, of unknown etiology, mainly manifested as cardiac enlargement. Not accompanied by pericarditis and endocarditis, may be accompanied by ventricular wall thrombus formation, with progressive heart failure as the main clinical manifestation.

(7) Metabolic diseases: Vitamin B1 deficiency.

(8) Keshan disease: Has obvious regional characteristics, mainly manifested as heart failure, myocardial enzymes are generally not elevated.

(9) Hyperthyroid myocardiopathy: Has manifestations of hyperthyroidism.

2. Do not easily diagnose when evidence is insufficient: If only a small number of premature contractions or mild T-wave changes occur within 3 weeks after a viral infection, it is not appropriate to easily diagnose as acute viral myocarditis. Sometimes, when a definite diagnosis cannot be made, long-term follow-up can be performed, treated as myocarditis, and endomyocardial or myocardial biopsy can be performed for viral gene detection and pathological examination if conditions permit. Be strict in diagnosis and broad in treatment.

3. Can viral myocarditis be cured?

Most cases of viral myocarditis can self-heal. Severe viral myocarditis can be fatal during the acute phase due to severe arrhythmia, acute heart failure, or cardiogenic shock. In some patients, the condition may stabilize after several weeks to several months, but there may be a certain degree of cardiac enlargement, reduced cardiac function, with or without arrhythmia or electrocardiographic abnormalities, which persist for a long time, forming chronic myocarditis and evolving into dilated cardiomyopathy.

VII Consultation Process for Chief Resident

1. Assess the patient's vital signs. If there are signs of life instability such as decreased blood oxygen, shallow and rapid breathing, decreased blood pressure, or malignant arrhythmias, immediately administer emergency treatments such as vasopressors to maintain blood pressure, mechanical ventilation, temporary pacemaker, balloon counter-pulsation, extracorporeal membrane oxygenation, etc.

2. Supplement key medical history, such as whether there was a history of respiratory, urinary, or gastrointestinal prodromal infections 1-3 weeks before the onset, whether there was a history of hyperthyroidism, whether there was a history of other infectious diseases (syphilis), whether there was a long history of alcohol consumption, whether there was poisoning, allergy, etc.

3. Pay attention to important physical examinations, such as rapid breathing, even orthopnea, enlarged heart borders, tachycardia (including various arrhythmias), systolic murmur at the apex, and moist rales in both lungs, etc.

4. Auxiliary examinations, such as routine blood tests, blood gas analysis, renal function, electrolytes, electrocardiogram, chest X-ray, BNP or NT-proBNP, D-dimer, echocardiography, etc. If conditions permit, further improve virological tests, endomyocardial and myocardial biopsies, etc.

5. Etiological treatment after a clear diagnosis, such as bed rest and restriction of physical activity in the later stage; integrated traditional Chinese and Western medicine and antiviral therapy; for patients with heart failure, administer diuretics and vasodilators, and if necessary, give positive inotropic drugs or device therapy; for high-degree conduction block, implant a temporary pacemaker; high-dose intravenous immunoglobulin and nutritional support therapy.

6. After excluding the above urgent and life-threatening causes and common causes, investigate some rare diseases, such as Keshan disease and isolated myocarditis.

Section 3 Infective Endocarditis

I Definition

Infective endocarditis (IE) is a microbial infection of the endocardial surface of the heart, accompanied by the formation of vegetations. Vegetations are platelet and fibrin clumps of varying sizes and shapes, containing large numbers of microorganisms and a small number of inflammatory cells. Patients with organic heart disease are a high-risk and susceptible population for IE, and bacteremia is a necessary condition for the occurrence of IE. During bacteremia, bacteria in the blood adhere to and multiply within the vegetations. Valves are the most commonly affected sites, but IE can also occur at the site of septal defects, chordae tendineae, or endocardium of the heart wall.

The incidence of IE in China still lacks exact epidemiological data. Based on case reports, streptococci and staphylococci are the main pathogenic microorganisms causing IE.

II Classification

There is no unified classification for IE. According to the differences in pathogenic microorganisms and clinical characteristics, IE can be classified into the following types.

1. Acute Infective Endocarditis: Severe toxic symptoms; rapid progression of the disease course, causing valvular destruction within a few days to a few weeks; frequent metastatic infections; the main pathogen is Staphylococcus aureus.

2. Subacute Infective Endocarditis: Mild toxic symptoms; disease course lasting for several weeks to several months; rare metastatic infections; the main pathogen is Streptococcus viridans, followed by Enterococcus.

3. Prosthetic Valve Endocarditis (PVE): IE is prone to occur after cardiac surgery, especially after prosthetic valve replacement, accounting for 10%-15% of the total number of IE cases. Early infections often occur within 60 days after surgery, usually with an acute and fulminant onset. Late infections are endocarditis occurring more than 2 months after surgery, commonly presenting with subacute manifestations. Fever is a common clinical manifestation, which can

lead to the rupture and insufficiency of prosthetic bioprosthetic valves, causing perivalvular abscesses, dehiscence, myocardial abscesses, and paravalvular leakage.

4. Right-sided infective endocarditis mainly occurs in intravenous drug users, after intravenous catheter placement, or after abortion. It presents with sepsis, characterized by recurrent multiple pulmonary embolisms without systemic embolism. It mostly affects normal heart valves, with the tricuspid valve being involved in more than 50% of cases, followed by the aortic and mitral valves. Acute onset is common and often accompanied by metastatic infections. Right heart failure occurs late and is rare.

5. Infective endocarditis associated with cardiac implantable electronic devices is mainly caused by direct contamination with pathogens during device implantation, followed by retrograde infection by pathogens along the lead, or hematogenous spread from other infectious foci involving the endocardium and leads.

Ⅲ Clinical Manifestations

The time interval from the occurrence of transient bacteremia to the onset of symptoms varies, mostly within 2 weeks, but many patients have no clear route of bacterial entry to be found. The clinical manifestations of IE are complex and diverse, and there are also significant differences in the manifestations among different populations. The clinical manifestations in elderly patients and immunosuppressed patients are often atypical, with a lower incidence of fever.

The main clinical manifestations of IE include fever; cardiac murmurs; unexplained embolism; unexplained sepsis; peripheral signs. Complications may include heart failure, myocardial abscess, acute myocardial infarction, purulent pericarditis, myocarditis, bacterial aneurysm, metastatic abscess, bacterial aneurysm or toxic encephalopathy of the nervous system, brain abscess, renal artery embolism, etc.

Fever accompanied by the following manifestations should be considered as IE: prosthetic materials in the heart; history of IE; history of valvular or congenital heart disease; other susceptibility factors for IE; recent procedures that may cause bacteremia in high-risk patients; evidence of chronic heart failure; new-onset conduction block; positive blood culture for typical IE pathogens or positive serological test for chronic Q fever; vascular or immunological manifestations such as embolism, Roth spots, splinter hemorrhages, petechiae, Osler's nodes, Janeway lesions; local or nonspecific neurological symptoms and signs; evidence of pulmonary embolism and infiltration; unexplained peripheral abscess.

Ⅳ Diagnosis

1. Laboratory and Other Examinations

(1) Routine examinations: ① Urine: Microscopic hematuria and mild proteinuria are common, and gross hematuria suggests renal infarction; ② Blood: Normochromic normocytic anemia is common in subacute cases, and white blood cell count is normal or mildly elevated; ③ Acute cases often have increased white blood cell count and significant left shift. Erythrocyte sedimentation rate is elevated in both cases.

(2) Immunohistochemical and molecular biological examinations: Pathological examination of valves or emboli is the gold standard for the diagnosis of IE. PCR can be used to detect pathogens in blood samples, and positive results can be used as an important diagnostic criterion for IE. Circulating immune complexes are present in 80% of patients. In subacute patients with a course of more than 6 weeks, 50% have positive rheumatoid factor.

(3) Blood culture: It is the most important method for diagnosing bacteremia and IE. Blood samples should be collected under strict aseptic conditions before starting antibiotic treatment. In patients who have not recently received antibiotic treatment, the positive rate of blood culture can be as high as over 95%, and more than 90% of patients have positive results obtained from specimens taken on the first day of admission. Bacteremia in IE is continuous, and blood samples do not need to be collected during fever spikes. If blood cultures are negative, the incidence of IE is 2.5%-31%, which often leads to delayed diagnosis and treatment, causing a significant impact on prognosis. The most common reasons are the use of antibiotics within 2 weeks before blood collection, improper culture techniques, or atypical pathogens such as fastidious microorganisms, which require timely adjustment of detection methods.

(4) Echocardiography: It helps confirm the diagnosis of IE by providing evidence supporting endocarditis, such as vegetations and perivalvular complications. Transthoracic echocardiography (TTE) can detect 50%-75% of vegetations, while transesophageal echocardiography (TEE) can detect vegetations $<$5 mm with a sensitivity of up to 95%. Generally, only TTE examination is required. TEE examination is needed only when prosthetic mechanical valves, right-sided heart lesions, or myocardial abscesses are present.

(5) X-ray examination: Multiple small patchy infiltrative shadows in the lungs suggest pneumonia caused by septic pulmonary embolism. In left heart failure, pulmonary congestion or pulmonary edema may be present. Aortic bacterial aneurysms can cause aortic dilation. Bacterial aneurysms can be diagnosed by angiography. CT is helpful in the diagnosis of cerebral infarction, abscess, and hemorrhage.

(6) Electrocardiogram: Occasionally, acute myocardial infarction or atrioventricular or intraventricular conduction block may be seen.

2. Duke Diagnostic Criteria for Infective Endocarditis

(1) Major criteria: ① Positive blood culture; ② Evidence of endocardial involvement: a. Echocardiographic findings, such as vegetations, abscess formation, or new dehiscence of a prosthetic valve; b. New valvular regurgitation.

(2) Minor criteria: ① Predisposing factors: presence of a cardiac condition predisposing to IE or intravenous drug users; ② Fever: temperature $>$38°C; ③ Vascular phenomena: major arterial emboli, septic pulmonary infarcts, mycotic aneurysm, intracranial hemorrhage, conjunctival hemorrhages, or Janeway lesions; ④ Immunologic phenomena: glomerulonephritis, Osler's nodes, Roth spots, or rheumatoid factor positivity; ⑤ Microbiological evidence: positive blood culture but not meeting major criteria or lack of serological evidence of infection with an IE pathogen.

(3) Definite IE is diagnosed if any of the following three conditions are met: ① Two major criteria are met; ② One major criterion and three minor criteria are met; ③ Five

minor criteria are met.

(4) Possible IE is diagnosed if either of the following two conditions is met: ① One major criterion and one minor criterion are met; ② Three minor criteria are met.

V Treatment

1. Anti-infective treatment: The key is to eliminate the pathogenic microorganisms in the vegetations and administer drugs according to pharmacokinetic indicators: use antimicrobial drugs; use a combination of two antimicrobial drugs with synergistic effects; use high doses to achieve effective drug concentrations at the infection site; administer intravenously; use long-term treatment, generally for 4-6 weeks, and for 6-8 weeks or longer in patients undergoing prosthetic valve repair.

2. Empirical treatment: Generally, empirical treatment is used before positive blood culture results are available, and it is suitable for patients with suspected IE who are relatively severe and unstable; empirical treatment regimens are formulated based on the severity of the infection, the type of affected heart valve, the presence of rare or resistant bacterial infections, etc.; treatment should cover common pathogens of IE.

3. Surgical treatment: Mainly applicable to left-sided valve IE. Indications for early surgery during the active phase include heart failure, uncontrollable infection, and prevention of embolic events.

4. Prescriptions:

(1) For infections caused by penicillin-sensitive streptococci, viridans streptococci, Streptococcus bovis, Streptococcus pyogenes, Streptococcus agalactiae, etc.

1) Penicillin 4 million U, intravenous injection / infusion, every 6 hours, for 4 weeks;

2) Ceftriaxone 2 g, intravenous or intramuscular injection, once daily, for 4 weeks, suitable for hospitalized patients allergic to penicillin;

3) Vancomycin 15 mg/kg, intravenous injection every 12 hours, for 4 weeks, suitable for patients allergic to both penicillin and cephalosporins.

(2) For infections caused by relatively penicillin-resistant streptococci, some viridans streptococci, or Streptococcus pneumoniae, etc.

1) Penicillin G 4 million U, intravenous injection, every 4 hours, for 4 weeks

(plus) Gentamicin 1 mg/kg, intravenous or intramuscular injection, every 12 hours, for 2 weeks;

2) Ceftriaxone 2 g, intravenous or intramuscular injection, once daily, for 4 weeks, suitable for hospitalized patients allergic to penicillin;

3) Vancomycin 15 mg/kg, intravenous injection every 12 hours, for 4 weeks, suitable for patients allergic to both penicillin and cephalosporins.

(3) For infections caused by penicillin-resistant streptococci, enterococci, and some other streptococci.

1) Penicillin G 18-30 million U, continuous intravenous infusion or divided doses, for 4-6 weeks

(plus) Gentamicin 1 mg/kg, intravenous or intramuscular injection, every 8 hours, for 2 weeks;

2) Ampicillin 12 g/day, continuous intravenous infusion or divided doses, for 4-6 weeks

(plus) Gentamicin 1 mg/kg, intravenous injection, every 8 hours, for 2 weeks;

3) Vancomycin 15 mg/kg, intravenous injection every 12 hours

(plus) Gentamicin 1 mg/kg, intravenous injection every 8 hours, for 4-6 weeks.

(4) For infections caused by methicillin-sensitive staphylococci.

1) Native valve

A. Nafcillin 2 g, intravenous injection, every 4 hours, for 4-6 weeks;

B. Cefazolin 2 g, intravenous injection, every 8 hours, for 4-6 weeks;

C. Vancomycin 15 mg/kg, intravenous injection, every 12 hours

(plus) Gentamicin 1 mg/kg, intravenous injection, every 8 hours, for 4-6 weeks;

2) Prosthetic valve or other prosthetic materials

Nafcillin 2 g, intravenous injection, every 4 hours

(plus) Gentamicin 1 mg/kg, intravenous injection, every 8 hours, for≥6 weeks;

Or based on drug susceptibility testing, cefazolin or vancomycin can be used to replace nafcillin.

(5) For infections caused by methicillin-resistant staphylococci.

1) Native valve

Vancomycin 15 mg/kg, intravenous injection, every 12 hours, for 4-6 weeks;

2) Prosthetic valve or other prosthetic materials

Vancomycin 15 mg/kg, intravenous injection, every 12 hours

(plus) Gentamicin 1 mg/kg, intravenous injection, every 8 hours

(plus) Rifampin 300 mg, oral, every 8 hours, for ≥6 weeks.

(6) For infections caused by the HACEK microorganism group: Haemophilus species, Actinobacillus actinomycetemcomitans, Cardiobacterium hominis, Eikenella species, Kingella kingae.

1) Ceftriaxone 2 g, intravenous or intramuscular injection, once daily, for 4 weeks;

2) Ampicillin 12 g/day, continuous intravenous infusion or divided doses, for 4-6 weeks

(plus) Gentamicin 1 mg/kg, intravenous injection, every 12 hours, for 2 weeks;

(7) For infections caused by Pseudomonas aeruginosa and other gram-negative bacilli.

Broad-spectrum penicillins or third-generation cephalosporins or imipenem, plus aminoglycosides, for 4-6 weeks. Combination therapy is recommended, and drugs are selected according to drug susceptibility testing.

(8) For infections caused by Neisseria, gonococci, etc.

1) Penicillin 2 million U, intravenous injection, every 6 hours, for 3-4 weeks;

Neisseria is highly sensitive to penicillin, but β-lactamase production tests must be performed. For most patients without complications, treatment for 3 weeks is sufficient.

2) Ceftriaxone 1 g, intravenous or intramuscular injection, once daily, for 3-4 weeks.

(9) For culture-negative cases, echocardiography-detected vegetations, or clinically highly suspected IE.

Vancomycin 15 mg/kg, intravenous injection, every 12 hours

(plus) Gentamicin 1 mg/kg, intravenous or intramuscular injection, every 8 hours, for 4-6 weeks;

(10) For prevention.

1) Dental treatment and oral or upper respiratory tract surgery;

Amoxicillin 3 g, oral, 1 hour before the procedure, followed by 1.5 g 6 hours later;

2) For high-risk endocarditis patients undergoing gastrointestinal or urinary tract examinations

Ampicillin 2 g, intravenous or intramuscular injection, half an hour before the procedure;

(plus) Gentamicin 1.5 mg/kg, intravenous or intramuscular injection, half an hour before the procedure;

6 hours later, ampicillin 1 g, intravenous or intramuscular injection, or amoxicillin 1 g, oral;

For penicillin-allergic patients: Vancomycin 1 g, intravenous infusion over 1-2 hours, plus gentamicin 1.5 mg/kg, intravenous or intramuscular injection, examination starts within 30 minutes after the completion of drug administration.

3) For penicillin-allergic patients receiving oral medication (oral and respiratory tract examinations): Clindamycin 600 mg, oral, 1 hour before the procedure;

4) Gastrointestinal or urinary tract endoscopy: Amoxicillin 3 g, oral, 1 hour before the procedure, followed by 1.5 g 6 hours later;

5) Cardiac surgery and valve replacement: Cefazolin 2 g, intravenous injection, starting at anesthesia induction, repeated at the same dose after 8-16 hours, or vancomycin 1 g, intravenous injection, starting at anesthesia induction, slowly infused over 1 hour, followed by 0.5 g repeated twice after 8-16 hours.

VI Common Issues Encountered in Consultation

1. Recommendations for antithrombotic therapy

(1) If major bleeding occurs, it is recommended to discontinue antiplatelet drugs.

(2) If intracranial hemorrhage occurs, it is recommended to discontinue all anticoagulant drugs.

(3) For ischemic stroke without bleeding, under close monitoring, it can be considered to switch oral anticoagulants to unfractionated heparin or low molecular weight heparin for 1-2 weeks.

(4) For patients with intracranial hemorrhage and prosthetic valves, after multidisciplinary consultation and discussion, unfractionated heparin or low molecular weight heparin should be resumed immediately.

(5) For endocarditis caused by Staphylococcus aureus, if no stroke occurs, under close monitoring, it can be considered to switch oral anticoagulants to unfractionated heparin or low molecular weight heparin for 1-2 weeks.

(6) Thrombolytic therapy is not recommended for patients with endocarditis.

2. How to treat IE secondary to cardiac implantable devices. Antibiotic treatment is listed in the prescription section. Remove the entire cardiac implantable electronic device system whenever possible; the method of transvenous lead removal is recommended; if it is difficult

to complete, there is severe tricuspid valve destruction, or the vegetation is >25 mm, surgical treatment can be considered. Remove necrotic tissue and locally newly formed granulation tissue as thoroughly as possible; achieve complete hemostasis, preferably using an electrocautery; for those with extensive local oozing, thrombin can be applied in the wound; after thorough debridement and hemostasis, perform pocket irrigation (hydrogen peroxide—metronidazole solution—gentamicin—normal saline, at least 2-3 times for each solution); drainage strips are generally not required.

3. When to consider surgical treatment. Emergency surgery for acute valvular regurgitation / obstruction causing refractory pulmonary edema or shock; emergency surgery for fistula into the heart chamber or pericardial refractory edema or shock; emergency surgery for acute valvular regurgitation or obstruction causing heart failure or hemodynamic instability; semi-elective surgery for focal uncontrollable infection; semi-elective surgery for persistent fever or positive blood culture results for more than 7-10 days; semi-elective surgery for vegetations that continue to grow after anti-infective treatment and one or more embolic events; semi-elective surgery for vegetations with a diameter >10 mm and other risk factors; semi-elective surgery for isolated vegetations with a diameter >15 mm.

4. How to treat IE complicated by pregnancy. High-risk pregnant women need prophylactic use of antibiotics when receiving dental treatment. The treatment principles are the same as those for ordinary patients, but in addition to selecting antibiotics based on the results of pathogenic examination and drug susceptibility, the toxicity of drugs to the fetus must be considered; surgical valve surgery and termination of pregnancy are only recommended for pregnant women when drug treatment fails to control the condition. The best timing for surgery is between 13 and 28 weeks of gestation; for pregnant women over 26 weeks of gestation who plan to undergo valve surgery under cardiopulmonary bypass, it is recommended to perform the surgery after cesarean section.

Ⅶ Consultation Process

1. Populations susceptible to IE include those with prosthetic materials in the heart; history of IE; history of valvular or congenital heart disease; other predisposing factors for IE; high-risk patients who have recently undergone procedures that cause bacteremia; evidence of chronic heart failure; new-onset conduction block; positive blood culture for typical IE pathogens or positive serological test for chronic Q fever; vascular or immunological phenomena such as embolism, Roth spots, splinter hemorrhages, petechiae, Osler's nodes, Janeway lesions; local or non-specific neurological symptoms and signs; evidence of pulmonary embolism and infiltration; unexplained peripheral abscess.

2. The clinical signs of patients presenting with IE are often complex and diverse. If a patient presents with fever accompanied by the following possible signs, IE should be suspected, such as cardiac murmurs; unexplained embolism; unexplained sepsis; peripheral signs.

3. Abnormalities on physical examination depend on the complications of IE: Simple infection of the endocardium may present with cardiac murmurs; cerebral embolism can lead to neurological symptoms; embolism to other sites can cause infection and ischemia in the

corresponding areas.

4. Pathological examination of valves or emboli is the gold standard for the diagnosis of IE; blood culture is the most important method for diagnosing bacteremia and IE; echocardiographic findings of vegetations and perivalvular complications provide evidence supporting endocarditis.

5. The treatment of IE is divided into anti-infective therapy and surgical treatment. The key to the selection of anti-infective therapy is based on the results of culture and drug susceptibility testing. If empirical treatment is used before culture results are available, the principles are: early, adequate dosage, and combination therapy; for patients with severe cardiac complications or ineffective antibiotic treatment, surgical treatment should be considered in a timely manner.

Section 4 Cardiac Valvular Diseases

I Aortic Stenosis (AS)

1. Etiology of AS

(1) Congenital valvular disease: Bicuspid, unicuspid, or tricuspid valve with commissural fusion.

(2) Degenerative aortic stenosis.

(3) Rheumatic heart disease.

(4) Radiation heart disease: May coexist with aortic regurgitation.

(5) Subvalvular aortic stenosis: Rare.

(6) Supravalvular aortic stenosis: Rare.

2. Clinical Manifestations of AS

Symptoms: Asymptomatic during the compensated period

Angina pectoris (without surgery)—5-year survival rate of 50%

Syncope (without surgery)—3-year survival rate of 50%

Heart failure (without surgery)—Average survival time <2 years

3. Main Physical Examination Findings. Systolic ejection murmur at the right upper sternal border, radiating to the neck. The intensity of the murmur does not necessarily correlate with the severity of valvular stenosis.

4. Diagnosis

(1) Electrocardiogram: Suggests left ventricular hypertrophy with strain, left atrial abnormality, intraventricular conduction block, occasionally third-degree atrioventricular block.

(2) Chest X-ray: Generally normal, no diagnostic value.

(3) Echocardiography: Including transesophageal echocardiography, is the gold standard.

Classification of AS severity:

1) Normal aortic valve area: 2-4 cm^2;

2) Mild aortic stenosis: >1.5 cm^2 or mean transvalvular gradient of 0-20 mmHg;

3) Moderate aortic stenosis: 1.0-1.5 cm^2 or mean transvalvular gradient of 20-40 mmHg;

4) Severe aortic stenosis: <1.0 cm^2 or mean transvalvular gradient >40 mmHg;

5) Critical severe aortic stenosis: <0.75 cm^2 or <0.5 cm^2/m^2 body surface area.

(4) Invasive assessment of AS: When clinical symptoms do not match echocardiographic data, invasive hemodynamic assessment is necessary.

5. Treatment. Surgical treatment is preferred. The risk of drug therapy is greater than surgical treatment in symptomatic patients. All patients require close observation and should avoid the use of vasodilators.

(1) Asymptomatic AS: Close observation, prophylaxis for endocarditis when necessary, maintenance of sinus rhythm, avoidance of vasodilators.

(2) Mild AS: Close observation, echocardiographic reassessment every 5 years, appropriate physical activity.

(3) Moderate AS: Close observation, echocardiographic reassessment every 2-3 years if clinically stable, no participation in competitive sports.

(4) Severe AS: Echocardiographic reassessment annually or at shorter intervals, avoidance of high-intensity exercise.

(5) AS patients with rheumatic fever usually require long-term secondary prevention, with monthly intramuscular injections of long-acting penicillin.

6. Surgical Treatment. Surgical treatment is shown in Tables 5-1 to 5-3.

Table 5-1 Four-Stage Classification of Valvular Heart Disease

Stage	Definition	Description
A	At risk	Patients with risk factors for progression to VHD
B	Progressive	Patients with progressive VHD (mild to moderate and asymptomatic)
C	Asymptomatic severe	Patients meeting criteria for severe VHD but asymptomatic: C1: Left or right ventricle still compensated C2: Left or right ventricle decompensated
D	Symptomatic severe	Patients with VHD who develop symptoms

Table 5-2 Treatment Recommendations Corresponding to AS Staging

Stage	Recommendation Class	Evidence Level
AVR is recommended for patients with symptomatic severe high-gradient AS (stage D1) as determined by history or exercise testing	I	B
AVR is recommended for asymptomatic patients with severe AS (stage C2) and LVEF <50%	I	B
AVR is recommended for patients with severe AS (stages C and D) undergoing other cardiac surgery	I	B
AVR is reasonable for asymptomatic patients with severe AS (stage C1, velocity ≥5 m/s) and low surgical risk	II_a	B
AVR is reasonable for asymptomatic patients with severe AS (stage C1), decreased exercise tolerance, and blood pressure decrease on exercise testing	II_a	B

(Continued)

Stage	Recommendation Class	Evidence Level
AVR is reasonable for symptomatic patients with low-flow, low-gradient severe AS (stage D1) and reduced LVEF if velocity ≥ 4 m/s (or mean gradient ≥40 mmHg) and valve area ≤1 mm² at any dose during low-dose dobutamine stress testing	II_a	B
AVR is reasonable for symptomatic patients with low-flow, low-gradient severe AS (stage D3), normal blood pressure, and LVEF ≥50% if clinical, hemodynamic, and anatomic data support valve obstruction as the cause of symptoms	II_a	C
AVR is reasonable for patients with moderate AS (stage B, velocity 3.0-3.9 m/s) undergoing other cardiac surgery	II_a	C
AVR may be considered for asymptomatic patients with severe AS (stage C1) with rapid disease progression and low surgical risk	II_a	C

Table 5-3 TAVR Recommendation Guidelines

Recommendation	Recommendation Class	Evidence Level
TAVR is recommended for patients with AS who meet indications for AVR but have contraindications to surgery and an expected post-procedural survival >12 months	I	A
Surgical AVR is recommended for patients with low to intermediate surgical risk who meet indications for AVR	I	B
For patients at high risk considering TAVR or surgical AVR, the heart valve team should closely communicate to determine the optimal treatment approach	I	C
TAVR can be considered as an alternative to surgical AVR for patients with AS who meet indications for AVR and have high surgical risk	II_a	B
Percutaneous aortic valve balloon dilation can be used as a transitional measure to surgical AVR or TAVR for patients with severe symptomatic AS	II_a	C
TAVR is not recommended for patients with complications that would prevent benefit from AS correction	Ⅲ: No Benefit	B

7. Preoperative Transition. In the intensive care unit, under invasive hemodynamic monitoring, vasodilators such as nitrates can be used. For rapid atrial fibrillation, actively manage to restore sinus rhythm. If necessary, aortic balloon counter-pulsation can help increase cardiac preload and improve coronary perfusion.

Ⅱ Aortic Insufficiency (AI)

1. Etiology of AI

(1) Primary valvular: ① Bicuspid aortic valve; ② Infective endocarditis; ③ Rheumatic heart disease; ④ Radiation heart disease; ⑤ Subvalvular aortic stenosis leading to leaflet damage; ⑥ Drugs: fenfluramine, phentermine, ergotamine, etc.

(2) Secondary aortic: ① Aortic root dilation: Marfan syndrome, syphilis, giant cell arteritis; ② Aortic dissection: Type A; ③ Ventricular septal defect: Supracristal type.

(3) Coexistence of both factors.

2. Clinical Manifestations of AI

(1) Acute AI: Hypotension, tachycardia, heart failure, acute pulmonary edema. Due to the lack of time for cardiac adaptation and compensation, the condition may rapidly deteriorate.

(2) Chronic AI: Can be asymptomatic for a long period. Typical symptoms are manifestations of right heart failure. Patients with severe regurgitation may experience angina pectoris, regardless of the presence of coronary artery obstruction.

(3) Clinical manifestations related to secondary causes.

3. Main Physical Examination Findings

(1) Decrescendo blowing diastolic murmur at the left sternal border. Austin-Flint murmur: A diastolic rumbling murmur at the apex. Blood pressure is normal in the early stage, with increased pulse pressure in the mid to late stages. Water-hammer pulse, capillary pulsation sign (nail bed or lips), pistol shot sound (over the large aorta).

(2) Physical signs related to secondary causes.

4. Diagnosis

(1) Electrocardiogram: Left ventricular hypertrophy, possibly left atrial abnormality. Atrial fibrillation is common. In endocarditis, severe atrioventricular conduction block may be present in the aortic valve.

(2) Chest X-ray: Extremely enlarged heart, possibly left atrial enlargement. In aortic abnormalities, dilatation of the ascending aorta may be seen.

(3) Echocardiography: The most commonly used non-invasive examination. It can assess left ventricular size, EF value, ascending aortic lesions, and aortic valve leaflet conditions. Multiple measurement methods are used to evaluate the severity of AI and generate a report.

5. Treatment

(1) Acute AI: Acute severe AI requires emergency surgery. Preoperatively, vasodilators can be selected to reduce afterload. Increased heart rate helps stabilize hemodynamics. IABP is an absolute contraindication.

(2) Chronic AI: For chronic AR with systolic blood pressure >140 mmHg, dihydropyridine calcium channel blockers or ACEI / ARB are recommended.

(3) Treatment of secondary causes.

(4) For patients with mild to moderate AI, if clinically stable, echocardiographic follow-up should be performed every 2 years. For patients with severe AR, echocardiographic follow-up should be performed every 6 months (Table 5-4).

Table 5-4 Surgical Indications for Chronic AR

Recommendation	Recommendation Class	Evidence Level
AVR is the preferred treatment for patients with symptomatic severe AI (Stage D)	I	B
AVR is the preferred treatment for asymptomatic patients with chronic severe AI and LVEF <50% (Stage C2)	I	B

(Continued)

Recommendation	Recommendation Class	Evidence Level
AVR is the preferred treatment for patients with severe AI (Stages C or D) undergoing other cardiac surgery	I	C
AVR is reasonable for asymptomatic patients with severe AI, LVEF >50%, and left ventricular end-systolic diameter >50 mm (Stage C2)	II_a	B
AVR is reasonable for patients with moderate AI undergoing other cardiac surgery	II_a	C
AVR may be considered for asymptomatic patients with severe AI, LVEF >50%, and left ventricular end-diastolic diameter > 65 mm (Stage C2)	II_b	C

Ⅲ Mitral Stenosis (MS)

1. Etiology of MS

(1) Rheumatic fever: More common in females. Recurrent streptococcal tonsillitis or pharyngitis may indirectly cause the disease. It can lead to four types of mitral valve structural fusion: commissural, leaflet tip, chordal, and mixed.

(2) Malignant carcinoid.

(3) Systemic lupus erythematosus.

(4) Rheumatoid arthritis.

(5) Mucopolysaccharidosis.

(6) Amyloidosis.

2. Clinical Manifestations of MS

(1) Dyspnea: Exertional dyspnea→Paroxysmal nocturnal dyspnea and orthopnea→Acute pulmonary edema.

(2) Hemoptysis: ① Sudden massive hemoptysis (severe MS); ② Blood-tinged sputum or sputum with blood streaks; ③ Large amount of pink frothy sputum; ④ Pulmonary infarction with hemoptysis.

(3) Cough: In winter.

(4) Hoarseness: Rare.

(5) Thromboembolism.

(6) Complication of infective endocarditis.

3. Main Physical Examination Findings. Malar flush (mitral facies). Apical impulse is normal or not prominent. Cardiac borders enlarged to the left.

Diastolic thrill. Accentuated S1 and opening snap (OS) may be heard. Low-pitched rumbling diastolic mid to late murmur at the apex, localized and not radiating. Accentuated and split P2. Graham Steell murmur. Blowing pansystolic murmur heard at L4-5.

4. Diagnosis

(1) Electrocardiogram: Suggests severe MS. May have "mitral P wave", P wave width >0.12 s, with notching. QRS complexes show right axis deviation and right ventricular hypertrophy.

(2) Chest X-ray: Left atrial enlargement, pear-shaped heart, double atrial shadow, pulmonary congestion. Enlarged left atrium compresses the lower esophagus posteriorly. Elevated left main bronchus. Right ventricular enlargement.

(3) Echocardiography: M-mode shows mitral valve wall-like changes (decreased EF slope, disappearance of A peak), anterior movement of the posterior leaflet, and thickened leaflets.

Classification of MS severity:

1) Normal mitral valve area: 4-6 cm^2;

2) Mild mitral stenosis: 1.6-2.0 cm^2;

3) Moderate mitral stenosis: 1.1-1.5 cm^2;

4) Severe mitral stenosis: $\leqslant$1.0 cm^2.

5. Treatment

(1) Prevention and treatment of rheumatic fever: Prophylactic antibiotics for patients under 30 years old. Prevention of infective endocarditis.

(2) Asymptomatic patients should avoid strenuous physical activity and have regular follow-up.

(3) Patients with dyspnea should reduce physical activity, restrict sodium, and take oral diuretics.

(4) For chronic patients with a course $<$1 year, left atrial diameter $<$60 mm, no high-degree or complete atrioventricular block, and no sick sinus syndrome, electrical or pharmacological cardioversion can be selected. Digoxin 0.125-0.25 mg/day, controlling ventricular rate at 70-90 beats/min (digoxin + diltiazem, digoxin + amiodarone; β-blockers).

(5) Prevention of embolism: Aspirin, warfarin.

(6) Acute hemoptysis: Sitting position, sedatives, diuretics, and lowering pulmon-ary venous pressure. For acute pulmonary edema, choose drugs that primarily dilate the veins and reduce cardiac preload. Diuretics, digitalis, ACEI for anti-heart failure treatment.

6. Surgical Treatment. Surgical treatment is shown in Tables 5-5 and 5-6.

Table 5-5 Indications for Mitral Valve Balloon Dilation

Recommendation	Recommendation Class	Evidence Level
Patients with symptomatic severe mitral stenosis (valve area $\leqslant$1.5 cm^2) and favorable valve morphology, without left atrial thrombus, and no moderate to severe mitral regurgitation	Ⅰ	A
Patients with asymptomatic very severe mitral stenosis (valve area $\leqslant$1.0 cm^2) and favorable valve morphology, without left atrial thrombus, and no moderate to severe mitral regurgitation (Class $Ⅱ_a$ recommendation, Evidence Level C)	$Ⅱ_a$	C
Patients with asymptomatic severe mitral stenosis (valve area $\leqslant$1.5 cm^2) and new-onset atrial fibrillation, with favorable valve morphology, without left atrial thrombus, and no moderate to severe mitral regurgitation	$Ⅱ_b$	C

(Continued)

Recommendation	Recommendation Class	Evidence Level
Symptomatic patients with a valve area >1.5 cm^2 and evidence indicating that mitral stenosis severely affects hemodynamic status (pulmonary capillary wedge pressure >25 mmHg or mean transvalvular gradient >15 mmHg during exercise)	II_b	C
Patients with severe mitral stenosis (valve area ≤1.5 cm^2), severe symptoms [New York Heart Association (NYHA) Class Ⅲ - Ⅳ], and unfavorable valve conditions but unsuitable for surgical treatment or at high surgical risk	II_b	C

Table 5-6 Surgical Indications for Mitral Stenosis

Surgical Indications	Recommendation Class	Evidence Level
Low-risk patients with severe mitral stenosis, valve area ≤1.5 cm^2, severe symptoms (NYHA Class Ⅲ - Ⅳ), unsuitable for mitral valve balloon dilation or with failed mitral valve balloon dilation	I	B
Patients with severe mitral stenosis (valve area ≤1.5 cm^2) who require cardiac surgery for other reasons	I	C
Patients with severe mitral stenosis (valve area ≤1.5 cm^2), severe symptoms (NYHA Class Ⅲ - Ⅳ), combined with other diseases (aortic valve disease, coronary heart disease, tricuspid valve disease, aneurysm, etc.) requiring simultaneous surgical treatment	II_a	C
Patients with other cardiac lesions requiring surgical treatment combined with moderate mitral stenosis (valve area 1.6-2.0 cm^2)	II_b	C
Patients with severe mitral stenosis (valve area ≤1.5 cm^2) and recurrent thromboembolism despite adequate anticoagulation therapy may be considered for concomitant mitral valve surgery and left atrial appendage resection	II_b	C

Ⅳ Mitral Insufficiency (MI)

1. Etiology of MI

(1) Acute: Mainly caused by mitral valve annulus, leaflet, papillary muscle lesions, chordae tendineae rupture, and prosthetic valve dehiscence. Main causes include infective endocarditis, acute rheumatic fever, myxomatous degeneration, amyloidosis, systemic lupus erythematosus, acute myocardial infarction, trauma (including cardiac valve surgery), and prosthetic valve mechanical failure.

(2) Chronic: Main causes include rheumatic heart discasc, infective endocarditis, mitral valve prolapse, degenerative valve disease, mitral annular and sub-annular calcification, infective endocarditis, significant left ventricular enlargement, systemic lupus erythematosus, scleroderma, and congenital malformations.

2. Clinical Manifestations of MI

(1) Acute MI: Mild MI causes milder symptoms. Severe regurgitation can rapidly lead to acute left heart failure, acute pulmonary edema, or cardiogenic shock.

(2) Chronic MI: Mild MI may be asymptomatic for life. Patients with severe regurgitation may experience chest pain, palpitations, fatigue, and dizziness in the early stage, and develop paroxysmal nocturnal dyspnea, orthopnea, pulmonary edema, and pulmonary hypertension in the late stage.

3. Main Physical Examination Findings. Cardiac borders are displaced downward and to the left. The first heart sound may be decreased. P2 is accentuated. The regurgitant murmur at the apex terminates before the second heart sound. Abnormalities of the anterior leaflet may present with a blowing holosystolic murmur, loudest at the apex. The murmur may radiate to the left axilla and left infrascapular region.

In posterior leaflet abnormalities, the murmur radiates to the left sternal border and cardiac base.

4. Diagnosis

(1) Electrocardiogram: In acute MI, the electrocardiogram is normal without significant changes. In chronic MI, left atrial enlargement, left ventricular hypertrophy, and non-specific ST-T changes are present. A few cases show signs of right ventricular hypertrophy.

(2) Chest X-ray: In acute MI, the cardiac silhouette is normal or shows mild left atrial enlargement. In chronic severe regurgitant MI, left atrial and left ventricular enlargement are common.

(3) Echocardiography: Mild regurgitation: Maximum jet area in the left atrium <4 cm^2.

Moderate regurgitation: Maximum jet area in the left atrium 4-8 cm^2.

Severe regurgitation: Maximum jet area in the left atrium >8 cm^2.

5. Treatment

(1) Acute MI: Nitroprusside, furosemide, digitalis, etc. Surgical options include emergency, elective, or selective surgery (prosthetic valve replacement or repair).

(2) Chronic MI

1) Medical treatment: Prevention of infective endocarditis and rheumatic fever; regular follow-up for asymptomatic patients with normal cardiac function; for atrial fibrillation, cardioversion, ventricular rate control, and long-term anticoagulation with warfarin; for heart failure patients, sodium restriction, diuretics, ACEIs or ARBs, β-blockers, and digitalis.

2) Surgical treatment: See Tables 5-7 and 5-8.

Table 5-7 Surgical Indications for Mitral Regurgitation

Surgical Indications	Recommendation Class	Evidence Level
Symptomatic patients with severe chronic primary mitral regurgitation and left ventricular ejection fraction (LVEF) $>30\%$	I	B
Asymptomatic patients with severe chronic primary mitral regurgitation, LVEF 30%-60%, and/or left ventricular end-systolic diameter ≥ 40 mm	I	B

(Continued)

Surgical Indications	Recommendation Class	Evidence Level
Patients with severe chronic primary mitral regurgitation combined with other cardiac lesions requiring surgical treatment	Ⅰ	B
Patients with chronic moderate mitral regurgitation combined with other cardiac diseases requiring surgical treatment	$Ⅱ_a$	C
Patients with chronic severe primary mitral regurgitation and LVEF ≤30%	$Ⅱ_b$	C

Table 5-8 Indications for Mitral Valve Repair

Surgical Indications	Recommendation Class	Evidence Level
For patients with severe primary mitral regurgitation limited to posterior leaflet lesions, mitral valve repair is preferred over mitral valve replacement	Ⅰ	B
For patients with primary mitral regurgitation with anterior leaflet lesions or combined anterior and posterior leaflet lesions, if mitral valve repair can be successfully performed and durability can be ensured, mitral valve repair is preferred	Ⅰ	B
For asymptomatic patients with mitral regurgitation and preserved left ventricular function (LVEF >60%, left ventricular end-systolic diameter <40 mm), if mitral valve repair can be successfully performed and durability can be ensured, with 95% of patients having no residual regurgitation and a mortality rate <1%, mitral valve repair is recommended in experienced centers	$Ⅱ_a$	B

V Tricuspid Valve Stenosis (TS)

1. Etiology of TS. Rheumatic heart disease, congenital tricuspid atresia, carcinoid syndrome, systemic lupus erythematosus, right atrial myxoma, endomyocardial fibrosis, implanted pacemaker, and ergotamine.

2. Clinical Manifestations of TS. Fatigue, systemic venous congestion, atrial fibrillation, and pulmonary embolism.

3. Main Physical Examination Findings. Jugular venous distention, tricuspid valve opening snap at the lower left sternal border, diastolic rumbling murmur at the left sternal border between the 4th and 5th intercostal spaces or near the xiphoid process, hepatomegaly, ascites, and generalized edema.

4. Diagnosis

(1) Electrocardiogram: Suggests right atrial enlargement.

(2) Chest X-ray: Prominent right atrium and superior vena cava, right atrial margin >5 cm from the midline.

(3) Echocardiography: Thickened tricuspid leaflets with restricted motion. In the four-chamber view, the normal opening distance is about 4 cm. If <2 cm, stenosis should be considered. Spontaneous contrast in the right atrium, right atrial thrombus, significant right atrial

enlargement, and occasionally small right ventricle and pulmonary artery.

1) Normal: Tricuspid valve area 6-8 cm^2; valve orifice diameter >4 cm.

2) Stenosis: Tricuspid valve area <1.5 cm^2; valve orifice diameter <2 cm.

5. Treatment

(1) Medical treatment: Treatment of right heart failure and control of arrhythmias.

(2) Surgical treatment: For patients with a diastolic trans-tricuspid pressure gradient >5 mmHg or a valve area <2.0 cm^2, percutaneous balloon tricuspid valvuloplasty can be performed, but the indications are not clear.

Ⅵ Tricuspid Regurgitation (TR)

1. Etiology of TR. Common causes include primary or various secondary pulmonary hypertension; obstruction of the right ventricular outflow tract and pulmonary artery; right ventricular myocardial infarction; and dilated right ventricular cardiomyopathy.

(1) Functional regurgitation: Common. Due to increased right ventricular systolic pressure or right ventricular dilatation, causing annular dilatation and regurgitation, without organic lesions of the tricuspid valve itself.

(2) Organic regurgitation: Rare. Congenital causes include tricuspid valve dysplasia, tricuspid valve prolapse, endocardial cushion defect (tricuspid valve cleft), tricuspid valve displacement malformation, and ventricular septal tumor (Tables 5-9 and 5-10).

Table 5-9 Semi-Quantitative Assessment of Regurgitation Severity

Length Method	Mild	Length <1/2 of the right atrium
	Moderate	Length >1/2 of the right atrium
	Severe	Regurgitant jet reaches the inferior vena cava or hepatic veins
Area Method	Mild	<20%
	Moderate	20%-40%
	Severe	>40%

Table 5-10 Semi-Quantitative Assessment of Regurgitant Pressure

Normal	Gradient	<30 mmHg
Mild Pulmonary Hypertension	Gradient	30-60 mmHg
Moderate Pulmonary Hypertension	Gradient	60-90 mmHg
Severe Pulmonary Hypertension	Gradient	>90 mmHg

Acquired / secondary causes include rheumatic disease, chest trauma, right atrial myxoma, right ventricular myocardial infarction or ischemia leading to right ventricular papillary muscle dysfunction, and late-stage right heart failure due to systemic venous hypertension and right ventricular overload.

(3) Physiological regurgitation: Present in 90% of people, with normal tricuspid valve

morphology and no right heart enlargement.

2. Clinical Manifestations of TR. Hemodynamic manifestations include systolic hepatic congestion, ascites, and edema. Diastolic right heart failure.

3. Main Physical Examination Findings. Signs of right heart failure, atrial fibrillation, and pulmonary embolism; jugular venous distention; increased right ventricular pulsation, third heart sound at the lower left sternal border, and high-pitched blowing holosystolic murmur, with a short diastolic rumbling murmur in severe regurgitation; systolic click in tricuspid valve prolapse; systolic hepatic pulsation; signs of systemic venous congestion.

4. Diagnosis

(1) Electrocardiogram: Suggests right atrial enlargement, incomplete right bundle branch block, and atrial fibrillation.

(2) Chest X-ray: Right atrial enlargement, dilated right ventricle and superior vena cava, possibly pleural effusion.

(3) Echocardiography: ① Functional regurgitation: Enlarged right atrium and right ventricle, increased tricuspid annular diameter, normal morphology of leaflets and subvalvular apparatus. ② Organic regurgitation: Involvement of tricuspid leaflets and subvalvular apparatus, such as shortening, prolapse, displacement, cleft, thickening, abnormal motion, vegetations, etc. Enlarged right atrium and right ventricle, weakened or enhanced right ventricular wall motion.

5. Treatment

(1) Medical treatment: In the absence of pulmonary hypertension, control right heart failure and arrhythmias.

(2) Surgical treatment: For TR secondary to mitral or aortic valve disease, mild regurgitation does not require surgery. Moderate to severe TR requires annuloplasty or valve replacement. For tricuspid valve dysplasia, carcinoid syndrome, infective endocarditis, etc., valve replacement should be performed.

Ⅶ Pulmonary Valve Stenosis (PS)

1. Etiology of PS. Congenital malformation; rheumatic heart disease; carcinoid syndrome.

2. Clinical Manifestations of PS. Mild cases may be asymptomatic. Moderate cases have dyspnea and fatigue. Severe cases may experience syncope or even sudden death.

3. Main Physical Examination Findings. The type of murmur is related to the degree of stenosis: In valvular type, L2 is loudest; in infundibular type, L3-L4 is loudest; in mixed type, L2-4 is widely present. Systolic ejection murmur at the left sternal border, may radiate to the neck or even the back, often with a click and thrill. P2 can be normal, diminished, or absent, reflecting the degree of stenosis.

4. Diagnosis

(1) Electrocardiogram: Mild stenosis may be normal; moderate or severe stenosis may show right axis deviation, right ventricular enlargement, incomplete conduction block, and tall peaked P waves.

(2) Chest X-ray: Fine pulmonary vascular markings, prominent pulmonary artery segment, small pulmonary vessels, clear lung fields, increased left pulmonary hilum pulsation, decreased or

static right pulmonary hilum pulsation. Enlarged right ventricle and right atrium. In mild stenosis, heart size may be normal.

(3) Echocardiography: Accelerated blood flow at the pulmonary valve orifice.

5. Treatment. Percutaneous balloon pulmonary valvuloplasty (PBPV)

Surgical treatment: For patients with unsuccessful dilation or unsuitable for dilation.

Mild stenosis does not require treatment; PBPV and surgical treatment have similar short-term and long-term efficacy.

Ⅷ Pulmonary Insufficiency (PI)

1. Etiology of PI. Common: Pulmonary artery trunk dilatation secondary to pulmonary hypertension, such as rheumatic mitral stenosis, Eisenmenger syndrome, idiopathic and Marfan syndrome pulmonary artery dilatation. Rare: Primary pulmonary valve lesions.

2. Clinical Manifestations of PI. Prominent clinical manifestations. Even moderate to severe reflux hemodynamic changes can be well tolerated. Often incidentally discovered during auscultation. Right heart enlargement and heart failure may occur in late stages.

3. Main Physical Examination Findings. Pulsation palpable at the left sternal border in the 2nd intercostal space, possibly accompanied by systolic or diastolic thrills. Right ventricular systolic ejection murmur, most pronounced at the left sternal border in the 2nd intercostal space. Third and fourth heart sounds often present at the left sternal border in the 4th intercostal space, enhanced on inspiration. Accentuated and split P2, Graham-Steell murmur.

4. Diagnosis

(1) ECG: Suggestive of right ventricular hypertrophy.

(2) Chest X-ray: Right ventricular and pulmonary trunk enlargement.

(3) Echocardiography: Doppler ultrasound is highly sensitive for the definitive diagnosis of pulmonary insufficiency and can semi-quantitatively assess the degree of regurgitation. Two-dimensional echocardiography helps to clarify the etiology.

5. Treatment. Primarily focuses on treating the primary disease-causing pulmonary hypertension, such as relieving mitral stenosis. Surgical treatment of the valve is only considered when severe pulmonary valve regurgitation leads to refractory right heart failure.

Ⅸ Consultation Process

1. Each type of valvular heart disease has common etiologies, requiring a detailed history. For example: Aortic stenosis (AS) is common in congenital valve disease, degenerative aortic stenosis, rheumatic heart disease, etc. Aortic regurgitation (AR) is common in bicuspid aortic valve, infective endocarditis, rheumatic heart disease, aortic root dilatation, etc. Mitral stenosis (MS) is common in rheumatic fever, malignant carcinoid, systemic lupus erythematosus, rheumatoid arthritis, mucopolysaccharidosis, amyloidosis, etc. Mitral insufficiency (MI) is common in infective endocarditis, acute rheumatic fever, myxomatous degeneration, amyloidosis, systemic lupus erythematosus, acute myocardial infarction, traumatic (including valvular heart surgery), prosthetic valve mechanical failure, infective endocarditis, mitral valve prolapse, degenerative valve disease. Tricuspid stenosis (TS) is common in rheumatic heart

disease, congenital tricuspid atresia, carcinoid syndrome, systemic lupus erythematosus, right atrial myxoma, endocardial fibrosis, etc. Tricuspid regurgitation (TR) is common in primary or various secondary pulmonary hypertension, right ventricular outflow tract and pulmonary artery obstruction, right ventricular myocardial infarction, right ventricular dilated cardiomyopathy. Pulmonary stenosis (PS) is common in congenital malformations, rheumatic heart disease, carcinoid syndrome. Pulmonary insufficiency (PI) is common in rheumatic mitral stenosis, Eisenmenger syndrome, etc.

2. Valvular heart disease presents with different symptoms based on the characteristics of each valve: the most common are heart failure, angina pectoris, and syncope; summarize and analyze according to the characteristics of each valve.

3. Physical examination: Different valvular lesions cause cardiac murmurs with varying periods, locations, and sounds.

4. Auxiliary examinations: Chest X-ray, ECG, echocardiography, among which echocardiography is the most important diagnostic tool.

5. Identify stenosis or regurgitation of each valve, then combine with the severity to determine the treatment plan.

Key Points of Valvular Disease Consultation:

1) Identify the etiology and severity of the lesion.

2) Distinguish the treatment differences between single valve disease and multi-valve combined lesions.

3) Clearly indicate the treatment contraindications for the patient.

4) Be familiar with (or at least review) whether the patient already has surgical indications.

Section 5 Pulmonary Hypertension

Pulmonary hypertension (PH) is a broad category of malignant pulmonary vascular diseases characterized by elevated pulmonary artery pressure, with or without pulmonary arteriolar lesions, often leading to right heart failure and even death. Pulmonary hypertension has become a common disease that seriously threatens human physical and mental health.

I Several Definitions

1. Pulmonary hypertension refers to hypertension in the pulmonary circulation system, including pulmonary arterial hypertension (PAH), pulmonary venous hypertension, and mixed pulmonary hypertension. Any systemic or localized lesion that causes an increase in pulmonary circulatory blood pressure throughout the entire pulmonary circulation can be referred to as pulmonary hypertension (abbreviated as PH). Currently, it can be divided into five major categories: pulmonary arterial hypertension, pulmonary hypertension associated with left heart disease, pulmonary hypertension associated with respiratory system diseases or hypoxia, chronic thromboembolic pulmonary hypertension, and pulmonary hypertension with unclear multiple factors.

2. Pulmonary arterial hypertension refers to isolated pulmonary arterial pressure elevation while pulmonary venous pressure is normal, mainly caused by primary small artery lesions or other related diseases leading to increased pulmonary arterial resistance. Pulmonary capillary wedge pressure (PCWP) is needed for diagnosis.

3. Idiopathic pulmonary arterial hypertension is a type of pulmonary arterial hypertension, referring to a specific disease without a history of PAH gene mutations and clear risk factor exposure, corresponding to the English term "idiopathic pulmonary arterial hypertension, IPAH".

4. Heritable pulmonary arterial hypertension refers to familial pulmonary arterial hypertension patients with known gene mutations and idiopathic pulmonary arterial hypertension patients with gene mutations. The "Guidelines" have eliminated the diagnostic term familial pulmonary arterial hypertension.

5. The latest clinical classification of pulmonary hypertension is shown in Table 5-11.

Table 5-11 Clinical Classification of Pulmonary Hypertension

1. Pulmonary Arterial Hypertension
(1) Idiopathic
(2) Heritable
Bone morphogenetic protein receptor 2
Activin receptor-like kinase 1, endoglin. Unknown genetic factors
(3) Drugs or toxins
(4) Disease-associated pulmonary arterial hypertension
Connective tissue diseases
Human immunodeficiency virus infection
Portal hypertension
Congenital heart disease (left-to-right shunt of heart or great vessels)
Schistosomiasis
Chronic hemolytic anemia
(5) Persistent pulmonary hypertension of the newborn
(6) Pulmonary veno-occlusive disease, pulmonary capillary hemangiomatosis
2. Pulmonary Hypertension Due to Left Heart Disease
(1) Systolic dysfunction
(2) Diastolic dysfunction
(3) Valvular heart disease
3. Pulmonary Hypertension Due to Lung Diseases and/or Hypoxia
(1) Chronic obstructive pulmonary disease
(2) Interstitial lung disease
(3) Other pulmonary diseases with mixed restrictive and obstructive pattern
(4) Sleep-disordered breathing

(Continued)

(5) Alveolar hypoventilation disorders
(6) Chronic exposure to high altitude (chronic mountain sickness)
(7) Developmental lung diseases
4. Chronic Thromboembolic Pulmonary Hypertension
5. Pulmonary Hypertension with Unclear Multifactorial Mechanisms
(1) Hematologic disorders: Myeloproliferative disorders, splenectomy
(2) Systemic disorders: Sarcoidosis, pulmonary Langerhans cell histiocytosis, lymphangioleiomyomatosis, neurofibromatosis, vasculitis
(3) Metabolic disorders: Glycogen storage disease, Gaucher disease, thyroid disorders
(4) Others: Tumoral obstruction, fibrosing mediastinitis, chronic renal failure on dialysis

II Several Diseases Commonly Associated with Pulmonary Hyperten-sion in Consultation

1. Connective Tissue Disease-Associated Pulmonary Arterial Hypertension. In daily consultations, patients with connective tissue diseases (CTD) from the rheumatology and immunology department complicated by pulmonary arterial hypertension are commonly encountered. Approximately 3%-13% of CTD patients develop PHA, and severe PH significantly affects the prognosis of CTD patients, with PH being one of the important causes of death in CTD, usually due to circulatory failure. This should be given high attention in clinical practice. Once discovered, it should not be taken lightly or with an indifferent attitude during consultation. Necessary examinations and active treatment should be given early.

2. Pulmonary Hypertension Associated with Chronic Lung Diseases. Pulmonary hypertension related to respiratory system diseases and/or hypoxia is another very common type of pulmonary hypertension in clinical practice, which includes the following 7 categories in many guidelines: chronic obstructive pulmonary disease, interstitial lung disease, lung diseases with coexisting restrictive and obstructive ventilatory dysfunction, sleep-disordered breathing, alveolar hypoventilation syndrome, chronic mountain sickness, and alveolar-capillary dysplasia.

For patients with chronic lung diseases, the presence of pulmonary hypertension indicates a worse clinical prognosis. In fact, the clinical manifestations related to pulmonary hypertension often overlap with the manifestations of the underlying lung disease, making it difficult to strictly distinguish. In addition, echocardiography has a lower sensitivity for diagnosing pulmonary hypertension in these patients. Therefore, it is not easy to detect pulmonary hypertension in patients with lung diseases in the early stage. However, if there is a mismatch between the degree of decrease in arterial oxygen saturation and 6-minute walk distance and the degree of lung function impairment, one should be alert to the presence of pulmonary hypertension. Right heart catheterization is required for definitive diagnosis.

3. Chronic Thromboembolic Pulmonary Hypertension (CTEPH). Diagnosed when the mean pulmonary arterial pressure remains greater than 25 mmHg 6 months after acute pulmonary

embolism. About 2%-4% of patients with acute pulmonary embolism develop CTEPH, most commonly in female patients aged 40-50 years. The vast majority of patients do not seek medical attention until they develop dyspnea, hypoxemia, and right ventricular dysfunction. This disease should not be forgotten during emergency or surgical consultations to avoid missed diagnosis.

4. Thyroid Disease-Associated Pulmonary Arterial Hypertension. The diagnosis of thyroid disease-associated pulmonary arterial hypertension requires 4 conditions: ① The patient is clearly diagnosed with hyperthyroidism or hypothyroidism. There may be evidence of "autoimmune thyroid disease," such as positive thyroid-stimulating hormone receptor antibodies, anti-thyroglobulin antibodies, or anti-thyroid microsomal antibodies; ② Clinical manifestations such as chest tightness, shortness of breath, and dyspnea after activity; ③ Echocardiography or hemodynamic measurements suggest an elevated estimated pulmonary arterial pressure or actual measured right ventricular systolic pressure; ④ Exclusion of other diseases causing pulmonary arterial hypertension, mainly pulmonary vascular diseases, pulmonary parenchymal lesions, and other connective tissue diseases.

The characteristic of this type of pulmonary arterial hypertension is a good prognosis, especially hyperthyroidism-associated pulmonary arterial hypertension. After thyroid function returns to normal, pulmonary arterial hypertension can completely return to normal. "Reversibility" is its biggest feature. Therefore, in the diagnosis and treatment of pulmonary arterial hypertension, thyroid disease-associated pulmonary arterial hypertension must be excluded.

5. Congenital Heart Disease-Associated Pulmonary Arterial Hypertension. Pul-monary arterial hypertension is a common and serious complication of left-to-right shunt congenital heart disease, which has a decisive impact on the patient's clinical course, the feasibility and efficacy of surgical or interventional treatment, and prognosis. About 5% of adult patients with congenital heart disease eventually develop pulmonary arterial hypertension, of which 25%-50% have Eisenmenger syndrome. The main purpose of consultation for these patients is to determine the surgical indications, select the surgical method, perform necessary preoperative examinations and drug treatment, and improve cardiac function in cooperation with the surgical department.

6. Left Heart Disease-Associated Pulmonary Hypertension. Refers to pulmonary venous hypertension caused by left ventricular systolic dysfunction, left ventricular diastolic dysfunction, or mitral and aortic valve lesions, ultimately leading to increased pulmonary arterial pressure and right ventricular dysfunction. Although Doppler echocardiography can observe elevated left ventricular filling pressure, right heart catheterization to measure PCWP or left ventricular end-diastolic pressure is still necessary to determine left heart disease-associated pulmonary hypertension.

The right heart catheterization diagnostic criteria for left heart disease-associated pulmonary hypertension: mean pulmonary arterial pressure (mPAP) ≥25 mmHg and PCWP >15 mmHg, with normal or decreased cardiac output. It is divided into two types based on hemodynamic characteristics: reactive elevation refers to a transpulmonary gradient >12 mmHg; passive elevation refers to a transpulmonary gradient ≤12 mmHg.

7. Hemolytic Anemia-Associated Pulmonary Hypertension. Hemolytic anemia is an important associated factor and risk factor for pulmonary hypertension. With the significant prolongation of survival in patients with hemolytic anemia, pulmonary arterial hypertension has become the most common disabling and fatal complication in patients with sickle cell anemia, thalassemia, and hemoglobinopathies. When consulting outside, it is recommended that consulting physicians regularly screen for pulmonary hypertension in patients with hemolytic anemia using echocardiography and perform right heart catheterization to confirm the diagnosis in suspected patients. Intensifying the treatment of hemolytic anemia may be effective for mild pulmonary hypertension, delay the progression of pulmonary hypertension, reduce the incidence of severe pulmonary hypertension, and thus improve patients' quality of life and prognosis.

In addition, some rare diseases that cause pulmonary arterial hypertension, such as schistosomiasis, pulmonary veno-occlusive disease, and appetite suppressants, should also be understood to avoid misdiagnosis or difficulty in diagnosis during consultation.

Ⅲ Examination Methods

Medical history, physical examination, laboratory tests, and instrumental examinations are the basis for diagnosing pulmonary hypertension, among which instrumental examinations are indispensable and play a crucial role in the diagnosis, treatment, and prognosis of the disease. The main examinations include:

1. Electrocardiogram. Characteristic manifestations of pulmonary arterial hypertension include: ① Right axis deviation; ② S wave in lead I; ③ Pulmonary P wave; ④ Signs of right ventricular hypertrophy, with ST-T wave flattening or inversion in the right precordial leads. The electrocardiogram has certain importance in diagnosis but lacks specificity.

2. Chest X-ray. Characteristic manifestations of pulmonary arterial hypertension include dilatation of the main pulmonary artery and enlargement of the pulmonary hilum, thickening of the right lower pulmonary artery trunk, accompanied by peripheral pulmonary vascular sparseness ("pruning phenomenon"). The value of X-ray examination in diagnosing and evaluating pulmonary arterial hypertension is not as good as electrocardiography, but it can detect primary pulmonary diseases.

3. Echocardiography. It is the most important noninvasive examination method for screening pulmonary arterial hypertension. In the absence of pulmonary valve stenosis and outflow tract obstruction, the pulmonary arterial systolic pressure is equal to the right ventricular systolic pressure, which can be estimated by measuring the systolic pressure gradient between the right ventricle and right atrium using echocardiography. According to the modified Bernoulli equation, the difference between the right ventricle and right atrium is approximately equal to $4V^2$, where V is the maximum tricuspid regurgitation velocity (m/s). Currently, the internationally recommended echocardiographic diagnostic criterion for pulmonary arterial hypertension is a pulmonary arterial systolic pressure $\geqslant$40 mmHg. In addition to tricuspid regurgitation and estimating pulmonary arterial systolic pressure, the presence of concurrent right ventricular dilatation and hypertrophy provides more evidence for a definitive diagnosis.

Echocardiography is the most important method for screening pulmonary arterial hypertension and can assess disease severity and prognosis. Current prognostic indicators include: tricuspid annular plane systolic excursion (TAPSE), left ventricular eccentric index (LVEI), Tei index (myocardial performance index), presence of pericardial effusion, etc. Additionally, the important value of echocardiography is also reflected in its ability to detect intracardiac and great vessel malformations. Therefore, echocardiography is an essential tool in every consulting physician's examination plan during consultation.

4. Right Heart Catheterization. It is not only the gold standard for diagnosing pulmonary arterial hypertension but also an indispensable examination method for diagnosing and evaluating pulmonary arterial hypertension. The following can be obtained: ① Superior and inferior vena cava pressure and blood oxygen saturation; ② Right atrial and right ventricular systolic pressure, diastolic pressure, mean pressure, and blood oxygen saturation; ③ Pulmonary arterial systolic pressure, diastolic pressure, mean pressure, and blood oxygen saturation; ④ Cardiac output and cardiac index; ⑤ Total pulmonary vascular resistance; ⑥ Small pulmonary arterial resistance; ⑦ Systemic vascular resistance; ⑧ Pulmonary capillary wedge pressure.

5. Acute Vasodilator Testing. For various types of pulmonary arterial hypertension patients, especially idiopathic pulmonary arterial hypertension patients, pulmonary vasospasm may be involved in the development of pulmonary arterial hypertension. Acute vasodilator testing is an effective means to screen these patients. Patients with positive test results can have significantly improved prognosis with calcium channel blocker therapy.

Positive criteria for acute pulmonary vasodilator testing: The patient's mean pulmonary arterial pressure decreases to within 40 mmHg; the decrease in mean pulmonary arterial pressure exceeds 10 mmHg; the cardiac output remains unchanged or increases. All three conditions must be met simultaneously to diagnose a positive test result.

Studies from abroad have shown that among patients with an initial positive acute pulmonary vasodilator test, about 46% have a negative test result one year later after treatment with calcium channel blockers. Therefore, it is recommended that patients with an initial positive test who receive calcium channel blocker therapy undergo a repeat acute pulmonary vasodilator test one year later. If the result is still positive, it indicates that the patient remains sensitive and can continue calcium channel blocker therapy.

6. Pulmonary Function Evaluation. A routine examination. If there are no contraindications, all pulmonary arterial hypertension patients need to complete pulmonary function tests to understand whether the patient has various ventilatory disorders and provide diagnostic evidence for excluding chronic obstructive pulmonary disease, interstitial lung disease, etc. Most pulmonary arterial hypertension patients have mild ventilatory or diffusion dysfunction on pulmonary function tests. Some patients with connective tissue diseases combined with interstitial lung disease and pulmonary veno-occlusive disease often have a significant decrease in diffusion function.

7. Sleep Monitoring. About 15% of the patients with obstructive sleep apnea have concurrent pulmonary arterial pressure elevation. Therefore, this examination should be routinely performed in patients with pulmonary arterial hypertension.

8. Pulmonary Angiography. Not all pulmonary hypertension patients need this examination. It is

only indicated in the following five situations: ① Clinically suspected thromboembolic pulmonary hypertension but noninvasive examinations cannot provide sufficient evidence; ② Clinically considered central chronic thromboembolic pulmonary hypertension with indications for surgery, requiring preoperative pulmonary angiography to guide surgery; ③ Clinically diagnosed pulmonary vasculitis, requiring understanding of the extent of pulmonary vascular involvement; ④ Preoperative diagnosis of pulmonary artery tumors; ⑤ Under-standing the presence of pulmonary vascular malformations. It should be performed in experienced centers, using iso-osmolar contrast agents as much as possible and reducing the injection rate.

9. Pulmonary Ventilation-Perfusion Scintigraphy. Similar to CT pulmonary angiography, it is one of the main means for the differential diagnosis of pulmonary embolism.

10. Cardiovascular Magnetic Resonance Imaging. It is one of the most promising noninvasive examination methods, but due to some technical reasons, not many hospitals in China carry out this examination.

11. Others. In addition to the above-mentioned instrumental examinations, the 6-minute walk distance test for functional evaluation must be introduced.

The 6-minute walk distance test is the most important examination method for assessing the activity endurance status of pulmonary arterial hypertension patients. It calculates the distance the patient walks in 6 minutes, and the results have a significant correlation with prognosis. The result report is shown in Table 5-12. Additionally, the 6-minute walk distance test is also a key method for evaluating the effectiveness of treatment. Almost all clinical studies of new drugs for pulmonary arterial hypertension use the 6-minute walk distance test results as the main observation endpoint. After completing the test, the Borg dyspnea rating (Table 5-13) also needs to be performed. The 6-minute walk test results are currently recommended to be compared using their absolute value changes (e.g., an increase of 50 m in distance) rather than comparing each result with the normal value.

Table 5-12 6-Minute Walk Distance Test Result Report Form

Name		Gender		Age		Ward		Case Number	
Current Diagnosis									
Cardiac Function Classification									
Test Date									
Walking Distance									
		Before Test				After Test			
Heart Rate									
Blood Pressure									
Fingertip Oxygen Saturation									
Borg Dyspnea Rating									
Symptoms Experienced by the Patient During the Test									
Remarks									

Table 5-13 Borg Dyspnea Rating Scale

Rating Index	Degree of Dyspnea
0 point	No dyspnea or fatigue symptoms at all
0.5 point	Very slight dyspnea symptoms (barely noticeable)
1 point	Very slight dyspnea symptoms
2 points	Slight dyspnea symptoms (mild)
3 points	Moderate dyspnea symptoms
4 points	Dyspnea symptoms are slightly heavy
5 points	Severe dyspnea symptoms (heavy)
6 points	
7 points	Very heavy dyspnea or fatigue
8 points	
9 points	
10 points	Extremely severe dyspnea (heaviest)

Ⅳ Treatment

1. General Treatment

(1) Avoid pregnancy.

(2) Immunize against influenza and pneumococcal infections.

(3) Social and psychological support therapy.

(4) Exercise training based on drug therapy.

(5) Provide continuous oxygen therapy for patients with WHO functional Class Ⅲ and Class Ⅳ and arterial oxygen partial pressure <8 kPa (60 mmHg).

(6) Use epidural anesthesia instead of general anesthesia for pulmonary arterial hypertension patients undergoing elective surgery.

(7) High-intensity exercise is not recommended for pulmonary arterial hypertension patients.

2. Supportive Treatment

(1) PAH patients with right heart failure and fluid retention should receive diuretic therapy.

(2) Oral anticoagulant therapy is recommended for patients with idiopathic PAH, heritable PAH, and PAH caused by polycyclic aromatic hydrocarbons.

(3) Angiotensin-converting enzyme inhibitors, angiotensin-2 receptor antagonists, and beta-receptor blockers are not recommended for PAH patients unless they have concomitant hypertension, coronary heart disease, or left heart failure.

3. Several Commonly Used Selective Pulmonary Vasodilators for the Treatment of Pulmonary Arterial Hypertension

(1) Calcium channel blockers: In cases of positive acute vasodilator testing, nifedipine and amlodipine can be used for patients with bradycardia, while diltiazem can be used for patients with tachycardia. Calcium channel blocker therapy is recommended for patients with a strong response to acute vasodilator testing. It is recommended to closely follow up and re-evaluate patients with idiopathic PAH, heritable PAH, and drug-induced PAH after 3-4 months of high-

dose calcium channel blocker therapy.

(2) Phosphodiesterase Type Ⅴ inhibitors: Sildenafil (Viagra), usual dose 20 mg, three times daily. Additionally, there are vardenafil and tadalafil.

(3) Prostaglandin analogues: Including intravenous epoprostenol, subcutaneous treprostinil (Remodulin), oral beraprost (Dorna), and inhaled iloprost (Ventavis). The efficacy and safety of this class of drugs have been confirmed by evidence-based medicine and extensive clinical practice and are recommended by guidelines in multiple countries.

(4) Endothelin receptor antagonists: Bosentan (Tracleer), initial dose 62.5 mg, twice daily for 4 weeks, then increased to a maintenance dose of 125 mg, twice daily. Additionally, there are ambrisentan and sitaxsentan available internationally.

The above drugs can be used alone or in combination, depending on the patient's specific condition and disease progression.

4. Atrial Septostomy. If the patient's symptoms do not significantly improve after adequate medical treatment, atrial septostomy can be recommended to reduce right ventricular preload, increase left ventricular filling pressure and stroke volume, thereby improving hemodynamics and clinical symptoms. However, this surgery is less commonly performed in China.

5. Lung Transplantation. According to the 2010 Chinese Guidelines for Pulmonary Hypertension, single lung transplantation, double lung transplantation, and combined heart-lung transplantation can be used to treat end-stage PAH patients.

V Key Points for the Treatment of Several Common Types of PH

1. Pulmonary Hypertension Associated with Left Heart Disease

(1) Currently, there is a lack of specific drugs for the treatment of PH associated with left heart disease.

(2) The main goal of treating PH associated with left heart disease should be to treat the primary disease.

(3) Due to the lack of evidence-based medicine, the use of PAH-targeted drugs is currently not recommended in patients with PH associated with left heart disease.

2. Pulmonary Hypertension Associated with Lung Disease and/or Chronic Hypoxia

(1) For patients with PH associated with chronic obstructive pulmonary disease and interstitial lung disease who have long-term hypoxia, long-term oxygen therapy is an optional treatment.

(2) Endothelin receptor antagonists should be the first choice for PH patients with confirmed interstitial lung disease.

(3) Oral sildenafil can be used for PH in patients with chronic obstructive pulmonary disease, but it may cause a decrease in oxygen saturation.

(4) For patients with severe sleep-disordered breathing, long-term treatment with noninvasive ventilation.

3. Pulmonary Hypertension Associated with CTEPH

(1) Long-term anticoagulation therapy, usually using warfarin to adjust the INR to 2-3.

(2) Hospitals with the capability can perform pulmonary endarterectomy.

(3) PAH-targeted drugs may be effective for some patients.

(4) Percutaneous pulmonary artery balloon dilation and stent placement can be considered as a treatment option for some patients who cannot undergo pulmonary endarterectomy.

4. Pulmonary Arterial Hypertension Associated with Congenital Heart Disease

(1) Use bosentan in patients with WHO functional Class Ⅲ and Eisenmenger syndrome.

(2) Oral anticoagulants can be considered for patients with pulmonary artery thrombosis or signs of heart failure in the absence of significant hemoptysis.

(3) If supplemental oxygen can continuously increase oxygen saturation and alleviate symptoms, supplemental oxygen should be considered.

(4) If symptoms of hyperviscosity are present, usually when the hematocrit is >65%, replacement of blood with equal volume of fluid should be considered.

(5) Iron supplementation can be given to patients with low plasma ferritin levels.

(6) Calcium channel blockers are not recommended for patients with Eisenmenger syndrome.

5. Pulmonary Arterial Hypertension Associated with Connective Tissue Diseases

(1) The treatment principles for pulmonary arterial hypertension associated with connective tissue diseases should be the same as those for idiopathic pulmonary arterial hypertension.

(2) Right heart catheterization is recommended for all patients suspected of having pulmonary arterial hypertension associated with connective tissue diseases.

(3) Oral anticoagulants are administered based on individual circumstances for patients with a tendency for thrombosis.

Ⅵ Consultation Process

1. Patients often present with right heart failure, with symptoms mainly including exertional dyspnea and gastrointestinal symptoms (abdominal distension, loss of appetite, nausea, vomiting, etc.); physical signs include edema, jugular venous distention, hepatomegaly, etc.

2. Supplement key medical history information, such as the presence of connective tissue diseases, chronic lung diseases, history of chronic thromboembolism, thyroid diseases, congenital heart diseases, hemolytic anemia, valvular heart diseases, etc.

3. Pay attention to important physical examinations, such as the presence of anemia, barrel chest, lip cyanosis, increased cardiac dullness on percussion, the presence of dry or wet rales, jugular venous distention, lower limb edema (unilateral or bilateral), jugular venous distention, cardiac murmurs, and hepatomegaly, etc.

4. Auxiliary examinations: electrocardiogram, chest X-ray, echocardiography, right heart catheterization, acute vasodilator testing, pulmonary function evaluation, sleep monitoring, pulmonary angiography, pulmonary ventilation-perfusion scintigraphy, cardiovascular magnetic resonance imaging. Among them, right heart catheterization is the gold standard for diagnosing pulmonary arterial hypertension and an indispensable examination method for diagnosing and evaluating pulmonary arterial hypertension.

5. Treatment of pulmonary arterial hypertension: ① The most important aspect is to clarify the underlying cause. For patients presenting with heart failure, give diuretics and symptomatic

supportive treatment, while for critically ill patients, provide endotracheal intubation and assisted ventilation; ② Take relevant measures according to different etiologies. Calcium channel blockers can be used for patients with positive acute vasodilator testing. Currently, there are other pulmonary vasodilators: phosphodiesterase Type Ⅴ inhibitors: sildenafil (Viagra), prostaglandin analogues, endothelin receptor antagonists: bosentan (Tracleer); atrial septostomy and lung transplantation can be performed if medical treatment is ineffective.

Section 6 Progress in Transcatheter Aortic Valve Replacement Technology

Ⅰ Overview

With the extension of human life expectancy and the aging population, the incidence of aortic valve disease is increasing. In developed countries, the incidence of aortic valve stenosis is 4%-5% among the elderly over 75 years old. For a long time, surgical aortic valve replacement (SAVR) has been the main treatment for aortic valve stenosis. However, due to the large trauma of surgery, the need for extracorporeal circulation, and the high surgical risk, 30%-50% of patients are unable to undergo surgery due to advanced age, poor cardiac function, severe complications, or fear of surgery.

Transcatheter aortic valve replacement (TAVR) is a minimally invasive valve replacement surgery that refers to the placement of an assembled aortic valve into the aortic root through a catheter to replace the original aortic valve, functionally completing aortic valve replacement, becoming a new treatment for these patients. TAVR is one of the fastest-developing technologies in the medical field. Since Cribier et al. completed the world's first TAVR in 2002, after more than a decade of rapid development, TAVR has become the main treatment for aortic valve stenosis patients who cannot tolerate or are at high risk for surgical surgery. In China, since Academician Ge Junbo and others performed the first TAVR in October 2010, this technology has been gradually promoted in China. With the continuous development of equipment and the continuous advancement of technology, TAVR technology is becoming increasingly mature, and related clinical research has made great progress. It is being increasingly used to treat intermediate-risk and even low-risk patients for surgical surgery.

Ⅱ Indications: From High-Risk to Low-Risk

1. Currently, the two guidelines in Europe and the United States suggest similar indications for TAVR. Class Ⅰ indications: surgical contraindications, life expectancy over 1 year, and symptomatic calcific severe AS. Class Ⅱ_a indications: high surgical risk, life expectancy over 1 year, and symptomatic calcific severe AS. Surgical contraindication refers to the risk of death or irreversible complications >50% within 30 days after surgery. High surgical risk mainly refers to patients with a score of ≥8 from the American Society of Thoracic Surgeons. The Chinese expert consensus on transcatheter aortic valve replacement (TAVR) proposes that the absolute indications for TAVR are surgical contraindications, life expectancy over 1 year, and symptomatic calcific severe AS; relative indications are high surgical risk, life expectancy over 1 year, and

symptomatic calcific severe AS.

2. The PARTNER Ⅱ a study enrolled 2032 patients with intermediate-risk surgical risk and severe aortic stenosis. Based on the patient's clinical characteristics and imaging examination, they were divided into the femoral artery (1550 cases) and transapical access group (482 cases), and each group was further randomly divided to receive TAVR or SAVR treatment. The study endpoint was the incidence of death or disabling stroke. After 2 years of follow-up, the incidence of major endpoint events in the TAVR group was 19.3%, and in the SAVR group was 21.1% [*HR*=0.89 (95% *CI*, 0.73-1.09), *P*=0.25]. The study showed that the effect of TAVR was not inferior to SAVR in intermediate-risk patients. The femoral artery access subgroup of TAVR was even superior to SAVR [16.8% vs 20.4%, *HR*=0.79 (95% *CI*, 0.62-1.00), *P*=0.05]. Compared with the TAVR group, the SAVR group had a larger aortic valve area, lower acute kidney injury, lower incidence of severe bleeding and new-onset atrial fibrillation; the SAVR group had a lower incidence of severe vascular complications and aortic valve regurgitation. The "2017 ACC Valvular Disease Management Guidelines" listed intermediate-risk patients as a Class ⅡA indication for TAVR.

3. In February 2016, the U. S. FDA approved the first large-scale, randomized clinical trial (PARTNER Ⅲ) of TAVR for the treatment of low-risk patients. The PARTNER Ⅲ trial, using the Sapien 3 valve (Edwards Lifesciences), will enroll approximately 1,300 elderly patients: STS score <4, age >65 years, severe, symptomatic aortic stenosis.

Ⅲ Diversification of Surgical Approaches

Currently, there are 7 surgical approaches available for TAVR, but the main approach is the femoral artery, followed by the transapical approach. Other approaches such as the subclavian artery, carotid artery, thoracic aorta, abdominal aorta, iliac artery, and axillary artery have also been reported in a small number of cases. Studies of the transfemoral approach, especially in high-risk and intermediate-risk patients, have shown that transfemoral TAVR is significantly superior to SAVR. As the diameter of the delivery sheath continues to decrease, more patients will be able to undergo TAVR through the femoral artery approach, and the incidence of vascular complications will continue to decrease, thereby further improving the prognosis of TAVR patients. Studies have shown that the transcarotid approach is a new access route for performing TAVR, which is safe and feasible. Its advantages include a short and straight access route, easy control of the delivery system, easy adjustment of the valve position, and superficial and thick blood vessels that are easy to separate and suture, allowing the use of a larger sheath. Overall, the transfemoral approach is simpler to operate and is currently the first choice. If it cannot be satisfied, other surgical approaches can be used.

Ⅳ Promotion of Minimalist TAVR

Traditional TAVR is performed in a hybrid operating room, under general anesthesia, with transesophageal echocardiography, surgeons, and even extracorporeal circulation standby. In 2014, Babaliaros et al. first proposed the concept of minimalist TAVR. Minimalist TAVR surgery can be performed in a regular catheterization room, using local anesthesia with mild sedation, transthoracic echocardiography monitoring, through the femoral artery approach, subcutaneous puncture, vascular suture device suturing, and a urinary sheath, without the need for surgeons to be present on standby. It greatly simplifies the traditional, tedious, and complex TAVR, and even eliminates the need for professional anesthesiologists to be present. Simple, safe, effective, and low-cost minimalist TAVR has been accepted by more and more centers.

V Reconsideration of TAVR Valve Degeneration

In the initial use of TAVR, elderly, high-risk patients with infective endocarditis who could not tolerate surgical surgery became the first batch of subjects, and there is still a lack of long-term durability data at this stage. A report on the long-term durability of early TAVR valves released at the 2016 European Cardiovascular Course (EuroPCR) showed that within 5-7 years after TAVR, the valve degeneration rate increased significantly; at 8 years, about 50% of patients had valve degeneration. This study is the longest follow-up study to date for the assessment of TAVR valve function. Under current conditions, caution should be exercised in applying TAVR to younger patients with longer life expectancy. If the patient is $<$70 years old and has a low risk of surgical surgery, surgical surgery should still be the first choice.

VI Development of TAVR in China

Although TAVR in China started relatively late, with the continuous efforts of the government, doctors, patients, and manufacturers, progress will be made in many aspects in the future, and the gap with Western countries is continuously narrowing. Venus A, the first domestically designed valve with completely independent intellectual property rights, has taken the lead in completing clinical trials, with 268 cases completed, and will be launched in the near future. The J-Valve and VitaFlow valves have also completed enrollment and entered the follow-up phase; with the introduction of new-generation valves into clinical practice, the success rate of surgery will continue to improve, and complications will continue to decrease.

VII Common Questions in Consultation

1. What are the common complications of TAVR? The common complications of TAVR include stroke, paravalvular leak, arrhythmia, vascular complications, and bleeding. Less common complications include coronary artery obstruction, annular rupture, subacute endocarditis, etc. Stroke mainly occurs within 3 days after the procedure, and the occurrence of early stroke is clearly related to intraoperative manipulation, while the occurrence of late stroke is mainly related to the patient. Paravalvular leak is a common complication after TAVR, and even mild paravalvular leak can increase the mortality and readmission rate 1 year after the procedure. Pacemaker implantation is a common complication after TAVR, especially after self-expanding valve implantation. High-risk factors include low implantation height, large calcification volume of the left ventricular outflow tract, right bundle branch block, and patient-prosthesis mismatch. The choice of anticoagulant drugs needs to take into account the risk of bleeding and thrombosis. With the continuous reduction of the diameter of the new-generation valve sheath, the occurrence of vascular complications has decreased.

2. How to evaluate the expansion of TAVR indications? The Chinese expert consensus proposes that the absolute indications for TAVR are surgical contraindications, life expectancy over 1 year, and symptomatic calcific severe AS; the relative indications are high surgical risk, life expectancy over 1 year, and symptomatic calcific severe AS. The PARTNER II_a study provides evidence-based medicine evidence for intermediate-risk patients, while low-risk patients are still in the clinical research stage.

3. What is the anticoagulation strategy after TAVR? The current anticoagulation treatment after TAVR is still recommended as a dual antiplatelet therapy with clopidogrel and aspirin for 3-6 months, followed by lifelong aspirin therapy.

4. How to evaluate the issue of valve degeneration? Within 5-7 years after TAVR, the valve degeneration rate increases significantly; at 8 years, about 50% of the patients have valve degeneration. If the patient is 70 years old and the surgical risk is low, surgical treatment should still be the first choice.

Ⅷ Consultation Process

1. Although TAVR has developed rapidly and widely abroad, the technology is still in its initial stage in China. Therefore, strict control is required when selecting suitable cases, and the indications for TAVR application in China must be mastered: the Chinese expert consensus proposes that the absolute indications for TAVR are surgical contraindications, life expectancy over 1 year, and symptomatic calcific severe AS; the relative indications are high surgical risk, life expectancy over 1 year, and symptomatic calcific severe AS.

2. For suitable patients, it is necessary to inform them of the risks and benefits of both SAVR and TAVR and compare their advantages and disadvantages. The advantages of TAVR are minimal trauma and rapid recovery; for some populations that are considered contraindicated or extremely high-risk from a surgical perspective, TAVR can bring hope to patients; of course, the high price, related surgical complications, and valve degeneration rate are also concerns for most patients.

3. Due to the high valve degeneration rate of TAVR, SAVR is recommended for young patients (<70 years old) with long life expectancy and low surgical risk.

Chapter 6

Pregnancy-Related Diseases

Section 1 Hypertension in Pregnancy

I Overview

Hypertension disorders in pregnancy refer to abnormally elevated blood pressure in pregnant women. During pregnancy, a series of pathophysiological and hemodynamic changes can occur in the mother's body, such as sympathetic activation, increased blood volume, increased cardiac output, and fluctuations in peripheral vascular resistance, all of which are important factors in the development and exacerbation of hypertension. The incidence of hypertension in pregnancy is 6%-10% in Western populations and similar in China at 5.6%-9.4%. Hypertensive disorders in pregnancy can increase the risk of fetal growth restriction, placental abruption, disseminated intravascular coagulation, cerebral edema, acute heart failure, and even acute renal failure, and are important causes of maternal and fetal mortality.

II Classification

Hypertensive disorders in pregnancy include pre-existing hypertension before pregnancy and hypertension that develops during pregnancy, preeclampsia, and eclampsia. Due to differences in pathophysiological mechanisms and clinical features, the principles of prevention and treatment are significantly different from those of chronic hypertension in non-pregnant individuals. According to the standards of the American College of Obstetricians and Gynecologists (ACOG) and the American Hypertension Education Program Working Group, hypertensive disorders in pregnancy are classified into four categories:

1. Chronic hypertension: Systolic blood pressure ≥140 mmHg and/or diastolic blood pressure ≥90 mmHg before pregnancy or before 20 weeks of gestation, or blood pressure does not return to normal 12 weeks postpartum. According to the ACOG grading standards, systolic blood pressure of 140-179 mmHg and/or diastolic blood pressure of 90-109 mmHg is considered mild hypertension, while systolic blood pressure ≥180 mmHg and/or diastolic blood pressure ≥ 180 mmHg, especially when accompanied by target organ damage, is considered severe hypertension.

2. Gestational hypertension: New onset of hypertension after 20 weeks of gestation. The diagnosis of this hypertension requires two measurements, both meeting systolic blood pressure ≥ 140 mmHg and/or diastolic blood pressure ≥90 mmHg (taking the 5th Korotkoff sound as the reading), at least 6 hours apart. The patient's urine protein is negative, and blood pressure

gradually returns to normal within 12 weeks postpartum. This condition may progress to preeclampsia. Some patients with gestational hypertension whose blood pressure does not return to normal 12 weeks after delivery should be diagnosed with chronic hypertension.

3. Preeclampsia / eclampsia: Preeclampsia is a pregnancy-specific disease characterized by new-onset hypertension and proteinuria after 20 weeks of gestation, often accompanied by edema and hyperuricemia. Preeclampsia is further divided into mild and severe forms. Mild preeclampsia is defined as systolic blood pressure≥140 mmHg and/or diastolic blood pressure≥90 mmHg, with urine protein≥300 mg/24 h. Severe preeclampsia is defined as systolic blood pressure ≥ 160 mmHg and/or diastolic blood pressure≥110 mmHg, 24-hour urine protein ≥2.0 g and/ or qualitative test (++), serum creatinine>106 μmol/L or increased from baseline, platelet count<100,000/mm^3, or the presence of microangiopathic hemolytic anemia, elevated lactate dehydrogenase or liver enzymes, accompanied by headache or other cerebral or visual symptoms, or persistent upper abdominal discomfort. Patients with preeclampsia who develop seizures can be diagnosed with eclampsia. Seizures can occur before, during, or after delivery, or even in women without preeclampsia.

4. Preeclampsia / eclampsia with chronic hypertension: Systolic blood pressure ≥ 140 mmHg and/or diastolic blood pressure ≥90 mmHg before pregnancy or before 20 weeks of gestation, and the development of preeclampsia or eclampsia during pregnancy.

Ⅲ Clinical Manifestations

1. Clinical manifestations of general hypertension: Similar to general hypertension, the clinical manifestations of hypertension in pregnancy also include blood pressure fluctuations, dizziness, fatigue, proteinuria, and other symptoms.

2. Unique clinical manifestations in pregnant women: Obstetric specialty symptoms include irritability, tension, poor sleep, blurred vision, abdominal distension, vomiting, poor appetite, shortness of breath, chest tightness, varicose veins in the lower extremities, etc. The most unique and dangerous symptom is seizures. Once seizures occur, eclampsia should be considered. During pregnancy, fetal-related clinical manifestations include placental abruption, low birth weight, intrauterine growth restriction, and perinatal death, which require close attention from obstetricians and cardiologists.

Ⅳ Diagnosis and Assessment

-10870981221. Diagnostic Criteria: The diagnostic standards for the previously mentioned classifications have been detailed. Refer to the respective categories in the aforementioned classification section for the diagnostic criteria of each of the four types of pregnancy-induced hypertension.

-10870981212. Diagnostic Steps:

-10870981222.1 Medical History: Confirm whether the high blood pressure was pre-existing before pregnancy, i. e., chronic hypertension, as per the diagnostic criteria outlined in Section 2.1. Additionally, inquire about any history of renal disease and instances of snoring at night. If affirmative, further details should be gathered about the onset of these conditions and any current or past use of antihypertensive medication.

-10870981212.2 Physical Examination: A thorough and systematic physical examination of pregnant women or women planning to conceive is required, covering the following aspects:

(1) Measure blood pressure according to standard procedures. Pregnant women, especially in the middle and late stages of pregnancy, may experience shortness of breath and palpitations after activity. Therefore, it is necessary to wait 5-10 minutes after the patient is at rest before measuring blood pressure. In some pregnant women, due to increased blood volume or coexisting hyperthyroidism or aortic valve insufficiency, the fifth Korotkoff sound (disappearance sound) may not be detected when measuring blood pressure. In this case, the diastolic blood pressure reading should be taken at the fourth Korotkoff sound (muffling sound). If elevated blood pressure is found, repeat the measurement at least once after 6 hours. If the repeated blood pressure measurement remains elevated, hypertensive disorders in pregnancy are suspected.

(2) Monitor heart rate and, if necessary, check orthostatic blood pressure and four-limb blood pressure. Measure body mass index, waist circumference, and hip circumference. Observe for the presence of Cushingoid appearance, neurofibromatosis skin spots, thyroid eye signs, and lower extremity edema. Listen for vascular bruits, including the carotid arteries, femoral arteries, renal arteries, and abdominal aorta. Inspect, palpate, percuss, and auscultate the whole body and individual organs, such as the thyroid gland, abdomen, heart and lungs, and extremities.

(3) Further Evaluation. For patients with suspected hypertensive disorders in pregnancy, further investigate the presence of symptoms and signs of hypertension and/or preeclampsia and perform necessary auxiliary examinations to assess for target organ damage. Examination items generally include: ambulatory blood pressure monitoring, complete blood count, urinalysis, coagulation function, liver function, kidney function, blood glucose, serum uric acid, and 24-hour urine collection for quantitative protein measurement. Perform cardiac ultrasound, hepatobiliary and pancreatic ultrasound, bilateral renal and urinary system ultrasound, pelvic ultrasound, and even transvaginal ultrasound.

(4) Hypertension Risk Stratification and Cardiac Function Classification. If the patient has chronic hypertension, further comprehensive assessment of hypertension risk stratification and clinical cardiac function is required. Cardiac function assessment is based on the New York Heart Association (NYHA) functional classification, as shown in Figure 6-1.

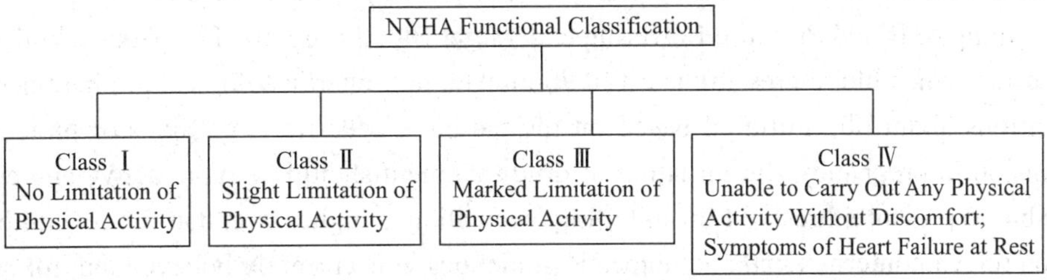

Figure 6-1 NYHA Functional Classification

In addition, due to the unique physiological characteristics of pregnant women, such as higher baseline heart rate and chest tightness and shortness of breath in late pregnancy caused by weight gain, these factors may interfere with the accurate assessment of cardiac function. This requires clinicians to carefully analyze the patient's condition in conjunction with the opinions of obstetricians, neither overemphasizing the physiological changes of pregnancy and overlooking heart disease and decreased cardiac function, nor over-diagnosing and causing unnecessary tension. A simple method to assess cardiac function in pregnant women is to compare with the common feelings of normal pregnant women of the same age group, which requires clinicians to repeatedly experience and discern in practice (Figure 6-2).

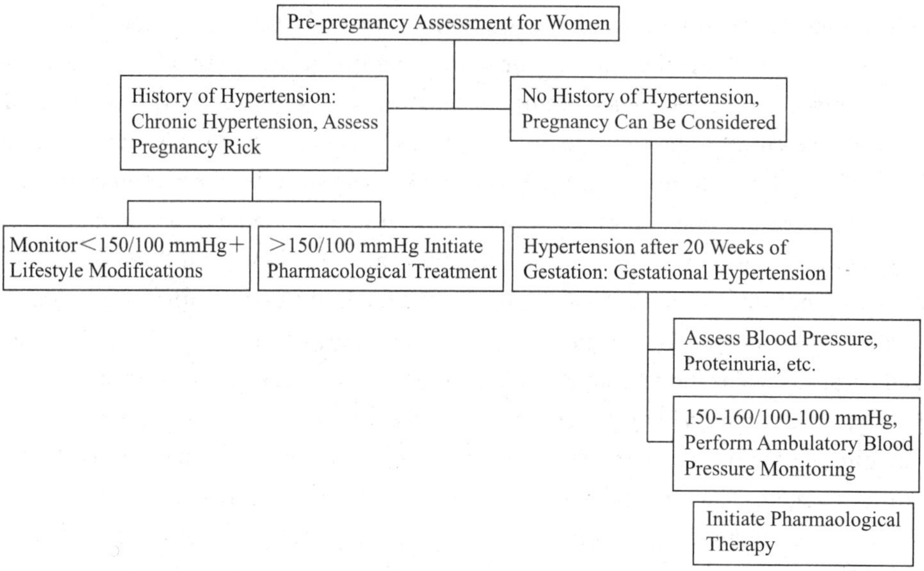

Figure 6-2 Diagnostic Steps for Hypertension in Pregnancy

V Treatment

So far, no antihypertensive drug is absolutely safe for pregnant women. Most drugs are classified as Category C in the US FDA's safety rating (i. e., risk to the mother and fetus cannot be ruled out). Both pregnant women's families and doctors have varying degrees of concern about antihypertensive drugs. Therefore, when choosing drugs for patients with hypertensive disorders in pregnancy, careful initiation and weighing of risks and benefits are necessary.

1. Timing of Blood Pressure Lowering and Target Blood Pressure. For patients with general hypertension, when blood pressure is ≥140/90 mmHg, non-pharmacological or pharmacological interventions should be initiated based on the patient's specific situation. For patients with hypertension in pregnancy, the initiation of drug treatment should be more active and cautious, and the blood pressure threshold for initiating medication is higher than that for general patients. Based on relevant international and domestic guidelines, it is currently believed that for pregnant women with significantly elevated blood pressure but no target organ damage, it is reasonable to control blood pressure below 150/100 mmHg. For pregnant women with mildly elevated blood pressure (blood pressure <150/100 mmHg), close observation can be performed, and medication may not be necessary for the time being. Only when systolic blood pressure is ≥150

mmHg and/or diastolic blood pressure is ≥100 mmHg or target organ damage occurs should drug therapy be considered. For chronic hypertensive patients who have already received drug treatment and become pregnant, blood pressure should be controlled at an appropriate level to avoid the occurrence of unexpected postural hypotension (PH) or supine hypotensive syndrome (SHS) due to excessively low blood pressure.

2. Non-pharmacological Treatment. Proper blood pressure monitoring, healthy lifestyle and dietary habits, appropriate exercise, participation in prenatal classes, online education, stress reduction, and psychological counseling are important components of blood pressure control in early pregnancy and throughout the entire pregnancy. For pregnant women with blood pressure < 150/100 mmHg, non-pharmacological methods should be used as much as possible to control blood pressure, and close monitoring should be performed. Unlike the treatment of hypertension in non-pregnant patients, strict control of salt intake during pregnancy may reduce blood volume and have adverse effects on the fetus, so only moderate salt restriction is recommended. Abdominal circumference, waist circumference, and leg circumference also need to be closely monitored, and weight gain should be maintained within the recommended reasonable range during pregnancy.

3. Selection of Antihypertensive Drugs

(1) α-adrenergic agonists: Methyldopa is an α-adrenergic receptor agonist. A large-sample randomized controlled study with a follow-up of 7.5 years confirmed that this drug can control hypertension in pregnancy and is relatively safe. Therefore, in 2000, it was recommended as the first-line treatment for hypertension in pregnancy by the US National High Blood Pressure Education Program. However, this drug is difficult to obtain in China.

(2) Beta-receptor blockers

1) Labetalol: It is a drug with both α and β receptor blocking effects, has a significant antihypertensive effect, and has fewer adverse reactions, so it can be considered as a priority.

2) Metoprolol sustained-release: It has little effect on the fetus and can also be considered for use. Fetal monitoring should be strengthened to be alert for bradycardia and hypoglycemia.

3) Propranolol and atenolol: Neither is recommended for use because they can cause premature delivery and intrauterine growth restriction in pregnant women.

(3) Calcium channel blockers

1) Nifedipine: Studies have found that nifedipine does not have adverse effects on the fetus in early and mid-pregnancy and can be used in patients in early and mid-pregnancy. There is no clear clinical evidence for late pregnancy.

2) Amlodipine, felodipine, diltiazem, verapamil: Currently, there are no reports of these four types of drugs causing fetal malformations, and their safety for the fetus remains to be verified. Recent studies have found that nicardipine also has good efficacy and safety for patients with hypertension in pregnancy. In addition, the use of calcium channel blockers by pregnant women may weaken uterine contractions, which also requires careful observation and response in clinical practice.

(4) Diuretics: Their value in the treatment of hypertensive disorders in pregnancy remains controversial. A meta-analysis including 9 randomized trials and 7,000 pregnant women

showed that diuretics do not have adverse effects on the fetus. Based on this, the 2016 Chinese Hypertension Consensus recommends that pregnant women who have been treated with thiazide diuretics before pregnancy can continue to use them, and those who develop systemic edema, acute heart failure, or pulmonary edema during pregnancy can also choose to use them. Due to the fact that diuretics can cause insufficient blood volume in pregnant women and lead to electrolyte disturbances, caution should be exercised when using diuretics in patients with no or mild edema. If complicated by preeclampsia, diuretics should be discontinued. During the use of diuretics, attention should be paid to monitoring indicators such as blood volume and electrolytes.

(5) Angiotensin-converting enzyme inhibitors (ACEIs) and angiotensin receptor blockers (ARBs): Because they may cause fetal cardiovascular malformations, polydactyly, hypospadias, spontaneous abortion, and lead to decreased placental blood perfusion in pregnant women in the middle and late stages of pregnancy, oligohydramnios, intrauterine growth restriction, renal failure, low birth weight, fetal lung hypoplasia, cranial and facial bone underdevelopment, and other risks, ACEIs and ARBs have become drugs that are contraindicated during pregnancy. Women with chronic hypertension who are currently taking these drugs should discontinue them before planning pregnancy.

(6) Selection of intravenous antihypertensive drugs

1) Calcium channel blockers such as labetalol and nicardipine, α-blockers such as urapidil and phentolamine are all used for intravenous injection in severe hypertension and even eclampsia. It is generally recommended to start with a low dose and strengthen monitoring to avoid causing a hypotensive response. However, phentolamine has been reported to have adverse reactions that affect uterine blood flow distribution, and its use in the treatment of hypertension in pregnancy is still controversial. It is not routinely used in cases of non-emergency sudden blood pressure elevation.

2) Sodium nitroprusside may increase the risk of fetal cyanide poisoning and is not recommended unless other drugs are ineffective.

3) In patients with preeclampsia or eclampsia, intravenous magnesium sulfate is often used, taking advantage of its anticonvulsant, antispasmodic, sedative, and fetal lung maturation-promoting effects. It has now been confirmed that magnesium sulfate is superior to sedatives in preventing seizures and recurrence and reducing maternal mortality.

4) The above drugs are commonly used in patients with severe hypertension during pregnancy (blood pressure＞180/110 mmHg). The optimal blood pressure-lowering strategy for patients with hypertensive disorders in pregnancy still requires further exploration through large-scale, well-designed clinical trials (Tables 6-1 and 6-2).

Table 6-1 Medications for Hypertension in Pregnancy

Drug	Dosage	Adverse Reactions to Pregnant Women
Methyldopa	0.5-3.0 g/d, 2 times/d	Peripheral edema, anxiety, nightmares, drowsiness, dry mouth, hypotension, maternal liver damage, no serious adverse effects on the fetus
Labetalol	200-1, 200 mg/d, 2-3 times/d	Persistent fetal bradycardia, hypotension, neonatal hypoglycemia

(Continued)

Drug	Dosage	Adverse Reactions to Pregnant Women
Hydrochlorothiazide	12.5-25 mg/d	Fetal malformations, electrolyte disturbances, insufficient blood volume
Nifedipine	30-120 mg/d	Hypotension, inhibition of labor (especially when used with magnesium sulfate)
Hydralazine	50-300 mg/d, 2-4 times/d	Hypotension, neonatal thrombocytopenia
ACEI	Contraindicated in pregnancy	Oligohydramnios, intrauterine growth retardation, renal failure, low birth weight, major cardiovascular malformations, polydactyly, hypospadias
ARB		Spontaneous abortion, fetal lung hypoplasia, craniofacial bone underdevelopment

Table 6-2 Use of Intravenous Antihypertensive Drugs

Drug	Specification	Preparation	Initial Dose	Maximum Dose
Nicardipine	2 mg/2 mL	10 mg+NS 40 mL or 30 mL+NS 100 mL	10 mL/h (2 mg/h)	30 mg/h
Magnesium Sulfate	25%/10 mL (2.5 g)	Eclampsia: Loading: 10 mL+10 mL solution, iv bolus <5 min Maintenance: 4.0+NS (GS) 250 mL	Loading: 1-3 mL/min Maintenance: 1-2 g/h	1-8 mg/min
		Torsades de pointes ventricular tachycardia: Loading: 1-2 g diluted slowly intravenous push, e. g., 4 mL+NS 6 mL or 8 mL diluted to 40 mL iv Maintenance: 20 mL add NS to 50 mL (100 mg/mL)	Maintenance: 5 mL/h (about 8 mg/min)	
		or Maintenance 2, 500 μg (10 ampoules)+ NS to 50 mL	5 mL/hour (250 μg/h)	
Nitroglycerin	5 mg/mL	50 mg+NS 40 mL	0.6 mL/h (10 μg/min)	200 μg/min
		or 30 mg+NS 24 mL	3 mL/h (5 μg/min)	
		or 5 mg+GS (NS) 49 mL		
		or 25 mg+GS250 mL		
Sodium Nitroprusside	50 mg/vial (powder)	50 mg+5% GS 50 mL	0.6 mL/h (10 μg/min)	200-300 μg/min
Urapidil (ebrantil)	25 mg/5 mL	5 mg+NS 20 mL slowly push over 5 minutes, 50 mg+NS 40 mL	6 mL/h (100 μg/min)	400 μg/min
		or 250 mg stock solution	1.2 mL/h (100 μg/min)	
		or 100 mg+5% GS 500 mL iv drip	1 mL/min (200 μg/min)	
		or 50 mg+250 mL solution, 25 mL/h equivalent to 5 mg/h iv drip	5-15 mg/h	

(Continued)

Drug	Specification	Preparation	Initial Dose	Maximum Dose
Labetalol	50 mg/5 mL/vial	Loading dose: 0.25 mg/kg iv 5 min or 50 mg po 200 mg+NS (GS) 30 mL then adjust: 100 mg+NS (GS) 250 mL	Start infusion at 6 mL/h 1-4 mL/min	20-160 mg/h

Ⅵ Common Questions in Consultation

1. Pay attention to seemingly non-specific early symptoms and initiate timely blood pressure monitoring to observe fluctuations.

Due to increased blood volume, limited activity, and other reasons, pregnant women have relatively poor ability to self-regulate blood pressure. When non-specific symptoms such as irritability, tension, poor sleep, blurred vision, abdominal distension, vomiting, as well as poor appetite occur, blood pressure and even heart rate monitoring should be initiated promptly. Early detection and treatment, timely blood pressure monitoring, and prevention of preeclampsia and eclampsia are essential. Conduct a comprehensive risk assessment of hypertension throughout pregnancy.

(1) Pre-pregnancy assessment: It is recommended that patients with hypertension assess their blood pressure level, target organ damage, and currently used antihypertensive drugs and their efficacy before pregnancy. It is best to reassess whether pregnancy is feasible after drug treatment. For patients with severe refractory hypertension, it should be clearly informed to postpone pregnancy. Guide patients to actively improve their lifestyle, such as appropriate salt restriction, control body mass index within the ideal range (18-24 kg/m^2) through diet control and increased physical activity and abandon the outdated notion of "the fatter the better" for pregnant women.

(2) Early pregnancy assessment: Inform the patient of pregnancy risks and potential serious complications, guide them to receive standardized prenatal care at the corresponding level of hospital, and regularly monitor blood pressure, cardiac function, and liver and kidney function.

(3) Mid-late pregnancy assessment: Some hypertensive patients have insufficient awareness of the severity of their condition and pregnancy risks. Some patients miss the diagnosis of heart disease due to the absence of clinical symptoms. A small number of patients with a strong desire for pregnancy conceal their medical history and engage in risky pregnancies, and they are already in the mid-late stage of pregnancy when seeking medical attention. For these patients, whether to continue the pregnancy should be comprehensively judged and managed in a stratified manner based on blood pressure level, degree of target organ damage, pregnancy risk classification, cardiac function status, medical technology level and conditions of the hospital, the willingness of the patient and family members, their understanding and tolerance of disease risks, etc.

2. Prevention and treatment of severe hypertension and related complications during pregnancy.

(1) Initiation of a multidisciplinary treatment (MDT) model: For hypertensive pregnant

women with grade 3 or higher hypertension, high-risk hypertension, complications such as acute or chronic heart failure, renal insufficiency, stroke, or even aortic dissection, preeclampsia and/or eclampsia, the MDT should be actively initiated, and joint consultations should be arranged with doctors from related departments such as obstetrics, cardiology, neurology, psychological counseling, and nutrition. Assess the respective weights of pregnancy, maternal safety, childbirth, and breastfeeding, and determine whether to continue the pregnancy and use medications.

(2) Adjustment of antihypertensive drugs: For those whose blood pressure cannot be reduced to normal with lifestyle intervention measures, drug treatment is required. It is recommended to switch to nifedipine and/or labetalol to control blood pressure 6 months before the planned pregnancy. If the blood pressure still cannot be reduced below 150/100 mmHg after treatment with these two drugs, or if there is mild hypertension but accompanied by proteinuria, it is recommended to postpone pregnancy.

(3) Consultation guidance for hypertensive pregnant women during delivery: Obstetric blood pressure-related consultations mostly occur during sudden acute blood pressure elevations during the delivery process. At this time, intravenous antihypertensive treatment can be initiated after sedation, analgesia, and reassurance measures. The drugs are as mentioned above. Hemodynamic changes during delivery will cause blood pressure fluctuations and increased cardiac load; if combined with adverse factors such as anemia, hypoproteinemia, and infection, it can lead to decreased cardiac function. Obstetric factors such as twin pregnancy, polyhydramnios, and preeclampsia can also exacerbate heart disease, and serious cardiac complications that endanger the lives of the mother and child, such as heart failure, malignant arrhythmia, pulmonary hypertension crisis, cardiogenic shock, and embolism, may occur, which require attention from the consulting physicians.

Ⅶ Consultation Process

1. Clarify whether the patient had hypertension before pregnancy, i. e., chronic hypertension, and inquire about the history of kidney disease and snoring at night. If present, further investigate the time of onset and whether the patient has ever taken or is currently taking antihypertensive medications.

2. Perform a thorough and systematic physical examination on pregnant women or women planning to become pregnant. Measure blood pressure according to standard procedures. Pregnant women, especially in the middle and late stages of pregnancy, may experience shortness of breath and palpitations after activity, so it is necessary to wait 5-10 minutes after the patient is at rest before measuring blood pressure. If elevated blood pressure is found, repeat the measurement at least once after 6 hours. If the repeated blood pressure measurement remains elevated, hypertensive disorders in pregnancy are suspected.

3. Pay attention to important physical examination findings, such as orthostatic blood pressure and four-limb blood pressure. Measure body mass index, waist circumference, and hip circumference. Observe for the presence of Cushingoid appearance, neurofibromatosis skin spots, thyroid eye signs, and lower extremity edema. Listen for vascular bruits, including the carotid arteries, femoral arteries, renal arteries, and abdominal aorta. Inspect, palpate, percuss, and

auscultate the whole body and individual organs, such as the thyroid gland, abdomen, heart and lungs, and extremities.

4. Perform rapid auxiliary examinations. For patients with suspected hypertensive disorders in pregnancy, further investigate the presence of symptoms and signs of hypertension and/or preeclampsia and assess for target organ damage. These examinations include: ambulatory blood pressure monitoring, complete blood count, urinalysis, coagulation function, liver function, kidney function, blood glucose, serum uric acid, and 24-hour urine collection for quantitative protein measurement. Perform cardiac ultrasound, hepatobiliary and pancreatic ultrasound, bilateral renal and urinary system ultrasound, pelvic ultrasound, and even transvaginal ultrasound.

5. When choosing drugs for patients with hypertensive disorders in pregnancy, careful initiation and weighing of risks and benefits are necessary. Drug therapy should be considered when systolic blood pressure is ⩾150 mmHg and/or diastolic blood pressure is ⩾100 mmHg or when target organ damage occurs. For drug therapy selection, methyldopa, labetalol, nifedipine, etc., can be used. Pay attention to rationally selecting the type and dosage of antihypertensive drugs according to the patient's condition.

6. Conduct a comprehensive risk assessment of hypertension throughout pregnancy, monitor blood pressure, and prevent and treat preeclampsia and eclampsia.

Section 2 Pregnancy Complicated by Arrhythmia

I Overview

Pregnancy complicated by arrhythmia, including arrhythmias that occur for the first time during pregnancy and recurrent arrhythmias in pregnant women with a history of arrhythmia, is the most common complication during pregnancy. Epidemiological studies have shown that most arrhythmias have a good prognosis. Among pregnant women without organic heart disease, the incidence of ventricular premature beats is 56%, the incidence of atrial premature beats is 59%, and the incidence of pathological arrhythmias is low, often secondary to congenital or organic heart disease. Since a small number of arrhythmias can rapidly deteriorate hemodynamics in a short period of time, endangering the lives of both mother and child, this is a clinical issue that requires high attention from obstetricians and cardiologists in consultation.

II Classification

According to the type of onset, pregnancy arrhythmias can be divided into two categories: rapid and slow arrhythmias. Among them, rapid arrhythmias include supraventricular arrhythmias (atrial and junctional premature beats, supraventricular tachycardia, atrial flutter, and atrial fibrillation) and ventricular arrhythmias (such as ventricular premature beats, paroxysmal ventricular tachycardia). Slow arrhythmias include sinus-origin slow arrhythmias, atrioventricular junctional bradycardia, ventricular autonomous rhythm, and conduction block (including sinoatrial block, intra-atrial block, and atrioventricular block), characterized by a slow heart rate. Common clinical conditions include sinus bradycardia, sick sinus syndrome, and atrioventricular block, etc.

Ⅲ Diagnosis and Assessment

1. The diagnosis of pregnancy arrhythmia mainly relies on symptoms and electrocardiogram (ECG). Other auxiliary examinations such as thyroid function, dynamic ECG, echocardiography, BNP, blood electrolytes, as well as sleep monitoring and anxiety / depression scales from psychological specialists, can also provide auxiliary diagnostic clues.

(1) When pregnant women experience symptoms such as palpitations, chest tightness, dizziness, or blackouts, the above-mentioned ECG and other auxiliary examinations should be completed as soon as possible.

(2) After discovering arrhythmia, the nature of the arrhythmia should be immediately clarified: malignant or benign, atrial or ventricular, rapid or slow.

(3) Combine the pregnant woman's symptoms, ventricular rate, and previous underlying heart disease to perform risk stratification and assess the severity of the condition.

(4) Actively search for and remove reversible triggers or underlying causes. In addition to factors such as infection, anemia, electrolyte disturbances, drugs, and thyroid dysfunction, myocardial injury markers can be tested when necessary, especially the level and changes of cardiac troponin, which helps to detect myocardial injury caused by inflammation or ischemia. B-type natriuretic peptide (BNP) or N-terminal pro-B-type natriuretic peptide (NT-proBNP) can help assess ventricular volume load and wall tension, indirectly evaluating cardiac function.

(5) Dynamic ECG examination should be performed for frequently occurring or persistent arrhythmias to understand the characteristics of arrhythmia onset (such as frequency, onset time, duration, heart rate during onset, and whether there are other combined arrhythmias).

2. The key points of ECG diagnosis for common arrhythmias during pregnancy are as follows.

(1) Atrial premature beats

1) Premature appearance of P' wave (P' wave may overlap with the T wave of the previous sinus beat).

2) P'-R interval is normal or slightly prolonged.

3) The morphology of the P' wave is different from the sinus P wave.

4) The QRS complex after the P' wave can be normal or deformed. If there is a deformed QRS wave, it is called atrial premature beats with intraventricular aberrant conduction. If there is no QRS wave after the P wave, it is called a non-conducted atrial premature beat. If the morphology and coupling interval of P' are different in the same lead, it is called multifocal atrial premature beats.

5) There is often an incomplete compensatory pause, that is, the time between two normal P waves including atrial premature beats is shorter than twice the normal P-P interval.

(2) Paroxysmal supraventricular tachycardia

1) The heart rate is usually 130-250 beats/min, with a regular rhythm.

2) The QRS morphology is mostly normal, with a few cases being wide and deformed.

3) P waves are retrograde (inverted in Ⅱ, Ⅲ, aVF), often not visible, or retrograde P waves

are located at the end of the QRS complex.

(3) Atrial flutter

1) P waves disappear and are replaced by sawtooth-like flutter waves (F waves), with a frequency of generally 250-350 beats/min.

2) There is no isoelectric line between flutter waves.

3) The ventricular rate is irregular or regular, depending on whether the atrioventricular conduction ratio is constant.

4) The QRS morphology is mostly normal.

(4) Atrial fibrillation

1) P waves disappear and are replaced by small and irregular f waves.

2) The frequency of f waves is 350-600 beats/min.

3) The ventricular rate is absolutely irregular.

4) The QRS morphology is mostly normal.

(5) Complete atrioventricular block

1) P waves and QRS complexes each have their own rhythm, unrelated to each other.

2) The QRS frequency is slow, and the P wave frequency is faster than the QRS frequency.

3) The pacing site is below the block site, and the QRS complex can be normal or deformed.

(6) Ventricular tachycardia

1) The frequency is usually 140-200 beats/min.

2) The QRS complex is wide and deformed, with a duration >0.12 s.

3) There is no fixed P-R relationship (atrioventricular dissociation).

4) Ventricular fusion waves can be seen.

(7) Ventricular fibrillation: No identifiable QRS complexes, replaced by fibrillation waves with extremely irregular waveforms, amplitudes, and frequencies.

Ⅳ Safety of Antiarrhythmic Drugs During Pregnancy

1. Due to the lack of prospective or randomized studies in the field of cardiovascular diseases during pregnancy, most FDA and new guideline recommendations are only level C evidence, that is, it cannot be determined whether there is embryonic damage. Table 6-3 lists the FDA classification and safety summary of common antiarrhythmic drugs.

Table 6-3 FDA Safety Classification of Common Antiarrhythmic Drugs

FDA Classification	Definition of Classification	Related Drugs
A	Safety: Multiple randomized controlled trials have confirmed safety, and no adverse effects on the fetus have been found at any stage of pregnancy	Currently lacks randomized trials
B	No evidence of harm to humans: Although animal experiments have shown harm to the embryo, multiple randomized controlled trials have not found adverse effects on human fetuses; or animal experiments have not found harm, but there is a lack of human research evidence.	Lidocaine and sotalol

(Continued)

FDA Classification	Definition of Classification	Related Drugs
B	Theoretically, there is a possibility of causing harm to the fetus, but the probability is low	Lidocaine and sotalol
C	Harmfulness cannot be ruled out: There is a lack of randomized controlled studies in humans, but animal experiments have shown harm to the embryo or lack animal experimental data The use of medication during pregnancy may cause harm to the fetus, but the potential benefits outweigh the risks	Quinidine, procainamide, mexiletine, flecainide, propafenone, propranolol, metoprolol, disopyramide, ibutilide, dofetilide, dronedarone, verapamil, diltiazem, digoxin, and adenosine
D	Possibly harmful: Human studies have confirmed harm to the fetus. When absolutely necessary, the benefits of medication during pregnancy may still outweigh the risks	Phenytoin, amiodarone, and atenolol
X	Contraindicated during pregnancy: Both animal and human studies have shown significant embryotoxicity, and the harm far outweighs the potential benefits	

2. Common antiarrhythmic drugs are as follows.

(1) Class Ⅰ antiarrhythmic drugs (sodium channel blockers)

Class $Ⅰ_a$: These drugs have a strong pro-arrhythmic effect and are rarely used now.

Class $Ⅰ_b$: Lidocaine is mainly used to terminate ventricular tachycardia and is also used for local anesthesia. This drug has good maternal and fetal tolerance. Mexiletine is an oral preparation structurally similar to lidocaine. The safety evidence for its use during pregnancy is limited, but it seems to be well tolerated.

Class $Ⅰ_c$: Propafenone and flecainide are both broad-spectrum antiarrhythmic drugs and have good tolerance during pregnancy, but they should be avoided in patients with organic heart disease. Flecainide can also be used to treat fetal arrhythmias.

(2) Class Ⅱ antiarrhythmic drugs: Beta-blockers belong to Class Ⅱ antiarrhythmic drugs and are suitable for supraventricular and ventricular arrhythmias. These drugs may cause fetal growth restriction and should be avoided in the first 3 months of pregnancy as much as possible. The FDA classification of atenolol is Category D, and it is prohibited throughout pregnancy. Cardioselective β1 receptor blockers such as metoprolol have less impact on β2 receptor-mediated uterine relaxation and are thus more advantageous.

(3) Class Ⅲ antiarrhythmic drugs (potassium channel blockers): This class of drugs includes amiodarone, sotalol, dofetilide, ibutilide, and dronedarone, which are broad-spectrum antiarrhythmic drugs. Amiodarone can lead to a series of serious fetal safety issues, including fetal hypothyroidism, birth defects, etc. The FDA has listed this drug as Category D, only allowing its use when life-threatening arrhythmias occur, and other drugs are ineffective. The FDA classification of sotalol is tentatively Category B, and its overall safety data is relatively

limited. Dofetilide has a good effect in treating atrial fibrillation, but it can cause torsade de pointes ventricular tachycardia, so monitoring should be strengthened during use. Its FDA classification is Category C. Dronedarone has high fetal toxicity and is contraindicated during pregnancy.

(4) Class Ⅳ antiarrhythmic drugs (calcium channel blockers): They mainly include non-dihydropyridine calcium channel blockers verapamil and diltiazem. Verapamil has a good effect in terminating paroxysmal supraventricular tachycardia, but it should not be used when combined with hypotension. Overall, the safety of calcium channel blockers during pregnancy is relatively good.

(5) Adenosine: The safety of adenosine during pregnancy is good, and it has a significant effect in terminating supraventricular tachycardia. It is often used as the first-choice injection drug. Adenosine has a short half-life of only 2-3 seconds and must be administered by intravenous bolus injection. The starting dose is 6 mg, and it can be repeatedly injected while observing the effect. Adverse reactions such as transient bradycardia, transient dyspnea, and transient flushing resolve within a few minutes, but it is contraindicated in patients with atrioventricular block and bronchial asthma.

(6) Digoxin: Digoxin has good safety data in both the mother and fetus for the treatment of supraventricular tachycardia. However, it is also necessary to monitor blood drug concentrations during use. After 6 months of pregnancy, the presence of digoxin-like substances in the maternal plasma causes a significant increase in the blood drug concentration measured by radioimmunoassay.

V Treatment Principles and Consultation-Related Considerations

1. Most arrhythmias that occur during pregnancy are benign. Treatment methods for arrhythmias include drug therapy, electrical cardioversion, device implantation, and radiofrequency ablation. Currently, there are no absolutely safe antiarrhythmic drugs. When deciding on the treatment of arrhythmias during pregnancy, clinicians need to weigh the pros and cons and make a comprehensive assessment to avoid unnecessary adverse drug reactions and/or complications.

2. When analyzing an ECG of a pregnant woman, it is necessary to analyze the characteristics of "wide, narrow, fast, and slow" during onset. "Wide" and "narrow" refer to whether the width of the QRS complex exceeds 0.12 s, while "fast" and "slow" refer to the heart rate.

(1) When encountering a "wide" and "fast" ECG, immediate attention is required, and it should be treated according to the malignant arrhythmia protocol. Timely electrical cardioversion should be initiated to prevent sudden death.

(2) When encountering a "wide" and "slow" ECG, immediate attention is also required, and it should be treated according to the emergency bradyarrhythmia protocol. Actively investigate for reversible causes such as hyperkalemia and initiate temporary or permanent pacing if necessary.

(3) When encountering a "narrow" and "slow" ECG, close observation is required, and the necessity of temporary pacemaker implantation should be assessed.

3. Narrow QRS complex (duration less than 0.12 s) tachycardia. Sinus tachycardia, atrial tachycardia, and junctional tachycardia all belong to narrow QRS complex tachycardia. The first step is to treat the underlying heart disease and control the precipitating factors. For those with hemodynamic changes, antiarrhythmic drugs can be appropriately used according to the type of premature beats. For those without organic heart disease, no special treatment is needed. It is advisable to actively remove the triggering factors and use sedatives or low-dose β-blockers as appropriate.

4. For acute episodes of supraventricular tachycardia, vagal maneuvers should be performed first. If ineffective, drug treatment can be used, such as adenosine triphosphate, verapamil, or propafenone. If adenosine fails to terminate the tachycardia, intravenous metoprolol is recommended. Once the supraventricular tachycardia is terminated, the drug should be immediately discontinued. For recurrent episodes, oral medication should be given for maintenance. Considering the impact of radiation on the fetus, radiofrequency ablation is recommended to be postponed until after delivery.

5. Atrial flutter and atrial fibrillation

(1) Atrial flutter and atrial fibrillation are less common during pregnancy unless there is structural heart disease or hyperthyroidism. Rapid ventricular rate atrial flutter and atrial fibrillation can lead to severe hemodynamic changes in the mother and fetus, and prompt treatment is required. Direct current cardioversion with 50-100 J is the first choice. Among the cardioversion drugs, quinidine has the longest history of use and has good safety. Short-term use of other Class I_a/I_c antiarrhythmic drugs is also relatively safe. For patients with normal cardiac structure and stable hemodynamics, drug termination of atrial flutter and atrial fibrillation can be considered. Intravenous ibutilide or flecainide is often effective and can be considered, but experience with their use during pregnancy is very limited.

(2) Regardless of whether electrical or pharmacological cardioversion is used for atrial flutter and atrial fibrillation, anticoagulation and/or transesophageal echocardiography should be performed beforehand to exclude left atrial thrombus.

1) Studies have shown that warfarin can cross the placenta and cause miscarriage, bleeding, and malformations. It is relatively contraindicated in the first 3 months of pregnancy. Heparin or low molecular weight heparin can be used instead of warfarin in the first and last 3 months and should be used for at least 3 weeks before electrical cardioversion and continued for 4 weeks after cardioversion.

2) For patients with atrial fibrillation <48 hours and no risk of thrombus, intravenous heparin can be administered before cardioversion, and oral anticoagulants are not required after cardioversion.

3) The risk of thrombosis in patients with atrial fibrillation depends on risk factors. Thrombosis is rare in pregnant women without structural heart disease or risk factors (lone atrial fibrillation), and anticoagulation or antiplatelet therapy is not required.

4) Atrioventricular nodal blocking drugs such as digoxin, beta-blockers, and non-dihydropyridine calcium channel blockers can be used to control the ventricular rate. For patients with severe symptoms despite the use of rate-controlling drugs, preventive antiarrhythmic drugs

(sotalol, flecainide, or propafenone) can be used. Flecainide and propafenone should be used in combination with atrioventricular nodal blocking drugs. Dronedarone is contraindicated.

6. Ventricular tachycardia is a dangerous "wide" and "fast" ECG. Although its occurrence during pregnancy is not high, once it occurs, it will have a serious impact on the mother and fetus. Therefore, it is necessary to actively assess the risk and promptly treat it to prevent sudden death.

(1) Idiopathic ventricular tachycardia in pregnant women without organic heart disease mostly originates from the right ventricular outflow tract and left ventricular posterior septum. It manifests as short, non-sustained episodes and is less often persistent. It is generally well-tolerated. If the symptoms are not obvious or the hemodynamic state is stable, observation can be performed. The mechanism of right ventricular outflow tract idiopathic ventricular tachycardia is mostly increased automaticity, so if the ventricular tachycardia rate is relatively fast and the patient cannot tolerate it, beta-blockers can be the first choice. Left ventricular idiopathic ventricular tachycardia is mainly related to bundle branch reentry. Although its occurrence is not as common as right ventricular outflow tract ventricular tachycardia, it is prone to persistence and responds better to the calcium channel blocker verapamil.

(2) Ventricular tachycardia in pregnant women with organic heart disease is potentially dangerous. Regardless of whether the ventricular tachycardia is monomorphic or polymorphic, and regardless of whether the hemodynamics are stable, emergency treatment is required.

1) For hemodynamically unstable ventricular tachycardia, direct current cardioversion can be used regardless of the stage of pregnancy. It is currently believed that the magnitude of the energy used for direct current cardioversion has no significant impact on the mother and fetus.

2) For hemodynamically stable ventricular tachycardia, drug therapy can also be chosen. Procainamide and lidocaine are relatively safe and effective.

3) Class Ⅲ antiarrhythmic drug amiodarone has a good effect on ventricular tachycardia. However, for pregnant women, since it can cause fetal thyroid dysfunction and intrauterine growth retardation, it should be avoided during pregnancy as much as possible.

4) Sotalol is relatively safe, but it also has the risk of causing torsade de pointes ventricular tachycardia in pregnant women, especially in patients with decreased cardiac function. Therefore, for such patients, close monitoring should be provided, and factors that may induce arrhythmias, such as electrolyte disturbances, heart failure, and infection, should be avoided.

5) For torsade de pointes ventricular tachycardia caused by long QT syndrome, 1-2 g of magnesium sulfate can be administered by slow intravenous injection. Injecting too quickly can lead to maternal hypotension and fetal bradycardia. For bradycardia with long QT syndrome, a permanent pacemaker can be implanted.

7. Ventricular flutter and ventricular fibrillation. For ventricular flutter and ventricular fibrillation, direct current cardioversion with 100-360 J should be performed immediately. For long-term prevention of cardiac arrest, an ICD can be implanted. Currently, small-sample studies have shown that ICD treatment has no obvious adverse effects on pregnant women and fetuses. However, there are occasional reports of emergency cesarean section required after cardioversion, so close monitoring of the mother and fetus is necessary during the cardioversion process.

8. Bradyarrhythmias

(1) Sinoatrial node dysfunction: The incidence is low. If the pregnant woman's symptoms are not obvious and the vital signs are stable, observation and monitoring can be performed. If the symptoms are obvious, temporary pacing can be performed.

(2) Atrioventricular block: During pregnancy, there is no need for prophylactic pacing. Vaginal delivery generally does not increase additional risks for pregnant women with complete atrioventricular block, unless there are obstetric contraindications. For pregnant women with atrioventricular block, if there is bradycardia and blackout or syncope, temporary pacing can be performed during delivery. The risk of implanting a permanent pacemaker (preferably single-chamber) is very low. Pacemaker implantation is safe, especially after 8 weeks of gestation, and can be performed under ultrasound guidance.

Ⅵ Consultation Process

1. Actively inquire whether the pregnant woman has symptoms such as palpitations, chest tightness, dizziness, or blackouts, and complete the ECG examination as early as possible to clarify the nature of the arrhythmia: malignant or benign, atrial or ventricular, rapid or slow.

2. Supplement key medical history information, such as whether there is an underlying heart disease, history of diabetes or renal insufficiency, recent diarrhea, poor appetite, bloody stools, hematuria, and the possibility of poisoning. Perform risk stratification based on the pregnant woman's symptoms, ventricular rate, and previous underlying heart disease, and assess the severity of the condition.

3. Actively search for and remove reversible triggers or underlying causes, such as infection, anemia, electrolyte disturbances, drugs, and thyroid dysfunction. Rapid auxiliary examinations are required, such as thyroid function, dynamic ECG, echocardiography, BNP, blood electrolytes, and myocardial injury markers if necessary. If the arrhythmia leads to heart failure, cardiac ultrasound should be completed as soon as possible.

4. Most arrhythmias that occur during pregnancy are benign. Treatment methods for arrhythmias include drug therapy, electrical cardioversion, device implantation, and radiofrequency ablation. Based on the currently known type of arrhythmia, choose an appropriate antiarrhythmic regimen. If hemodynamic instability occurs, assess the use of electrical cardioversion, pacemakers, and other related rescue measures.

Section 3 Pregnancy Complicated by Coronary Heart Disease

I Overview

Clinical studies have shown that 0.2%-4% of pregnant women have cardiovascular diseases; in Western countries, cardiovascular diseases have become the main cause of death during pregnancy. In addition, due to the increase in childbearing age and the successful medical and surgical treatment of congenital heart diseases, the number of pregnant women with heart diseases is showing an upward trend. The occurrence of acute coronary syndrome (ACS) during pregnancy is very rare, with an incidence of only 3-6/100,000. In addition to traditional risk factors such as smoking, hypertension, hyperlipidemia, diabetes, and family history, preeclampsia, eclampsia, puerperal infection, severe postpartum hemorrhage, and spontaneous coronary artery dissection can also induce ACS. Although the incidence of ACS is low, the perinatal mortality rate is as high as 5%-10%.

Ⅱ Diagnosis

1. Common clinical manifestations: The common clinical manifestations of coronary heart disease during pregnancy are similar to those of non-pregnant patients. Evaluation is based on the location, nature, duration, and inducing factors of chest pain. If the pain lasts for a long time, accompanied by sweating and a sense of impending death, dynamic observation of ECG and myocardial injury markers should be performed to confirm the diagnosis of ACS.

2. Auxiliary examinations

(1) Myocardial enzyme spectrum and myocardial infarction-specific marker tests.

(2) ECG: There are often ST-segment and T-wave changes, and new bundle branch block may also occur, such as new-onset complete left bundle branch block. However, due to the elevated diaphragm and cardiac displacement in late pregnancy, abnormal Q waves and T wave changes may also appear on the ECG, which need to be combined with clinical manifestations; for patients with suspected cardiovascular disease, performing a sub-maximal exercise test to reach 80% of the maximum heart rate is safe.

(3) Echocardiography: Segmental ventricular wall motion reduction means that the amplitude of endocardial motion toward the heart during systole is 2-4 mm, or 50%-70% less than that of the normal ventricular wall. The wall thickness of the corresponding segment is normal, and some walls are slightly thinned. The three-layer structure of the myocardium is clear, and some endocardial echoes are enhanced. The ventricular wall motion is uncoordinated.

(4) Coronary angiography: It has extremely high diagnostic value. Although the impact of radiological examinations on the fetus depends on the radiation dose and the stage of pregnancy when exposed to radiation, guidelines recommend that the general principle is to avoid or reduce radiation exposure as much as possible.

During pregnancy, we need to consider the impact on the fetus, and radionuclide examinations are not suitable. Non-radiological examinations are often recommended. For the diagnosis of coronary heart disease during pregnancy, dynamic observation of ECG and myocardial enzyme spectrum changes is particularly important.

Ⅲ Diagnosis and Differential Diagnosis

The main differential diagnoses include preeclampsia, pulmonary embolism, and aortic dissection, but sometimes it also needs to be differentiated from acute abdomen, gastroesophageal reflux, intercostal neuralgia, and costochondritis. Preeclampsia often presents with hypertension, proteinuria, and symptoms such as headache, blurred vision, nausea, vomiting, and upper abdominal discomfort. Aortic dissection mainly manifests as sudden severe tearing pain in the chest and back, often with elevated blood pressure; in patients with severe dissection, cardiac ultrasound sometimes reveals an aortic intimal flap. For the diagnosis of pulmonary embolism, since the clinical manifestations of pulmonary embolism lack specificity, for patients with unexplained dyspnea, chest pain, syncope, or shock, especially when accompanied by unilateral or bilateral asymmetric lower limb swelling and pain, ECG, blood gas analysis, echocardiography, and lower limb vascular ultrasound should be performed. Based on these results, pulmonary embolism can be initially suspected or other diseases can be excluded. D-dimer testing should be routinely performed, and negative results can basically rule out pulmonary embolism.

Ⅳ Treatment

1. General management: Oxygen therapy, bed rest, and supportive symptomatic treatment.

2. Drug therapy: The "2011 ESC Guidelines on the Management of Cardiovascular Diseases during Pregnancy" lists more than 60 commonly used cardiovascular drugs according to FDA classification, placental passage, breast milk excretion, and adverse reactions. The US FDA classifies drugs into five categories:

Class A means that controlled studies in pregnant women have failed to demonstrate a risk to the fetus in the first trimester, and there is no evidence of risk in later trimesters.

Class B means that animal reproduction studies have failed to demonstrate a risk to the fetus, and there are no adequate and well-controlled studies in pregnant women, or animal reproduction studies have shown an adverse effect, but adequate and well-controlled studies in pregnant women have failed to demonstrate a risk to the fetus in any trimester.

Class C means that animal reproduction studies have shown an adverse effect on the fetus, and there are no adequate and well-controlled studies in humans, but potential benefits may warrant use of the drug in pregnant women despite potential risks.

Class D means there is positive evidence of human fetal risk based on adverse reaction data from investigational or marketing experience or studies in humans, but potential benefits may warrant use of the drug in pregnant women despite potential risks.

Class X means that studies in animals or humans have demonstrated fetal abnormalities, and/or there is positive evidence of human fetal risk based on adverse reaction data from investigational or marketing experience, and the risks involved in use of the drug in pregnant women clearly outweigh potential benefits.

The guidelines recommend that in emergency situations, drugs not recommended during pregnancy should not be prohibited, and the risks and benefits must be weighed for each patient's specific situation. Different recommendation grades have differences and shortcomings, such as the US FDA, online data, and pharmaceutical companies' recommendations. For clinicians, the guidelines provide a safety table for medication use during pregnancy to guide medication use during pregnancy.

(1) Antiplatelet therapy: Rupture of unstable plaques in the coronary arteries can induce local thrombus formation, and platelet activation plays a very important role in acute thrombus formation. Antiplatelet therapy has become a routine treatment for ACS.

1) Aspirin: FDA Class B, can be used safely.

2) Thienopyridines: Safety is unknown. If they must be used (such as after stent placement),

only clopidogrel can be used, and the duration of use should be shortened as much as possible. Other thienopyridines should be used with caution.

3) Ⅱb/Ⅲa receptor inhibitors: There is no safety evaluation for use in pregnant women.

(2) Anticoagulant therapy: Thrombin is a key factor in converting fibrinogen into fibrin and ultimately forming thrombi, so inhibiting thrombin is critical. It is recommended that all ACS patients receive anticoagulant therapy.

1) Heparin: FDA Class B, can be used safely.

2) Low molecular weight heparin: FDA Class B, can be used safely.

3) Danaparoid: FDA Class B, can be used safely.

4) Bivalirudin: There is no safety evaluation for use in pregnant women.

(3) Beta-blockers: These drugs reduce heart rate by blocking cardiac β1 receptors, inhibit myocardial contractility, and thus reduce myocardial oxygen consumption; by prolonging the effective refractory period of the myocardium and increasing the ventricular fibrillation threshold, they can reduce the incidence of malignant arrhythmias. Beta-blocker therapy can not only relieve symptoms of angina pectoris but also reduce patient mortality. Metoprolol can be used during pregnancy, FDA Class C.

(4) Nitrates: Used to relieve persistent ischemic chest pain, control hypertension, or alleviate pulmonary edema. Commonly used drugs include nitroglycerin and isosorbide dinitrate. They can be used during pregnancy, FDA Class B.

(5) Angiotensin-converting enzyme inhibitors (ACEIs)/angiotensin receptor blockers (ARBs): ACEIs / ARBs mainly reduce the incidence of congestive heart failure by affecting myocardial remodeling and reducing excessive ventricular dilation, thus reducing mortality. They should be used as early as possible in the general population without contraindications. They are contraindicated during pregnancy. ACEIs / ARBs can cause teratogenicity and fetal death, especially during the first 16 weeks of pregnancy.

(6) Aldosterone receptor antagonists: In the general population, they are usually used on the basis of ACEI treatment. For patients with LVEF <0.40 after STEMI, heart failure, or diabetes, without significant renal dysfunction, aldosterone receptor antagonists should be given. The commonly used drug is spironolactone; it is not recommended during pregnancy, FDA Class D.

(7) Statins: In addition to their lipid-lowering effects, statins also have multiple effects such as anti-infection, improving endothelial function, and inhibiting platelet aggregation. They need to be used as early as possible in the general population, regardless of cholesterol levels. They are contraindicated during pregnancy, FDA Class X.

3. Reperfusion therapy

(1) Thrombolytic therapy: Only used for life-threatening ACS when the patient cannot be transferred to a hospital for emergency PCI treatment. Although recombinant tissue-type plasminogen activator does not cross the placental barrier, it can still cause bleeding in pregnant women (subplacental hemorrhage).

(2) Interventional therapy: For patients with stable angina pectoris, drug therapy and continued observation are recommended. For all pregnant women with coronary heart disease, if the symptoms of coronary heart disease worsen, interventional therapy is required. Coronary

artery bypass grafting has a high mortality rate when used in pregnant women, and there is little data on similar cases, so it is not recommended (Table 6-4).

Table 6-4 Recommendations for the Treatment of Acute Coronary Syndrome (ACS) During Pregnancy

Recommendation	Recommendation Class	Level of Evidence
ECG and troponin level should be checked when pregnant women have chest pain	I	C
PCI is preferred over thrombolytic therapy for pregnant women with ST-segment elevation myocardial infarction	I	C
Non-surgical treatment is chosen for low-risk pregnant women with non-ST-segment elevation ACS	II_a	C
CAG+PCI is chosen for high-risk pregnant women with non-ST-segment elevation ACS	II_a	C

4. Maternal interventions during pregnancy: The recommended optimal time for interventional therapy is 4-7 months of pregnancy. This is because the development of various organs of the fetus has been completed at this stage, the fetal thyroid is not yet active, the uterine volume is still small, and the distance between the fetus and the chest is the largest, so the impact on the fetus is relatively small. It is also recommended that the X-ray exposure time should be shortened as much as possible during the procedure, and the pregnant uterus should be shielded to avoid direct exposure. Cardiac surgery is only recommended when medical or interventional procedures fail, and the mother's life is threatened. The optimal timing for surgery is 13-28 weeks of gestation. When the gestational age exceeds 28 weeks, delivery should be considered before surgery, and maternal corticosteroid management should be performed as much as possible within 24 hours before surgery. However, fetal heart rate and uterine tone should be monitored during cardiopulmonary bypass, and the cardiopulmonary bypass time should be shortened as much as possible.

5. Choice of delivery time and mode: For most patients, vaginal delivery has the advantages of less bleeding, lower risk of infection and thrombosis, and is the preferred mode of delivery. The guidelines recommend that cesarean section should be performed to deliver the fetus in the following situations:

(1) There are obstetric indications for cesarean section.

(2) Oral anticoagulants are taken until delivery.

(3) Marfan syndrome, aortic diameter >40 mm.

(4) Acute or chronic aortic dissection.

(5) Severe heart failure.

(6) Severe aortic stenosis or left ventricular outflow tract obstruction.

(7) Eisenmenger syndrome.

Whether vaginal delivery or cesarean section, maternal arterial blood pressure and heart rate should be closely monitored during and after delivery, and percutaneous oxygen saturation monitoring and continuous ECG monitoring should be performed. Routine prophylactic use of antibiotics is not recommended for either mode of delivery.

V Common Questions in Consultation

1. For patients with chest tightness and chest pain, first take a detailed medical history to rule out the possibility of aortic dissection, preeclampsia, pulmonary embolism, and other diseases. If the patient has no relevant history, but has tearing pain, be alert to the possibility of dissection; if accompanied by high blood pressure, proteinuria, and symptoms such as headache, blurred vision, nausea, vomiting, and upper abdominal discomfort, the diagnosis of preeclampsia needs to be clarified; for those with unexplained dyspnea, chest pain, syncope, or shock, especially when accompanied by unilateral or bilateral asymmetric lower limb swelling and pain, pulmonary embolism should be excluded.

2. According to the medical history and clinical manifestations, if the diagnosis of coronary heart disease is clear, we need to perform risk stratification and fully evaluate the patient and choose an appropriate treatment plan based on the condition.

For stable angina pectoris, non-surgical drug therapy is preferred, and PCI is not recommended. For ST-segment elevation myocardial infarction, emergency PCI is preferred within the specified time window, and thrombolytic therapy is not recommended. For low-risk non-ST-segment elevation myocardial infarction patients, non-surgical drug therapy is preferred, and PCI is not recommended; for high-risk non-ST-segment elevation myocardial infarction patients, PCI treatment is recommended.

VI Consultation Process

1. Assess the patient's vital signs and evaluate the location, nature, duration, and inducing factors of chest pain. If the pain lasts for a long time, accompanied by sweating and a sense of impending death, dynamic observation of ECG and myocardial injury markers should be performed to confirm the diagnosis of ACS.

2. Supplement key medical history information, such as whether there is an underlying heart disease, history of diabetes or hypertension, whether it is an acute onset, whether it is accompanied by chest tightness, chest pain, profuse sweating, whether there is cyanosis, hemoptysis, whether there is fever, cough, sputum, and whether there is a possibility of poisoning.

3. Rapid auxiliary examinations are required, such as ECG, troponin T, blood gas analysis, renal function, electrolytes, chest X-ray, BNP or NT-proBNP, D-dimer, etc. Arrange for cardiac ultrasound as soon as possible. Assess the possibility of coronary angiography based on the patient's condition. Guidelines recommend that the general principle is to avoid or reduce radiation exposure as much as possible. During pregnancy, we need to consider the impact on the fetus, and radionuclide examinations are not suitable. Non-radiological examinations are often recommended. For the diagnosis of coronary heart disease during pregnancy, dynamic observation of ECG and myocardial enzyme spectrum changes is particularly important.

4. In terms of differential diagnosis, it mainly needs to be differentiated from preeclampsia, pulmonary embolism, and aortic dissection, but sometimes it also needs to be differentiated from acute abdomen, gastroesophageal reflux, intercostal neuralgia, costochondritis, etc. Preeclampsia often presents with hypertension, proteinuria, and symptoms such as headache, blurred vision,

nausea, vomiting, and upper abdominal discomfort. Aortic dissection mainly manifests as sudden severe tearing pain in the chest and back, often with elevated blood pressure; in patients with severe dissection, cardiac ultrasound sometimes reveals an aortic intimal flap. For the diagnosis of pulmonary embolism, since the clinical manifestations of pulmonary embolism lack specificity, for those with unexplained dyspnea, chest pain, syncope, or shock, especially when accompanied by unilateral or bilateral asymmetric lower limb swelling and pain, ECG, blood gas analysis, echocardiography, and lower limb vascular ultrasound should be performed. Based on these results, pulmonary embolism can be initially suspected or other diseases can be excluded. D-dimer testing should be routinely performed, and negative results can basically rule out pulmonary embolism.

5. After the diagnosis is clear, treat the cause. For confirmed coronary heart disease, according to the patient's condition, provide secondary prevention drug therapy for coronary heart disease and interventional treatment: for patients with stable angina pectoris, drug therapy and continued observation are recommended, and PCI is not recommended. For ST-segment elevation myocardial infarction, emergency PCI is preferred within the specified time window, and thrombolytic therapy is not recommended. For low-risk non-ST-segment elevation myocardial infarction patients, non-surgical drug therapy is preferred, and PCI is not recommended; for high-risk non-ST-segment elevation myocardial infarction patients, PCI is recommended. The recommended optimal time for interventional therapy is 4-7 months of pregnancy. When the gestational age exceeds 28 weeks, delivery should be considered before surgery, and maternal corticosteroid management should be performed as much as possible within 24 hours before surgery.

Section 4 Pregnancy Complicated by Aortic Disease

Common aortic diseases include bicuspid aortic valve malformation, aortic coarctation, aortic atherosclerosis, Marfan syndrome, familial aortic dissection, aortic aneurysm, aortic arch dilation, tetralogy of Fallot, aortic valve stenosis, connective tissue disease, Ehlers-Danlos syndrome, Turner syndrome, trauma, aortitis, hypertension, etc.

Pregnancy is a high-risk period for patients with aortic disease, and aortic disease is one of the main causes of maternal death. This is due to hemodynamic changes: when the aorta is affected, it can manifest as aortic dilation, aortic valve regurgitation, heart failure, cardiac tamponade, etc. In severe cases, death often occurs due to acute cardiac tamponade, coronary artery occlusion, or rupture of the adventitia of the dissection. Therefore, the possibility of aortic disease should be considered in all pregnant women with chest pain during pregnancy, and the high-risk factor for aortic disease is aortic dissection.

The incidence of aortic dissection is 0.5-2.0/100,000, and about 50% of aortic dissections in young women occur during pregnancy, especially in the middle and late stages of pregnancy. Various factors leading to aortic wall degeneration and hemodynamic changes within the aortic lumen are the internal and external causes of aortic dissection formation. Pregnancy is an independent risk factor for aortic dissection in young women, which may be related to changes in hormone levels and increases in blood volume, cardiac output, and blood pressure during pregnancy. The increase in blood volume during pregnancy leads to an increase in left ventricular output and an increase in the impact force of blood flow on the aortic wall. Estrogen can inhibit the deposition of collagen and elastic fibers in the aortic wall; progesterone can promote the deposition of non-collagen proteins in the aortic wall, reducing the elasticity and increasing the brittleness of the vessel wall, both of which are prone to cause the formation and rupture of aortic dissection. 90% of aortic dissections during pregnancy are accompanied by hypertension or Marfan syndrome.

I Early Recognition and Diagnosis

1. Symptoms and signs: Typical clinical manifestations include the following aspects.

(1) Chest pain is the most common clinical symptom, with an incidence of up to 80%-90%, mostly sudden severe tearing pain that lasts for a long time and exacerbates in paroxysms. It is located behind or beside the sternum, and some patients have radiating pain to the back. As the pain location migrates and radiates, it indicates that the range of aortic dissection is expanding. Atypical symptoms include chest tightness, upper abdominal discomfort, neck pain, and breast distension.

(2) 65%-75% of patients have difficult-to-control blood pressure elevation, especially when painless shock occurs and blood pressure does not decrease, which is one of the main clinical features.

(3) 40%-75% of patients with Stanford type A dissection have aortic valve regurgitation, and the sudden onset of aortic valve insufficiency murmur after pain is one of the characteristics of this disease. Severe acute aortic valve regurgitation can lead to heart failure and cardiogenic shock.

(4) 15%-30% of patients have asymmetric blood pressure in the limbs or disappearance of pulse in one limb.

(5) Hematoma compression and intimal tearing can lead to dysphagia, hemoptysis, hematemesis, pericardial effusion, cardiac tamponade, etc. 10%-15% of patients develop myocardial ischemia or myocardial infarction.

(6) When the blood supply of aortic branch vessels is affected, dizziness, headache, disturbance of consciousness and speech, syncope, hemiplegia, paraplegia, acute renal failure, etc., may occur accordingly.

2. Auxiliary examinations: The confirmation of aortic dissection relies on imaging techniques. Mastering the clinical characteristics of the disease and choosing appropriate auxiliary examinations are the keys to early diagnosis.

(1) D-dimer: In patients with aortic dissection, D-dimer rapidly increases to a peak, while in other diseases, it gradually increases. Therefore, the D-dimer value within the first hour of onset in patients with chest pain has extremely high diagnostic value. *The 2014 European Society of Cardiology (ESC) Guidelines* first proposed: ① In patients with a low clinical probability of aortic dissection, negative D-dimer can be considered to exclude dissection (II_a B); ② In

patients with a moderate clinical probability of aortic dissection, positive D-dimer should prompt consideration of further examination (II_a B); ③ In patients with a high clinical probability of aortic dissection, D-dimer testing has no additional significance and is not recommended for routine examination (Ⅲ C).

(2) ECG: Lacks specific changes. When aortic dissection affects the coronary arteries, ECG changes such as ST-T changes, myocardial ischemia, and even myocardial infarction may occur, mostly in the posterior wall.

(3) Chest X-ray (there is radiation injury, so it needs to be used with caution during pregnancy): Aortic widening, localized bulging, tortuosity, or mediastinal widening suggests abnormalities.

(4) Echocardiography: ① Widening of the anterior, posterior, or both walls of the aorta; ② Changes in the cardiac cycle, with contradictory movements of the aorta; ③ Intimal flap sign and true and false double-lumen sign of aortic intimal separation; ④ Aortic dilation. Ultrasound is the preferred diagnostic method during pregnancy. It is superior to other examinations in assessing pericardial effusion, aortic valve insufficiency, and cardiac function status, but it is not as sensitive as CT in determining the location and extent of intimal rupture. Transesophageal echocardiography can accurately classify the disease and better show whether the left and right coronary arteries are affected, but it may cause nausea, vomiting, tachycardia, hypertension, etc.

(5) CT and MRI: Both of them have high sensitivity and specificity for the diagnosis of aortic dissection. CT has a strong ability to identify false lumens and can accurately show the degree of aortic dilation. It is easier to detect the sign of intimal tearing due to calcification moving centrally. It can quickly diagnose life-threatening primary diseases that cause acute chest pain and has a high negative predictive value. The advantage of MRI is that there is no risk of arterial catheterization and no radiation injury, making it suitable for pregnancy. Its sensitivity and specificity are both close to 100%, and it can determine the extent of the lesion, identify branch vessel lesions, and detect thrombi. It has a tendency to replace angiography as the gold standard for diagnosis. However, MRI scanning takes a long time and has certain difficulties in examining emergency patients with unstable circulation or consciousness. Multi-slice spiral CT angiography can quickly confirm the diagnosis and differential diagnosis, but it has radiation injury and nephrotoxicity, so it needs to be used with caution during pregnancy.

The clinical manifestations of acute aortic dissection are diverse and lack specificity. Atypical symptoms of aortic dissection are often misdiagnosed, especially in pregnant women. The incidence of preeclampsia and pulmonary embolism is much higher than that of aortic dissection, making it easier to be misled. However, aortic dissection is dangerous, progresses rapidly, and has a limited time for diagnosis. The mortality rate within 24 hours is 25% for those who are not treated in time. Therefore, in clinical practice, we must be highly alert to the "three inconsistencies", namely, the inconsistency between chest pain and ECG, the inconsistency between symptoms and signs, and the inconsistency between blood pressure and shock manifestations, and perform differential diagnosis.

II Treatment of Aortic Dissection

Individualized plans should be formulated based on the condition of the pregnant woman and fetus, with a multidisciplinary approach.

1. Pharmacological Treatment. The main purpose of medical treatment is to reduce blood pressure and myocardial contractility to decrease the shear stress at the aortic lesion site, prevent the progression of the dissection hematoma, and improve prognosis. In the acute onset period, drug control of pain and stabilization of hemodynamics are important. Once diagnosed, treatment should be initiated as soon as possible: ① Analgesia and sedation; ② Beta-blockers to control heart rate, with a target heart rate of 60-75 beats/min; ③ Sodium nitroprusside is the first choice for lowering blood pressure and dilating blood vessels. The dose should be adjusted to reduce blood pressure to the minimum required level for myocardial, cerebral, and renal perfusion. Generally, the systolic blood pressure is stably controlled at 100-120 mmHg, and the mean arterial pressure is maintained at 60-75 mmHg. Beta-blockers should be used before sodium nitroprusside; otherwise, the increased release of reactive catecholamines caused by vasodilators can lead to increased myocardial contractility and pulse amplitude, resulting in the progression of the dissection.

2. Surgical Treatment. For acute type I aortic dissection, regardless of early or late pregnancy, surgical treatment should be actively pursued. If the admitting hospital does not have cardiac surgical conditions, the patient should be immediately transferred to a hospital with cardiac and great vessel surgical capabilities.

The 2014 ESC Guidelines suggests that surgical intervention should be considered when the ascending aortic diameter is >50 mm or when there is dissection or moderate to severe heart failure caused by valvular regurgitation. Based on evidence-based research, it is currently believed that surgical treatment should be decisively adopted for pregnant patients with acute Stanford Type A aortic dissection. For patients who develop the condition before 28 weeks of gestation, aortic dissection repair surgery can be performed first while minimizing fetal injury, followed by close monitoring and expectant management until fetal maturity, and then elective cesarean section. For patients who develop the condition at 28 weeks of gestation, especially after 32 weeks, simultaneous cesarean section and aortic dissection repair surgery can be considered.

For Stanford Type B aortic dissection complicating pregnancy, there is currently no unified and clear treatment strategy. Since the cardiovascular load is not significant in early pregnancy, stable Stanford Type B aortic dissection occurring in early pregnancy is preferably treated with non-surgical pharmacological therapy. For pregnant women who develop the condition in mid to late pregnancy, it was previously believed that emergency surgical intervention was mainly targeted at patients with dissection rupture or combined organ malperfusion. However, pregnancy, childbirth, and the postpartum state themselves are independent risk factors for dissection rupture. With the maturation of endovascular repair techniques, more and more studies tend to appropriately expand the indications for surgical intervention for pregnancy-related aortic dissection to reduce the possibility of dissection rupture and save the mother and fetus. In general, for stable Stanford Type B aortic dissection with symptom relief after non-surgical pharmacological treatment, elective cesarean section can be performed first to terminate the pregnancy. If the condition further progresses after delivery, repair treatment can be considered. For acute Stanford Type B aortic dissection, non-surgical medical treatment + interventional endovascular stent-graft placement can be adopted. In the acute phase, non-surgical medical treatment is preferred. After the condition is stable, depending on the different pregnancy, delivery, and expected delivery dates, stent-graft placement can be performed before delivery, or it can be performed after delivery. If difficult-to-control hypertension, persistent chest pain, or aneurysm dilation still exist during the non-surgical treatment process, then emergency endovascular repair surgery should be performed first to treat the aortic dissection, maintain the hemodynamic stability of the pregnant woman, and then perform cesarean section to terminate the pregnancy.

The 2011 European Guidelines on the Management of Cardiovascular Diseases during Pregnancy make the following recommendations for the treatment of aortic diseases:

1. Women with pre-existing aortic disease and known aortic root dilation should be counseled about the risk of dissection during pregnancy and the risk of recurrence of aortic disease in offspring before conception (Class Ⅰ, Level C).

2. Patients with Marfan syndrome or other aortic diseases need to undergo a comprehensive aortic examination (CT / MRI) before pregnancy (Class Ⅰ, Level C).

3. Patients with Marfan syndrome and an aortic diameter >45 mm need to undergo surgery before pregnancy (Class Ⅰ, Level C).

4. Pregnant women with known aortic dilation, Type B aortic dissection (or a history of it), or a hereditary tendency for dissection need strict blood pressure control (Class Ⅰ, Level C).

5. Patients with aortic root dilation should have echocardiography every 4-8 weeks during pregnancy and 6 months postpartum (Class Ⅰ, Level C).

6. MRI monitoring is recommended for pregnant women with dilation of the distal ascending aorta, aortic arch, or descending aorta (Class Ⅰ, Level C).

7. Women with bicuspid aortic valves are recommended to have their ascending aorta examined (Class Ⅰ, Level C).

8. For those with an aortic diameter <40 mm, vaginal delivery is preferred (Class Ⅰ, Level C).

9. Women with aortic dilation or aortic dissection need to deliver in a hospital with cardiac surgery capabilities (Class Ⅰ, Level C).

10. Patients with an ascending aortic diameter >45 mm need to undergo cesarean section (Class Ⅱ_a, Level C).

11. Patients with aortic disease accompanied by bicuspid aortic valve and an aortic diameter >50 mm (or >27 mm/m^2 BSA) need to undergo surgery before pregnancy (Class Ⅱ_a, Level C).

12. Preventive surgery is recommended for patients with an aortic diameter >50 mm and continued enlargement during pregnancy (Class Ⅱ_a, Level C).

13. For patients with Marfan syndrome or other aortic diseases with an aortic diameter of 40-45 mm, epidural anesthesia and vaginal delivery should be considered, and the second stage of labor should be expedited (Class Ⅱ_a, Level C).

14. Cesarean section may be chosen for patients with Marfan syndrome or other aortic diseases with an aortic diameter of 40-45 mm (Class $Ⅱ_b$, Level C).

15. Pregnancy should be avoided in patients with Type B aortic dissection (or a history of it) (Class Ⅲ, Level C).

Ⅲ Prevention

Among patients with aortic diseases, those with aortic dissection must adopt long-term effective contraceptive measures after marriage and avoid pregnancy. If contraception fails and unintended pregnancy occurs, early artificial abortion should be performed to terminate the pregnancy. Patients with Marfan syndrome should avoid pregnancy. Actively and effectively controlling pregnancy-induced hypertension and treating primary diseases are effective methods to prevent aortic dissection during pregnancy.

Ⅳ Consultation Process

1. Assess the patient's vital signs, monitor bilateral upper limb blood pressure, and inquire about medical history, such as whether there is underlying heart disease, hypertension, a history of aortic dissection, a history of Marfan syndrome, whether it is accompanied by chest tightness, chest pain, profuse sweating, and whether the chest pain is sudden, severe, tearing, lasting for a long time, and paroxysmal, radiating to the back. Check for cyanosis, dysphagia, hemoptysis, hematemesis, etc.

2. Pay attention to important physical examination findings, such as asymmetric blood pressure in the limbs or disappearance of pulse in one limb, whether heart sounds are distant, whether the heart border percussion is enlarged, whether there is jugular venous distension, whether the patient is conscious, and whether there are neurological localization signs.

3. Rapid auxiliary examinations are required, such as ECG, echocardiography, chest X-ray, blood gas analysis, renal function, electrolytes, BNP or NT-proBNP, D-dimer, etc. Whole aorta CTA examination has high sensitivity and specificity for the diagnosis of aortic dissection. For highly suspected cases, whole aorta CTA should be completed as soon as possible to assist in the diagnosis, but it needs to be used with caution during pregnancy. MRI has no radiation injury and is suitable for pregnancy. Its sensitivity and specificity are both close to 100%, and it can determine the extent of the lesion, identify branch vessel lesions, and detect thrombi. It can be selected according to the situation.

4. The clinical manifestations of acute aortic dissection are diverse and lack specificity. In clinical practice, we must be highly alert to the "three inconsistencies", namely, the inconsistency between chest pain and ECG, the inconsistency between symptoms and signs, and the inconsistency between blood pressure and shock manifestations, and perform differential diagnosis. It needs to be differentiated from preeclampsia and pulmonary embolism.

5. Pharmacological treatment: ① Analgesia and sedation; ② Beta-blockers to control heart rate, with a target heart rate of 60-75 beats/min; ③ Sodium nitroprusside is the first choice for lowering blood pressure and dilating blood vessels. The dose should be adjusted to reduce blood pressure to the minimum required level for myocardial, cerebral, and renal perfusion. Generally,

the systolic blood pressure is stably controlled at 100-120 mmHg, and the mean arterial pressure is maintained at 60-75 mmHg. Beta-blockers should be used before sodium nitroprusside.

6. Surgical treatment: In the acute phase, non-surgical medical treatment is preferred. After the condition is stable, depending on the different pregnancy, delivery, and expected delivery dates, stent-graft placement can be performed before delivery, or it can be performed after delivery. For stable Stanford Type B aortic dissection with symptom relief after non-surgical pharmacological treatment, elective cesarean section can be performed first to terminate the pregnancy. If the condition further progresses after delivery, repair treatment can be considered. For acute Stanford Type B aortic dissection, non-surgical medical treatment + interventional endovascular stent-graft placement can be adopted. If difficult-to-control hypertension, persistent chest pain, or aneurysm dilation still exist during the non-surgical treatment process, then emergency endovascular repair surgery should be performed first to treat the aortic dissection, maintain the hemodynamic stability of the pregnant woman, and then perform cesarean section to terminate the pregnancy.

Section 5 Pregnancy Complicated by Congenital Heart Disease

I Overview

Congenital heart disease refers to heart disease with structural abnormalities of the heart and great vessels present at birth, including non-shunt types (aortic or pulmonary valve stenosis, Ebstein's anomaly, etc.), left-to-right shunt types (atrial septal defect, ventricular septal defect, patent ductus arteriosus, etc.), and right-to-left shunt types (tetralogy of Fallot, Eisenmenger syndrome, etc.). Mild cases may have no symptoms, while severe cases may have clinical manifestations of hypoxia or heart failure in the mother and child.

Currently, more than 50% of heart diseases during pregnancy are congenital heart diseases, and this proportion will continue to increase. With the rapid development of cardiac surgery, the number of pregnant women with congenital heart disease after surgery has significantly increased, and pregnancy complicated by congenital heart disease has become the leading type of pregnancy complicated by heart disease. Therefore, the rational management of pregnant women with congenital heart disease to reduce maternal and perinatal mortality and protect the health of mothers and infants is an important issue currently faced by obstetricians.

II Classification

(i) Left-to-Right Shunt Types

1. Atrial septal defect

(1) Clinical manifestations: Generally, patients with a defect area $<1\ cm^2$ are mostly asymptomatic and are only discovered during physical examination. Symptoms gradually become apparent with increasing age, with exertional dyspnea being the main manifestation, followed by supraventricular arrhythmias, especially atrial flutter and atrial fibrillation, which aggravate the symptoms. If the defect area is large, during pregnancy and delivery, due to increased pulmonary

vascular resistance, pulmonary hypertension, increased right atrial pressure, decreased systemic vascular resistance during pregnancy, and blood loss and reduced blood volume during delivery, right-to-left shunting may occur, leading to cyanosis and a high possibility of heart failure. The most typical sign on physical examination is a fixed split second heart sound with accentuation in the pulmonary valve area, and a Grade Ⅱ - Ⅲ systolic ejection murmur may be heard.

(2) Diagnosis: ① ECG: Findings may include right axis deviation, right ventricular hypertrophy, right bundle branch block, etc. ② X-ray examination: Enlargement of the right atrium and right ventricle, prominence of the pulmonary artery segment, and increased pulmonary vascular markings may be seen. However, because X-rays are an adverse factor affecting embryonic development, they are contraindicated in early pregnancy, should be used with caution in mid-pregnancy, and the abdomen should be protected with a lead apron when imaging is necessary for severe conditions. ③ Echocardiography: Two-dimensional echocardiography can show the absence of atrial septal echoes and right heart overload; color Doppler echocardiography can show shunting at the atrial level; transesophageal echocardiography can more accurately measure the size and location of the atrial septal defect. ④ Cardiac catheterization: It is the "gold standard" for the diagnosis of congenital heart disease, especially complex cardiac malformations.

With the development of non-invasive examination techniques such as echocardiography, it is currently only applicable to congenital heart diseases that cannot be clearly diagnosed by non-invasive examinations, for calculating left-to-right shunt volume and pulmonary vascular resistance, and for evaluating whether pulmonary hypertension is dynamic or resistive in combination with vasodilation tests, and for distinguishing whether there are other combined malformations. Because it needs to be performed under direct X-ray guidance, during pregnancy, it must be performed by skilled technical personnel, with the abdomen protected by a lead apron, and the operation time should be shortened as much as possible to reduce the radiation dose received by the mother and child.

(3) Management: For those with an atrial septal defect area $>2\ cm^2$, closure should be performed before pregnancy. In cases without surgery, the incidence of heart failure is quite high, and death may occur due to heart failure, embolism, pulmonary infection, or sepsis. In patients with atrial septal defect without complications, the maternal mortality rate is extremely low, and the fetal mortality rate is about 15%; if combined with pulmonary hypertension and right-to-left shunting occurs, termination of pregnancy is required.

2. Ventricular septal defect

(1) Clinical manifestations: Generally, according to the degree of hemodynamic impact and the severity of symptoms, ventricular septal defects are clinically divided into large, medium, and small types. ① Small ventricular septal defect: There is a significant pressure gradient between the left and right ventricles during systole, but the left-to-right shunt volume is large, with a pulmonary-to-systemic blood flow ratio (Qp/Qs) <1.5, and normal right ventricular and pulmonary artery pressures. Such patients are usually asymptomatic, and a grade Ⅳ - Ⅵ holosystolic murmur with thrill can be heard along the left sternal border in the 3rd-4th intercostal space, and the second heart sound may have a slight split without significant accentuation. ② Medium ventricular septal defect: The shunt volume between the left and right ventricles is

relatively large, with a Qp/Qs of 1.5-2.0, but the right ventricular systolic pressure is still lower than the left ventricle. On auscultation, in addition to a holosystolic murmur with thrill along the left sternal border, a mid-diastolic reflux murmur may also be heard in the apical area, and the second heart sound may be slightly accentuated. Some patients have exertional dyspnea. ③ Large ventricular septal defect: There is no longer a pressure gradient between the left and right ventricles during systole, and the left-to-right shunt volume is large, with a Qp/Qs>2.0. Due to the severe hemodynamic impact, few patients survive to adulthood, and secondary pulmonary vascular obstructive changes often occur, leading to right-to-left shunting and cyanosis, as well as dyspnea and reduced exercise capacity; the systolic murmur along the left sternal border often weakens to around grade Ⅲ, and the second heart sound is accentuated; sometimes a diastolic murmur caused by secondary pulmonary valve insufficiency can be heard.

(2) Diagnosis: ① ECG: In small ventricular septal defects, the ECG may be normal or show left axis deviation; in larger defects, left ventricular or biventricular hypertrophy may be present. ② X-ray examination: In adults with small ventricular septal defects, the X-ray film may show no abnormalities; in medium ventricular septal defects, increased pulmonary blood flow and slight enlargement of the cardiac silhouette to the left may be seen; in large ventricular septal defects, the main manifestation is marked dilation of the pulmonary artery and its main branches, but the vascular markings in the outer 1/3 of the lung fields suddenly decrease, and the size of the cardiac silhouette varies, manifesting as enlargement of the left atrium and left ventricle, or enlargement of the left atrium, left ventricle, and right ventricle, or mainly enlargement of the right ventricle, and upward lifting of the cardiac apex suggests right ventricular hypertrophy. Because of radiation injury, it should be used with caution during pregnancy. ③ Echocardiography: It is used to confirm the diagnosis and can also determine the size and location of the defect, assess ventricular hypertrophy and chamber size, and clearly identify intraventricular shunting and indirectly measure pulmonary artery pressure. Echocardiography is the main non-invasive examination for the definitive diagnosis of this disease. ④ Cardiac catheterization: It can measure the shunt volume at the ventricular level and pulmonary vascular resistance. It should be used with caution during pregnancy.

(3) Management: Changes in defect size and pulmonary artery pressure directly affect hemodynamic changes. Patients with a defect area <1.25 cm^2, no history of heart failure, and no other complications are less likely to develop pulmonary hypertension and heart failure and can generally pass through pregnancy and delivery smoothly. In adults with a large unrepaired defect, pulmonary hypertension and heart failure are likely to occur, and the incidence of bacterial endocarditis is also higher. Pregnancy can tolerate mild to moderate left-to-right shunting. When the pulmonary artery pressure approaches or exceeds the systemic level, it will develop into right-to-left shunting or Eisenmenger syndrome, at which point the maternal mortality rate will be as high as 30%-50%. The latter should be prohibited from pregnancy; if contraception fails, therapeutic abortion should be performed in early pregnancy.

3. Patent ductus arteriosus

(1) Clinical manifestations: Adults with patent ductus arteriosus may have different clinical manifestations depending on the size of the shunt volume.

Those with a very small shunt volume may have no subjective symptoms clinically, and the prominent sign is a continuous machinery-like murmur heard in the second intercostal space at the left sternal border and below the left clavicle. Those with a moderate shunt volume often have symptoms such as fatigue, palpitations after exertion, shortness of breath, and chest tightness. The nature of the murmur on cardiac auscultation is the same as above, often accompanied by a thrill, with a wide range of transmission. In patent ductus arteriosus with a large shunt volume, secondary severe pulmonary hypertension is often present, which can lead to right-to-left shunting. The diastolic component of the above-mentioned typical murmur is reduced or disappears, followed by the disappearance of the systolic murmur, and only a diastolic murmur caused by pulmonary valve insufficiency can be heard. At this time, patients often have cyanosis and severe clinical symptoms.

(2) Diagnosis: ① ECG: Common findings include enlargement of the left atrium and left ventricle, and enlargement of the right atrium and right ventricle may occur in pulmonary hypertension. ② X-ray examination: The characteristic change seen on fluoroscopy is the pulmonary hilar dance sign. The chest film may show prominence of the pulmonary artery segment, increased pulmonary blood flow, and enlargement of the left atrium and left ventricle. In the late stage, when right-to-left shunting occurs, the left-to-right shunt volume decreases, and the cardiac silhouette becomes smaller than before, and signs of right ventricular hypertrophy appear. It should be used with caution during pregnancy. ③ Echocardiography: Two-dimensional echocardiography can show the patent ductus arteriosus and enlargement of the left ventricular internal diameter. Color Doppler can measure the systolic and diastolic left-to-right shunt existing between the aorta and pulmonary artery. ④ Cardiac catheterization: To understand pulmonary vascular resistance, shunt conditions, and exclude other complex malformations, right heart catheterization and retrograde ascending aortography sometimes need to be performed. It should be used with caution during pregnancy.

(3) Management: It can be surgically cured in childhood, so pregnancy complicated by patent ductus arteriosus is uncommon. In patent ductus arteriosus with a larger shunt, if surgical correction is not performed before pregnancy, due to a large amount of arterial blood flowing to the pulmonary artery, pulmonary hypertension causes blood flow reversal, resulting in cyanosis and heart failure. If pulmonary hypertension or right-to-left shunting is already present in early pregnancy, termination of pregnancy is recommended. In those with a smaller patent ductus arteriosus and normal pulmonary artery pressure, there are generally no symptoms during pregnancy and can continue until full-term pregnancy.

(ii) Right-to-Left Shunt Types

1. Tetralogy of Fallot

(1) Clinical manifestations: Progressive cyanosis and dyspnea occur from childhood, with easy fatigability, and patients often rest in a squatting position after exertion. Severe hypoxia can cause syncope, and long-term increased right heart pressure and hypoxia can lead to heart failure. In addition to obvious cyanosis, patients often have clubbing of the fingers and toes, and cardiac auscultation reveals a weakened or absent second heart sound in the pulmonary valve area, and a systolic ejection murmur is often heard along the left sternal border. Cerebrovascular accidents,

infective endocarditis, and pulmonary infections are common complications of this disease.

(2) Diagnosis: ① Complete blood count: It can show significantly increased red blood cell count, hemoglobin, and hematocrit. ② ECG: Right axis deviation and right ventricular hypertrophy can be seen. ③ X-ray examination: The main manifestation is right ventricular hypertrophy, with a concave pulmonary artery segment forming a boot-shaped appearance, and reduced pulmonary vascular markings, making the lung fields abnormally clear. It should be used with caution during pregnancy. ④ Echocardiography: It can show right ventricular hypertrophy, ventricular septal defect, and overriding aorta. Right ventricular outflow tract stenosis and the condition of the pulmonary valve can also be displayed. ⑤ Magnetic resonance imaging: It can further clearly show various anatomical structural abnormalities. Nonenhanced magnetic resonance imaging has no adverse teratogenic effects on the embryo. ⑥ Cardiac catheterization: Patients who plan to undergo surgical treatment should undergo cardiac catheterization to further determine the nature and extent of the malformation and whether there are other combined malformations based on hemodynamic changes, changes in oxygen saturation, and shunt conditions, providing a basis for formulating a surgical plan. It should be used with caution during pregnancy.

(3) Management: Due to the high maternal and fetal mortality rates, pregnancy is generally not advisable.

2. Eisenmenger syndrome

(1) Clinical manifestations: Mild to moderate cyanosis, which worsens after exertion, gradually leading to clubbing of the fingers and toes, often accompanied by symptoms such as shortness of breath, fatigue, and dizziness, and later, symptoms related to right heart failure may appear. Physical examination shows a significantly enlarged heart border, obvious pulsation in the 3rd-4th intercostal space to the left of the sternum, weakening or disappearance of the original left-to-right shunt murmur (the diastolic component of the continuous murmur in patent ductus arteriosus may disappear), accentuated and split second heart sound in the pulmonary valve area, and later, a diastolic murmur may appear, and a systolic regurgitant murmur can be heard in the area slightly to the left of the lower sternum.

(2) Diagnosis: ① ECG: Right ventricular hypertrophy and strain, right atrial hypertrophy. ② X-ray examination: Enlargement of the right ventricle and right atrium, dilation of the pulmonary artery trunk and left and right pulmonary arteries, mild or no pulmonary congestion, thinning of vascular markings, and the condition of the left heart depends on the primary malformation. It should be used with caution during pregnancy. ③ Echocardiography: In addition to the manifestations of the original malformation, pulmonary artery dilation and relative pulmonary valve and tricuspid valve insufficiency support the diagnosis of this condition. ④ Cardiac catheterization: In addition to the original malformation, it can confirm bidirectional shunting or right-to-left shunting, pulmonary artery pressure, and pulmonary vascular resistance. The reactivity of the pulmonary vasculature can be assessed through vasodilation tests.

(3) Management: Most patients have complex cardiovascular malformations, and few survive to childbearing age without surgical correction. Such patients have extremely poor tolerance to the increase in blood volume and hemodynamic changes during pregnancy, with a

maternal mortality rate as high as 36%; if the cyanosis is severe, the spontaneous abortion rate can be as high as 80%, and pregnancy is not advisable.

(iii) Non-Shunt Types

1. Pulmonary valve stenosis

(1) Clinical manifestations: Mild stenosis may be asymptomatic, moderate stenosis may cause dyspnea and fatigue during activity, and severe stenosis may lead to syncope or even sudden death due to strenuous activity. The typical sign is a loud systolic ejection murmur in the second intercostal space at the left sternal border, which is widely transmitted and can be heard in the neck, the entire precordial area, and even the back, often accompanied by a thrill; the second heart sound in the pulmonary valve area is weakened.

(2) Diagnosis: ① ECG: It may be normal in mild stenosis; in moderate or severe stenosis, right axis deviation, right ventricular hypertrophy, and right atrial enlargement may occur, and incomplete right bundle branch block may also be seen. ② X-ray examination: Prominence of the pulmonary artery segment may be seen, which is caused by post-stenotic dilation, the pulmonary vascular markings are fine, and the lung fields are abnormally clear; leftward and upward displacement of the cardiac apex is a manifestation of right ventricular hypertrophy. If right heart failure is already present, the cardiac silhouette may be significantly enlarged. It should be used with caution during pregnancy. ③ Echocardiography: Thickening of the pulmonary valve can be seen, and the valve orifice area can be quantitatively measured; subvalvular infundibular stenosis can also be clearly delineated; Doppler technology can be used to calculate the pressure gradient across the valve or stenosis. ④ Right heart catheterization and right ventricular angiography: Determine the location and type of stenosis and measure the pressures in the right ventricle and pulmonary artery. It should be used with caution during pregnancy.

(3) Management: Those with mild stenosis can go through pregnancy and delivery. In those with severe stenosis (valve orifice area reduced by more than 60%), due to the increase in blood volume and cardiac output during pregnancy and delivery, the right ventricular load is increased, and severe right heart failure may occur. Therefore, severe pulmonary valve stenosis should be surgically corrected before pregnancy.

2. Aortic coarctation

(1) Clinical manifestations: Adults are often asymptomatic, and some patients may present with exertional dyspnea, headache, dizziness, nosebleeds, lower limb weakness, numbness, coldness, or even intermittent claudication. The most obvious signs are varying degrees of increased upper limb blood pressure and decreased lower limb blood pressure. The brachial artery blood pressure is more than 20 mmHg higher than the popliteal artery blood pressure, the carotid and supraclavicular artery pulsations are enhanced, while the femoral artery pulsation is weak, and the dorsalis pedis artery may even have no pulsation. The apical impulse is enhanced, and the heart border often enlarges to the left and downward. A mid-to-late systolic ejection murmur can be heard along the left sternal border to the mid-upper abdomen, and sometimes it can be heard in the left back.

(2) Diagnosis: ① ECG: Left ventricular hypertrophy and/or myocardial strain are often present. ② X-ray examination: Enlargement of the left ventricle and widening of the ascending

aorta can be seen, and dilation of the vessels above and below the coarctation forms a "3" sign of the aortic arch. "Notch" changes formed by intercostal artery erosion can be seen near the cardiac end at the lower edge of the posterior ribs, which is an indirect sign of the formation of collateral circulation. It should be used with caution during pregnancy. ③ Echocardiography: Showing an increased left ventricular internal diameter; thickening of the left ventricular wall; the location of the coarctation ring and its dilation above and below can be seen in the long axis of the aorta in the suprasternal notch. Doppler ultrasound can measure the pressure gradient above and below the coarctation. ④ Magnetic resonance imaging: It can more satisfactorily display the anatomical configuration of the entire aorta and the collateral circulation. Non-enhanced magnetic resonance imaging has no adverse teratogenic effects on the embryo. ⑤ Cardiac catheterization and aortography: Cardiac catheterization measures oxygen saturation and performs pressure measurements. Aortography shows the location and length of the coarctation, the collateral circulation, and whether there is a patent ductus arteriosus.

(3) Management: This condition is rare in females, so pregnancy complicated by aortic coarctation is uncommon. This disease is often accompanied by other cardiovascular malformations and has a poor prognosis. Those with mild aortic coarctation and good cardiac compensatory function can continue pregnancy under close observation; those with moderate to severe coarctation, even if surgically corrected, should be advised to use contraception or terminate the pregnancy in early pregnancy.

3. Ebstein's anomaly

(1) Clinical manifestations: Depending on the degree of tricuspid valve regurgitation, the difference in right ventricular load capacity, and the presence or absence of right-to-left shunting, there may be palpitations, dyspnea, fatigue, dizziness, and right heart failure. Typical signs include a significantly enlarged heart border and weak precordial pulsation. Cardiac auscultation may reveal a quadruple rhythm, which is formed by the asynchronous closure of various valves, splitting of heart sounds, and the addition of atrial sounds. A holosystolic murmur of tricuspid regurgitation can be heard at the lower end of the left sternal border, and dilated carotid pulsation and hepatomegaly with dilated pulsation may also be present.

(2) Diagnosis: ① ECG: First-degree atrioventricular block, tall peaked P waves, and right bundle branch block are common, and some patients may present with a pre-excitation syndrome (right-sided atrioventricular bypass) pattern. ② X-ray examination: A spherical giant heart shadow is its characteristic, mainly due to right atrial enlargement, and in patients with cyanosis, the pulmonary vascular markings are reduced. It should be used with caution during pregnancy. ③ Echocardiography: It can show the downward displacement of the valve, a giant right atrium, an atrialized right ventricle, and a relatively small functional right ventricle; an atrial septal defect can also be visualized. ④ Cardiac catheterization: Right heart catheterization should be performed in those who plan to undergo surgical treatment. It should be used with caution during pregnancy.

(3) Management: Most patients with Ebstein's anomaly can survive to childbearing age and can successfully complete pregnancy, but right heart failure, infective endocarditis, and paradoxical embolism may occur. The incidence of maternal and fetal complications is increased

in patients with cyanosis.

Ⅲ Summary

To sum up, cardiovascular adverse events that occur in pregnant women with congenital heart disease include heart failure, arrhythmia, subacute infective endocarditis, venous thrombosis, pulmonary embolism, etc., with heart failure having the highest incidence. Compared with patients with NYHA cardiac function Class Ⅰ - Ⅱ, those with Class Ⅲ - Ⅳ have statistically significant differences in cesarean section rate, puerperal infection, maternal heart failure, maternal mortality, gestational age, preterm birth rate, fetal growth restriction incidence, perinatal mortality, congenital heart disease in offspring, and mean neonatal birth weight. The risk of severe complications in those with cardiac function Class Ⅲ - Ⅳ is 27.7 times that of Class Ⅰ - Ⅱ. Pregnant women with congenital heart disease should undergo fetal cardiac ultrasound examination at 19th-22nd weeks of gestation; if there is a family member with congenital heart disease, fetal congenital heart disease screening should be performed at 13th weeks of gestation. Early termination of pregnancy is required in patients with cardiac function Class Ⅲ - Ⅳ, severe pulmonary hypertension, Eisenmenger syndrome, cyanotic congenital heart disease, transposition of the great arteries combined with ventricular dysfunction and/or severe tricuspid regurgitation. The management of congenital heart disease patients during pregnancy should be strengthened, comprehensively assessing the pregnancy risk, timely identifying relevant risk factors, and reducing the occurrence of cardiovascular and obstetric adverse events.

Ⅳ Consultation Process

1. Assess the patient's vital signs. If there are signs of life instability such as decreased oxygen saturation, shallow and rapid breathing, decreased blood pressure, and malignant arrhythmias, immediately administer emergency treatment such as mechanical ventilation, diuretic use, electrical cardioversion, temporary pacemaker, antiarrhythmic drugs, and vasopressor drugs to maintain blood pressure.

2. Supplement key medical history information, such as whether there is underlying heart disease, acute onset, whether it is accompanied by chest tightness, chest pain, profuse sweating, whether there is cyanosis, or hemoptysis.

3. Pay attention to important physical examination findings, such as whether dyspnea is aggravated in the supine position, whether the respiratory sounds in both lungs are symmetrical (whether there is weakened respiratory sounds on one side), whether there is cyanosis of the lips, whether there are heart murmurs on cardiac auscultation, whether there is a thrill on cardiac palpation, whether the heart border is enlarged on percussion, whether there are dry or moist rales, whether there is jugular venous distension, whether there is edema in the lower limbs (unilateral or bilateral), and even whether the patient is conscious.

4. Rapid auxiliary examinations are required, such as cardiac ultrasound, blood gas analysis, renal function, electrolytes, ECG, chest X-ray, BNP or NT-proBNP, D-dimer, etc. Carefully consider whether to perform a chest X-ray examination based on the pregnant woman's condition.

5. Treat the cause after a clear diagnosis. For example, if there is heart failure, administer

diuretics and vasodilators, and if necessary, use positive inotropic drugs or mechanical treatment to correct heart failure. For the treatment of pregnancy complicated by congenital heart disease, it is necessary to combine the results of cardiac ultrasound examination, assess the condition, determine the type of congenital heart disease, and provide corresponding management, as described above. Early termination of pregnancy is required in patients with cardiac function Class Ⅲ - Ⅳ , severe pulmonary hypertension, Eisenmenger syndrome, cyanotic congenital heart disease, transposition of the great arteries combined with ventricular dysfunction and/or severe tricuspid regurgitation.

Chapter 7

Cardiovascular Risk Assessment for Non-Cardiac Surgery

The global incidence of overall complications in non-cardiac surgeries ranges from 7% to 11%, with a mortality rate of 0.8%-1.5%. Among these complications, cardiovascular events account for 42%. Therefore, during non-cardiac surgeries, perioperative cardiovascular monitoring and management are crucial for patients to safely navigate through the perioperative period.

Section 1 Preoperative Assessment

I Overview

The causes of increased cardiovascular events due to surgery and trauma are mainly the systemic stress response caused by tissue damage and the imbalance of the sympathetic-vagal nervous system. Factors such as blood loss and fluid loss further aggravate the systemic stress response. Moreover, the surgical process itself can cause an imbalance in the body's coagulation and fibrinolysis system. Both can lead to increased myocardial oxygen consumption, resulting in coronary artery thrombotic events, myocardial ischemia, and heart failure.

The preoperative assessment of cardiovascular risk in non-cardiac surgery includes patient-related risk factors (such as patient temperature, changes in body position, intraoperative blood loss, fluid loss, and type of anesthesia), type of surgery (whether it is open surgery or laparoscopic surgery), and the urgency of the surgery (divided into emergency surgery, urgent surgery, and elective surgery). All of the above situations can seriously affect the patient's perioperative cardiovascular risk. The cardiovascular risks of various types of surgeries are shown in Table 7-1.

Table 7-1 Cardiovascular Risk of Various Types of Surgeries

Low Risk (Cardiac Events <1%)	Moderate Risk (Cardiac Events 1%-5%)	High Risk (Cardiac Events >5%)
Superficial surgery	Intraperitoneal surgery (splenectomy, esophageal hiatal hernia repair, and cholecystectomy)	Aortic and major vascular surgery
Chest surgery	Symptomatic carotid surgery	Open lower limb vascular reconstruction
Oral surgery	Small intrathoracic surgery	Open lower limb amputation
Thyroid surgery	Peripheral arterial angioplasty	Open lower limb thromboembolectomy
Transplant surgery	Vascular malformation repair	Duodenalpancreatic surgery

(Continued)

Low Risk (Cardiac Events <1%)	Moderate Risk (Cardiac Events 1%-5%)	High Risk (Cardiac Events >5%)
Eye surgery	Head and neck surgery	Partial hepatectomy
Asymptomatic carotid surgery	Major neurosurgical, gynecological, plastic, and urological surgery	Biliary tract surgery
Low risk (cardiac events <1%)	Medium risk (cardiac events 1%-5%)	High risk (cardiac events >5%)
Small plastic surgery	Kidney transplantation	Esophagectomy
Small urological surgery		Intestinal perforation repair
		Adrenalectomy
		Cholecystectomy
		Lung resection
		Lung or liver transplantation

Ⅱ Consultation Considerations

According to the ACC / AHA guidelines for perioperative cardiovascular risk assessment, the preoperative assessment of patients should include the following aspects.

1. Surgical risk factors: In cardiovascular assessment, anesthesia and surgery duration are the most commonly overlooked factors. Generally, the longer the anesthesia and surgery time, the higher the risk. Therefore, during consultation, attention should be paid to communicating with the patient's attending physician to correctly assess the situation.

2. Patient risk factors: The cardiac risk index assessment is as follows:

· High risk

(1) Acute coronary syndrome: myocardial infarction (7-30 days), unstable or severe angina pectoris (Canadian Cardiovascular Society Grade Ⅲ - Ⅳ).

(2) Decompensated heart failure, NYHA functional Class Ⅳ; new-onset heart failure or worsening of heart failure.

(3) Severe arrhythmias: second-degree Type Ⅱ or higher atrioventricular block, symptomatic ventricular arrhythmias, supraventricular arrhythmias with uncontrolled ventricular rate (resting heart rate >100 beats/min), symptomatic bradycardia.

(4) Severe valvular disease: severe aortic valve stenosis with valve area <1.0 cm^2 or mean pressure gradient >40 mmHg, or significant symptoms; significant symptoms of mitral valve stenosis; dyspnea, syncope, or heart failure after activity.

· Medium risk

(1) Mild angina pectoris (Canadian Cardiovascular Society Grade Ⅰ - Ⅱ).

(2) History of myocardial infarction or Q wave abnormality.

(3) Compensated heart failure or history of heart failure.

(4) Diabetes (insulin-dependent).

(5) Renal insufficiency (creatinine >2 mg/dL).

· Low risk

(1) Age <70.

(2) ECG showing left ventricular hypertrophy, left bundle branch block, ST-T abnormalities.

(3) Non-sinus rhythm (atrial fibrillation).

(4) Poor exercise tolerance (<4 METs).

(5) History of cerebrovascular accident.

(6) Uncontrolled hypertension (systolic >180 mmHg, diastolic >110 mmHg).

3. Preoperative testing

(1) Non-invasive examinations: ECG, exercise ECG test, myocardial nuclear imaging, ambulatory ECG, echocardiography, stress echocardiography, cardiac CT. Among them, ECG and echocardiography are essential examination items.

(2) Invasive examinations: A normal resting ECG cannot rule out coexisting coronary heart disease. Coronary angiography has confirmed that in patients with 50% obstruction of the three coronary arteries, 15% can have a normal resting ECG. Therefore, invasive examinations are indispensable for some patients.

4. Perioperative management includes acute coronary syndrome, arrhythmias, hypertension, perioperative anticoagulation / antiplatelet therapy and coping strategies, and related management of patients with cardiac pacemakers and ICDs.

Section 2 Surgical Risk Classification

Most patients with stable heart disease can tolerate low-risk and medium-risk surgeries without additional assessment, but it is recommended to assess cardiovascular disease risk with the assistance of anesthesiologists and optimize treatment. For patients with known heart disease who plan to undergo high-risk non-cardiac surgery or high-risk cardiac patients, a multidisciplinary team of experts, including anesthesiologists, cardiologists, surgeons, and other physicians such as internists and intensive care unit physicians if necessary, should jointly assess the degree of cardiovascular risk before surgery.

I Preoperative Risk Stratification

Perioperative risks are concentrated in a small proportion of surgical patients. Early identification of these individuals through perioperative risk stratification is of great value. The European Society of Cardiology (ESC)/European Society of Anaesthesiology (ESA) recommends using risk indicators for preoperative risk stratification of patients.

1. Revised Cardiac Risk Index (RCRI): Also known as the Lee index, it is a simple and widely used indicator for predicting major cardiac complications. It has 6 risk factors for severe perioperative cardiac events, including coronary heart disease (angina pectoris and/or old myocardial infarction), heart failure, stroke or transient ischemic attack, renal insufficiency, insulin-treated diabetes, and high-risk surgery type. Each item scores 1 point. A score of 0-1 is low risk, with an event incidence of 0.4%-0.9%; a score of 2 is medium risk, with an event

incidence of about 7%; a score of 3 or more is high risk, with an event incidence of about 11%.

2. The NSQIP model is an interactive online perioperative risk event calculator launched by the American College of Surgeons. This risk event calculator performs a series of clinical prediction models developed by applying the National Surgical Quality Improvement Program (NSQIP) registry study. The accuracy of the NSQIP model ranges from moderate to good and can predict a range of postoperative events, such as death, cardiac complications, pneumonia, and acute kidney injury, thereby reducing additional cumbersome bedside calculations.

Risk indicators can help assess cardiovascular risk before surgery but should not replace the decision-making of clinicians.

II Functional Reserve Assessment

The patient's functional capacity (FC) is a key determinant in assessing perioperative cardiovascular risk and can be evaluated using metabolic equivalents (METs).

A 40-year-old male weighing 70 kg has a baseline oxygen consumption of 3.5 mL/(Kg·min) at rest, which is equivalent to 1 MET. Excellent is >10 METs, good is 7-10 METs, and moderate is 4-7 METs. If the patient's FC is <4 METs, it indicates a higher incidence of perioperative cardiovascular risk.

METs can be estimated using questionnaires (Table 7-2).

Table 7-2 MET Estimation Table

1 MET	Eating, dressing, desk work
2 METs	Showering, shopping, cooking, walking down 8 steps
3 METs	Walking 1-2 street blocks on level ground; doing moderate-intensity housework such as vacuuming, sweeping, or carrying objects
4 METs	Doing light work in the yard (pulling weeds, weeding, sweeping, or pushing a lawn mower), painting, or light woodworking
5 METs	Brisk walking, dancing, washing a car
6 METs	Carrying own golf clubs for 9 holes, doing heavy woodworking, mowing the lawn with a push mower
7 METs	Carrying 27 kg of objects, doing strenuous outdoor work (such as digging, shoveling, etc.), walking uphill
8 METs	arrying objects upstairs, moving heavy furniture, jogging on level ground, climbing stairs quickly
9 METs	Cycling at a moderate pace, sawing wood, jumping rope (slowly)
10 METs	Fast swimming, cycling uphill, jogging at a speed of 10 km per hour
11 METs	Climbing two flights of stairs while carrying a load (such as a child), cross-country skiing, continuous fast cycling
12 METs	Continuous running on level ground (13 kilometers per hour)
13 METs	Any competitive activity: racing, rowing, cycling, intermittent sprinting

III Consultation Process

Patients' conditions are often complex, and multiple different risk factors may coexist simultaneously, requiring a comprehensive and indexed assessment based on the patient's actual situation; using the clinical risk indicators recommended by ESC / ESA for preoperative risk stratification of patients; and using the revised Cardiac Risk Index (RCRI) to predict the probability of major cardiac complications.

Section 3 Perioperative Cardiovascular Risk Assessment Methods

1. Refer to the seven-step preoperative cardiovascular risk assessment by ESC / ESA.

Step 1: Assess the urgency of the surgery. Emergency surgery does not allow for further cardiac examination and treatment. Clinical risk factors that may affect perioperative treatment and surgical procedures should be identified, recommendations for perioperative pharmacological treatment should be provided, cardiac events should be monitored, and previous cardiovascular pharmacological treatment should be continued. If it is not an emergency surgery, proceed to Step 2.

Step 2: Determine whether the patient has an unstable cardiac condition (unstable angina, acute heart failure, severe arrhythmia, symptomatic valvular heart disease, myocardial infarction within 30 days, and residual myocardial ischemia). If present, cancel or postpone the surgery, and have a multidisciplinary team of experts jointly assess the cardiovascular risk and discuss the preoperative treatment plan together. If there is no unstable cardiac condition, proceed to Step 3.

Step 3: Assess the cardiovascular risk of the surgery type (Table 7-3). Low-risk surgeries can be performed directly and adopt the lifestyle and pharmacolo-gical treatment recommendations provided by the guidelines based on the patient's risk factors. If there are more than one clinical risk factors, ECG mon-itoring is required. Medium or high-risk surgeries require further assessment (Step 4).

Table 7-3 Perioperative Cardiovascular Risk Assessment

Step	Emergency	Cardiovas-cular Status	Surgery Type	Functional Capacity	Cardiac Event Risk Factors	ECG	Cardiac Ultraso-und	Stress Test	BNP and Troponin
1	Emergency	Stable					Ⅲ C	Ⅲ C	
2	Emergency	Unstable							
	Elective	Unstable				Ⅰ C	Ⅰ C	Ⅲ C	Ⅱ B
3	Elective	Stable	Low risk		None	Ⅲ C	Ⅲ C	Ⅲ C	Ⅲ C
					≥1	Ⅱ$_b$C	Ⅲ C	Ⅲ C	
4	Elective	Stable	Medium or high risk	Good or ex-cellent			Ⅲ C	Ⅲ C	Ⅲ C
5	Elective	Stable	Medium risk	Poor	None	Ⅱ$_b$C	Ⅲ C		Ⅲ C
					≥1	IC	Ⅲ C	Ⅱ$_b$C	
6	Elective	Stable	High risk	Poor	1-2	IC	Ⅱ$_b$C	Ⅱ$_b$C	Ⅱ$_b$B
					≥3	IC	Ⅱ$_b$C	IC	Ⅱ$_b$B

Step 4: Assess the patient's functional capacity. Patients with moderate or good exercise tolerance (>4 METs) have a good prognosis and can undergo surgery. For those with definite coronary heart disease or myocardial ischemia, titrate low-dose beta-blockers preoperatively; for those with heart failure or reduced contractile function, administer ACEIs preoperatively; if undergoing vascular surgery, administer statins preoperatively. Patients with poor exercise tolerance (<4 METs) proceed to Step 5.

Step 5: Reassess the cardiovascular risk of the surgery type (Table 7-4). Patients with medium surgical risk can undergo surgery. In addition to the recommendations in Step 4, if there are more than one clinical risk factors, non-invasive stress testing is required. High-risk surgeries require further assessment (Step 6).

Table 7-4 Perioperative Cardiovascular Risk Management

Step	Emergency	Cardiovascular Status	Surgery Type	Functional Capacity	Cardiac Event Risk Factors	β-blockers	ACEIs	Aspirin	Statins	Coronary Revascularization
1	Emergency	Stable				Ⅰ B	Ⅱ$_a$C	Ⅱ$_b$B	Ⅰ C	Ⅲ C
2	Emergency	Unstable								Ⅱ$_a$C
	Elective	Unstable								Ⅰ A
3	Elective	Stable	Low risk		None	Ⅲ B	Ⅱ$_a$C	Ⅰ C	Ⅱ$_a$B	Ⅲ B
					≥1	Ⅱ$_b$B	Ⅱ$_a$C	Ⅰ C	Ⅱ$_a$B	Ⅲ B
4	Elective	Stable	Medium or high risk	Good or excellent		Ⅱ$_b$B	Ⅱ$_a$C	Ⅰ C	Ⅱ$_a$B	Ⅲ B
5	Elective	Stable	Medium risk	Poor	None	Ⅱ$_b$B	Ⅱ$_a$C	Ⅰ C	Ⅱ$_a$B	Ⅲ B
					≥1	Ⅱ$_b$B	Ⅱ$_a$C	Ⅰ C	Ⅱ$_a$B	Ⅲ B
6	Elective	Stable	High risk	Poor	1-2	Ⅱ$_b$B	Ⅱ$_a$C	Ⅰ C	Ⅱ$_a$B	Ⅱ$_b$B
					≥3	Ⅱ$_b$B	Ⅱ$_a$C	Ⅰ C	Ⅱ$_a$B	Ⅱ$_b$B

Step 6: Assess the patient's cardiac event risk factors. These include coronary heart disease (angina and/or old myocardial infarction), heart failure, stroke or transient ischemic attack, renal insufficiency, and insulin-treated diabetes. If there are≤2 cardiac event risk factors, in addition to the recommendations in Steps 4 and 5, resting cardiac ultrasound and BNP assessment of left ventricular function are required. For those with more than 3 cardiac event risk factors, proceed to Step 7.

Step 7: Non-invasive stress testing. Patients with no or mild to moderate myocardial ischemia should continue to undergo elective surgery. For patients with severe myocardial ischemia, individualized perioperative management is recommended. These patients need to carefully weigh the potential benefits and adverse consequences of the surgery and carefully evaluate the role of pharmacological treatment and/or coronary revascularization. For interventional treatment, the impact of antiplatelet therapy on surgery needs to be considered.

Non-cardiac surgery can be performed 2 weeks after PTCA, 4 weeks after bare-metal stent implantation, 12 months after older-generation drug-eluting stent implantation, and 6 months after new-generation drug-eluting stent implantation.

The perioperative cardiovascular risk assessment methods and management are shown in Tables 7-3 and 7-4. The similarities and differences in perioperative cardiovascular risk assessment between European and American guidelines are shown in Figure 7-1.

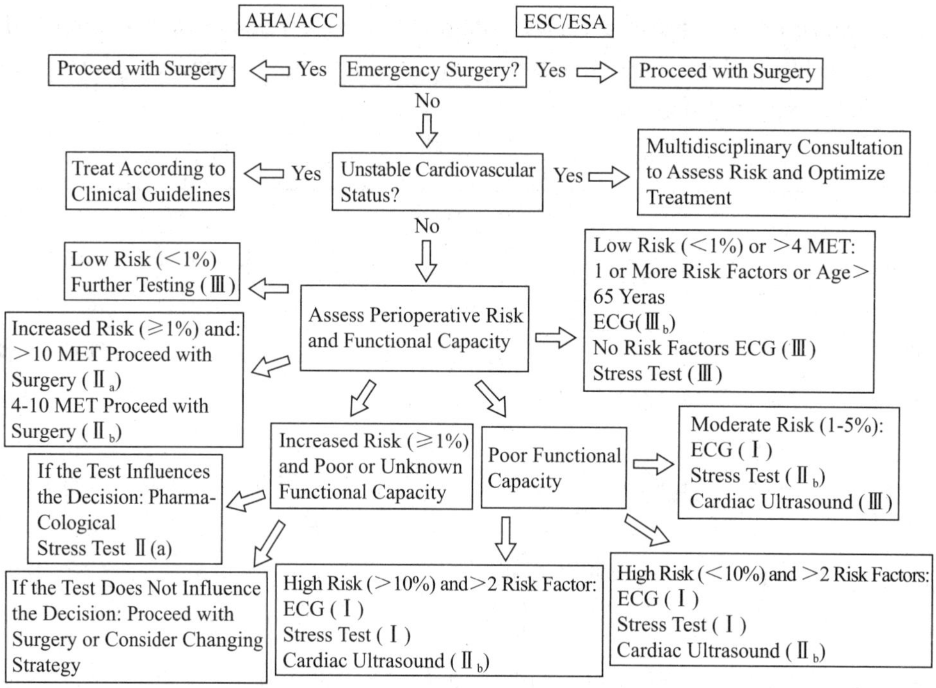

Figure 7-1 Similarities and Differences in Perioperative Cardiovascular Risk Assessment Between European and American Guidelines

2. Consultation Process. Some serious heart diseases can be identified through medical history, so correctable coronary heart disease risk factors and other comorbidities should be recorded. For patients who have been confirmed to have cardiovascular disease, any recent changes in symptoms should be clarified. While taking the medical history, an attempt should be made to determine the patient's functional capacity.

3. Assess perioperative-related risks using the seven-step preoperative cardiovascular risk assessment by ESC / ESA.

Section 4 Preoperative Assessment and Management of Com-bined Card-iovascular Diseases

I Coronary Heart Disease

For non-cardiac surgery, it is still unclear whether routine, preventive invasive coronary angiography and coronary revascularization can reduce coronary events. Therefore, the indications for perioperative coronary angiography and coronary revascularization are similar to those for non-surgical patients.

1. Coronary angiography

(1) No history of revascularization: Patients with ST-segment elevation myocardial infarction who are scheduled for non-emergency surgery should undergo urgent coronary angiography. Patients with NSTE-ACS who are scheduled for non-emergency surgery should undergo urgent or early interventional treatment based on risk assessment. Patients with myocardial ischemia who are scheduled for non-emergency surgery and still have unstable angina (CCS Grade Ⅲ - Ⅳ) after appropriate treatment should undergo coronary angiography. Coronary angiography is not recommended for patients with stable heart disease who are scheduled for low-risk surgery.

(2) History of revascularization and asymptomatic: Coronary angiography is not required for patients who have undergone CABG treatment within the past 6 years, unless the risk is high. If the patient has received bare-metal stent treatment, non-emergency surgery can be considered at least 4 weeks later, optimally 3 months later. If the patient has received drug-eluting stent treatment, non-emergency surgery should be performed at least 12 months after the procedure, and for second-generation drug-eluting stents, this period is 6 months. If the patient has recently undergone balloon angioplasty, surgery should be delayed for at least 2 weeks.

2. Coronary revascularization

(1) Preventive revascularization in stable / asymptomatic patients: For patients with stable coronary heart disease and indications for revascularization, late revascularization can be performed after successful non-cardiac surgery. For high-risk surgeries, preventive revascularization can be performed preoperatively based on the degree of stress-induced ischemia. Preventive revascularization is not recommended before low- and medium-risk surgeries.

(2) Revascularization in patients with NSTE-ACS: If non-cardiac surgery can be safely delayed in patients with NSTE-ACS, manage according to the NSTE-ACS guidelines. If it cannot be safely delayed, a team of experts needs to analyze and discuss the order of NSTE-ACS revascularization and non-cardiac surgery. For patients who have undergone non-cardiac surgery, enhanced pharmacotherapy and revascularization should be provided postoperatively according to the NSTE-ACS guidelines. If it is a semi-urgent non-cardiac surgery and there are indications for preoperative PCI, second-generation drug-eluting stents, bare-metal stents, or plain balloon angioplasty should be administered.

Ⅱ Chronic Heart Failure

Heart failure is a clear risk factor for perioperative and postoperative cardiac events. Left ventricular ejection fraction (LVEF) $\leqslant$35% is a strong predictor of postoperative cardiac events in vascular surgery. Although the impact of heart failure with preserved LVEF on morbidity and mortality is unclear, it is recommended to adopt management strategies similar to those for heart failure with reduced LVEF.

If the patient is diagnosed with heart failure and has recently undergone medium- or high-risk surgery, preoperative ultrasound assessment of left ventricular function and/or measurement of natriuretic peptide levels should be performed. beta-blockers, ACEIs or ARBs, mineralocorticoid receptor antagonists, and diuretics should be used according to guidelines. If heart failure is clinically suspected, left ventricular function should also be assessed and/or natriuretic peptide levels measured.

Beta-blockers should be used throughout the perioperative period, but high-dose preoperative use is not recommended. ACEIs or ARBs can be discontinued based on preoperative morning blood pressure levels. If continued, the patient's hemodynamics should be monitored and fluid resuscitation performed if necessary.

For newly diagnosed heart failure patients, heart failure treatment should be performed for at least 3 months, and medium- or high-risk surgery should be performed after improving cardiac function.

Ⅲ Hypertension

For newly diagnosed hypertensive patients, preoperative assessment of target organ damage and cardiovascular risk factors should be performed. Large fluctuations in blood pressure should be avoided preoperatively in hypertensive patients. Non-cardiac surgery should not be delayed in patients with systolic blood pressure $<$180 mmHg and diastolic blood pressure $<$110 mmHg.

Ⅳ Valvular Heart Disease

All patients with valvular heart disease undergoing medium- or high-risk surgery should have preoperative clinical and cardiac function assessment.

For patients with symptomatic severe aortic stenosis scheduled for elective low- or medium-risk non-cardiac surgery, or asymptomatic severe aortic stenosis scheduled for elective high-risk non-cardiac surgery, aortic valve replacement should be performed first after excluding high-risk surgical factors. For patients with symptomatic severe aortic stenosis and excessively high risk of valve surgery, aortic valve balloon valvuloplasty or transcatheter aortic valve implantation (TAVI) can be considered under the guidance of an expert team.

Elective non-cardiac surgery can be performed in patients with severe valvular regurgitation but without severe left ventricular dysfunction and heart failure. For patients with severe mitral stenosis and symptoms of pulmonary hypertension scheduled for elective medium- or high-risk non-cardiac surgery, percutaneous mitral commissurotomy should be performed first.

Ⅴ Arrhythmia

1. Ventricular arrhythmias: Oral antiarrhythmic drugs can be continued preoperatively, mainly used in patients with sustained ventricular tachycardia. It is not recommended for patients with ventricular premature beats.

2. Supraventricular arrhythmias: Oral antiarrhythmic drugs can be continued preoperatively. Electrical cardioversion is recommended for hemodynamically unstable patients, and stimulation of the vagus nerve or antiarrhythmic drugs are recommended to terminate supraventricular tachycardia in hemodynamically stable patients.

3. Bradyarrhythmias and pacing: The indications for temporary pacing during the

perioperative period are the same as those for permanent pacing. A dedicated person should be responsible for programming the patient's pacemaker before and after surgery. For patients with an implanted ICD, if the defibrillation function is turned off preoperatively, close ECG monitoring should be performed during surgery and an external defibrillator should be available.

Ⅵ Peripheral Diseases

All patients with peripheral arterial disease should receive antiplatelet and statin therapy and undergo blood pressure control. Preoperative clinical assessment of ischemic heart disease should be performed. If there are more than two risk factors, exercise ECG or stress imaging can be considered preoperatively. Routine preoperative use of beta-blockers is not recommended unless there is coexisting coronary heart disease or heart failure.

Ⅶ Pulmonary Vascular Diseases

Patients with chronic obstructive pulmonary disease should quit smoking for at least 2 months preoperatively. For high-risk patients with obesity hypoventilation syndrome, it is recommended to increase corresponding special examinations before elective surgery.

For patients with severe pulmonary hypertension undergoing elective surgery, a multidisciplinary team of experienced experts should intensify pharmacotherapy and continue using special drugs for treating pulmonary hypertension during the perioperative period, with close postoperative monitoring for 24 hours.

If right heart failure progresses postoperatively in patients with pulmonary hypertension, it is recommended that an experienced team of experts use diuretics and vasoactive drugs. For patients with severe right heart failure unresponsive to appropriate supportive treatment, it is recommended that an experienced team of experts temporarily use inhaled and/or intravenous pulmonary vasodilators preoperatively.

Ⅷ Congenital Heart Disease

Patients with simple defects, good compensation, and stable circulatory physiology can tolerate surgery. Preventive drugs should be used preoperatively to prevent infective endocarditis. However, for patients with complex congenital heart disease, it is recommended to consult relevant experts before surgery.

Ⅸ Consultation Process

1. Acute coronary syndrome: The incidence of perioperative acute myocardial infarction is 0.1%-0.4%, with a mortality rate of 10%, and the mortality rate of recurrent myocardial infarction is as high as 30%. The recurrence rate of myocardial infarction is 20% (5.7%) for surgery <3 months after myocardial infarction (most dangerous within 6 weeks), 10% (2.3%) for surgery 3-6 months after myocardial infarction, and 3%-5% for surgery >6 months after myocardial infarction. Whether non-cardiac surgery can be performed after myocardial infarction depends on the recovery of cardiac function and the degree of surgical risk. Non-emergency surgery should be postponed for patients with uncontrolled angina, ST-segment depression on ECG (≥0.2 mV),

or low left ventricular ejection fraction (<0.4). For patients with resectable malignant tumors, if it is a low-risk surgery, surgery can generally be considered 4-6 weeks after infarction; if it is a high-risk surgery, cardiac catheterization, echocardiography, or cardiac nuclear imaging should be performed first, and then it should be decided whether to perform PCI in advance.

Risk factors for recurrent myocardial infarction during the perioperative period include: ① The interval between myocardial infarction and surgery. Recent statistics show that the recurrence rate of myocardial infarction is 5.7% for patients undergoing surgery 0-3 months after myocardial infarction, which decreases to 2.3% for those undergoing surgery 3-6 months after myocardial infarction. This is related to the widespread use of acute thrombolysis and stent implantation after acute myocardial infarction, traumatic monitoring during the perioperative period, and increased means of hemodynamic regulation. Therefore, for patients with recent myocardial infarction, as long as their heart can tolerate it and there are active monitoring measures and other conditions, it is possible to tolerate emergency surgery outside the body cavity. *The 2002 ACC/AHA Guidelines* suggests that elective surgery should be performed 4-6 weeks after myocardial infarction. ② The location of myocardial infarction. Posterior wall myocardial infarction is often caused by right coronary artery occlusion, which can affect the blood supply to the sinoatrial node and atrioventricular node, so it is often accompanied by arrhythmia. ③ Age. The recurrence rate of myocardial infarction is higher in patients over 60 years old, especially between 65-74 years old. For patients with coronary heart disease over 70 years old, the perioperative mortality rate is 10 times higher than that of patients without coronary heart disease. ④ Surgery duration and location. The recurrence rate of myocardial infarction is 1.9% for surgeries shorter than 1 hour and 16.7% for surgeries longer than 6 hours. The recurrence rate of myocardial infarction is significantly increased in intrathoracic surgery, major vascular surgery, upper abdominal surgery, and emergency surgery.

2. Arrhythmias: Although some chronic arrhythmias are not contraindications for surgery, they still have surgical risks and should be treated as appropriate. For patients with severe atrioventricular block or sick sinus syndrome causing bradycardia, temporary pacing should be provided. For patients with frequent ventricular premature beats, the focus should be on assessing whether there is organic heart disease and the cardiac function status.

3. Management of hypertension: Patients with mild to moderate hypertension can undergo surgery as planned. If the baseline blood pressure is $>180/110$ mmHg, the surgery should be canceled. For those with blood pressure $>145/90$ mmHg, antihypertensive drugs should be given preoperatively. Blood pressure should be controlled at 130/80 mmHg for adults and 145/90 mmHg for the elderly. When it is difficult to control with oral medications, sodium nitroprusside or nitroglycerin intravenous infusion can be used (or in combination).

4. Perioperative anticoagulation / antiplatelet therapy and coping strategies: For patients requiring long-term anticoagulant therapy, such as after mechanical valve replacement surgery or atrial fibrillation with high-risk factors for stroke, long-term use of warfarin with an INR of 2-3 is more appropriate. If surgery is required, warfarin should be discontinued 3-5 days before surgery and replaced with heparin. Standard heparin should be discontinued 6 hours before surgery, and heparin replacement should be resumed 12 hours after surgery, or low-molecular-

weight heparin should be used as a replacement during the perioperative period. For patients after PCI, generally aspirin 100 mg/d and clopidogrel (Plavix, Taijia) 75 mg/d are used; for those with stent implantation: 6-12 months, if surgery is required, clopidogrel should be discontinued at least 5 days before surgery, preferably 2 weeks, for patients taking clopidogrel and aspirin.

5. Cardiac pacemakers: ① For patients with implanted cardiac pacemakers, electrosurgical knives can interfere with pacemaker function, leading to no pacing, increased pacing rate, lack of sensing, and other abnormalities. Consultation recommendations: For pacemaker-dependent patients, set to fixed-rate mode, turn off rate response function, and keep the electrosurgical knife's negative plate away from the pacemaker pocket. ② For patients with ICDs, electrosurgical knives can interfere with ICDs, leading to misperception and discharge. Consultation recommendations: Turn off the sensing function in ICD patients, apply external defibrillator electrode pads during surgery, and perform ECG monitoring after surgery.

Section 5 Perioperative Examinations

I Electrocardiogram

It is still unclear whether ECG monitoring is sensitive enough for the differentiation of myocardial ischemia, and the value of ECG monitoring is limited in the presence of intraventricular conduction block and ventricular pacing. The sensitivity of 24-hour dynamic monitoring for myocardial ischemia and ST-segment changes is 74%, and the specificity is 73%.

If the patient has risk factors, preoperative ECG can be considered. If the patient has no risk factors but is over 65 years old and undergoing medium- or high-risk surgery, preoperative ECG can be considered. If the patient has no risk factors and is undergoing low-risk surgery, ECG does not need to be a routine preoperative examination.

All surgical patients should undergo ECG monitoring during the perioperative period. When monitoring myocardial ischemia in the operating room, appropriate ECG leads should be selected, and 12-lead ECG monitoring can be performed for high-risk patients.

II Cardiac Color Doppler Ultrasound

Cardiac color Doppler ultrasound can measure the systolic and diastolic functions of the left and right ventricles, overall function, and segmental ventricular wall motion function, which is of great significance for the early diagnosis of heart failure in patients with heart disease, determining treatment plans, evaluating the efficacy of drug therapy, and indicating prognosis. Cardiac color Doppler ultrasound is non-invasive, simple in method, and can be repeated multiple times.

For low- and medium-risk surgeries, echocardiography does not need to be a routine preoperative examination. For heart failure patients with severe dyspnea or other changes in clinical status, left ventricular function should be assessed during the perioperative period. Left ventricular function assessment can be performed for patients with unexplained dyspnea and those with previous left ventricular dysfunction who have not been evaluated within 1 year.

For patients with a functional capacity <4 METs, cardiac event risk factors, and planned medium- or high-risk surgery, stress echocardiography can be performed. Preoperative stress echocardiography is not required for low-risk surgeries.

Ⅲ Transesophageal Echocardiography

Transesophageal echocardiography (TEE) has been widely used in cardiac surgery. TEE is quick, non-invasive, and can obtain rich information. TEE mainly reflects myocardial ischemia by observing segmental ventricular wall motion abnormalities. TEE examination is recommended for patients with acute severe and persistent hemodynamic instability during the perioperative period or during surgery. When ECG monitoring reveals significant ST-segment changes, the use of TEE to examine for severe myocardial ischemia should be considered.

Ⅳ CT Coronary Angiography

CT coronary angiography (CTA) has similar efficacy to coronary angiography (CAG) in diagnosing coronary artery lumen stenosis. The sensitivity of CTA for diagnosing obstructive coronary artery lesions is 98%, and the specificity is 88%. However, the assessment of lumen stenosis caused by lesions on CTA is not completely consistent with myocardial perfusion indicators. Therefore, CTA cannot replace the assessment and examination of myocardial and cardiac function indicators in moderate and severe lumen stenosis. The significance of performing CTA in low-risk acute chest pain patients is to exclude the possibility of coronary heart disease, screen patients with severe stenosis for CAG, and perform myocardial perfusion imaging for patients with moderate stenosis.

For patients with valvular heart disease, adult congenital heart disease, and low risk of coronary heart disease, preoperative CTA examination before non-cardiac surgery can accurately exclude the possibility of coronary heart disease, with a negative likelihood ratio of 0.01. More than 69% of patients can avoid invasive coronary angiography. For patients with a positive CTA diagnosis, conventional CAG still needs to be performed.

Ⅴ High-Sensitivity Cardiac Troponin (hs-cTn)

Compared with other biomarkers, cardiac troponin has higher sensitivity and tissue specificity in diagnosing myocardial infarction. High-sensitivity cardiac troponin (hs-cTn) refers to the detection of cTn using high-sensitivity methods. hs-cTn detection is not only more sensitive for the diagnosis of acute myocardial infarction but also very helpful for early risk stratification and prognostic assessment of ACS. Even a slight increase in hs-cTn during the perioperative period reflects associated myocardial injury and poor cardiac prognosis.

For the early diagnosis of acute myocardial infarction, guidelines recommend continuous testing for 3 hours with hs-cTn. The sensitivity of the second measurement within 3 hours for diagnosing myocardial infarction is close to 100%. Routine testing for risk stratification and cardiac event prevention is not recommended during the perioperative period. For high-risk surgical patients, testing of cardiac troponin can be considered preoperatively and within 48-72 hours after major surgery.

Ⅵ B-type Natriuretic Peptide (BNP)

B-type natriuretic peptide (BNP) and N-terminal pro-BNP (NT-ProBNP) are produced by cardiomyocytes due to increased myocardial wall tension. They can appear at any stage of heart failure and are independent of myocardial ischemia. NT-ProBNP and BNP are important predictors of many heart diseases.

NT-proBNP ⩾125 pg/mL and BNP ⩾35 pg/mL can be considered for chronic heart failure, while NT-proBNP ⩾300 pg/mL and BNP ⩾100 pg/mL can be considered for acute heart failure. However, this standard is not universally recognized, and the cutoff values of BNP and NT-proBNP for acute and chronic heart failure need to be adjusted according to age, weight, and renal function.

Routine testing of BNP and NT-proBNP for risk stratification and cardiac event prevention is not recommended during the perioperative period. For high-risk surgical patients, testing of NT-ProBNP and BNP can be considered to obtain information on the patient's perioperative and long-term postoperative prognosis.

Ⅶ Consultation Process

1. Inquire about cardiac-related medical history: Any chest tightness, chest pain, shortness of breath, palpitations, discomfort; any history of underlying heart disease, diabetes, or renal insufficiency, etc.

2. Cardiac-related physical examination to differentiate the presence of heart failure, valvular heart disease, arrhythmia, etc.

3. Basic items: BNP, myocardial enzymes, myocardial markers, D-dimer, ECG, exercise ECG test, dynamic ECG, echocardiography. For those with atrial fibrillation or atrial flutter, transesophageal echocardiography should be completed; for those with coronary heart disease, including ACS or unexplained cardiac enlargement, myocardial perfusion imaging and coronary CTA should be completed, and coronary angiography should be completed if necessary.

References

[1] Xue J, Pi L, Tan R, et al. Investigation on the time of emergency department visit and use of ambulances in patients with acute chest pain in Beijing [J]. *Chinese Journal of Emergency Medicine*, 2014, 23: 823-826.

[2] Nawar E W, Niska R W, Xu J. National hospital ambulatory medical care survey: 2005 emergency department summary [J]. *Adv Data*, 2007, 1-32.

[3] Li X, Murugiah K, Jian L, et al. 10 years trends in urban-rural disparities in treatments and outcomes after ST elevation myocardial infarction in China: insight from the CHINA PEACE Retrospective acute myocardial infarction [J]. *Lancet*, 2015, S2: 386.

[4] Editorial Board of Chinese Journal of Cardiovascular Diseases, Expert Group on Standardized Assessment and Diagnosis of Chest Pain. Chinese expert consensus on standardized assessment and diagnosis of chest pain [J]. *Chinese Circulation Journal*, 2014, S2: 42.

[5] Rittenberger J C, Beck P W, Paris P M. Errors of omission in the treatment of prehospital chest pain [J]. *Prehosp Emerg Care*, 2005, 9: 2-7.

[6] Yang X C, Zhang D P. Diagnosis and differential diagnosis of acute chest pain [J]. *Chinese Circulation Journal*, 2013, 28: 569-571.

[7] Anderson R T, Montori V M, Shah N D, et al. Effectiveness of chest pain choice decision aid in emergency department patients with low-risk chest pain: study protocol for a multicentre randomized trial [J]. *Trial*, 2014, 15: 166-177.

[8] Huo Y. Actively promote the demonstration of chest pain centers to improve the treatment level of ongoing myocardial infarction in China [J]. *Chinese Journal of Cardiovascular Diseases*, 2014, 42: 637-638.

[9] Li X, Sun J L, Dai G H, et al. Study on "one-stop imaging" of acute chest pain triad by 64-slice spiral CT [J]. *Clinical Radiology Journal*, 2011, 30: 974-978.

[10] Cheng S N, Zhao S H. Summary and interpretation of the 2015 ACR/ACC/AHA reasonable application of emergency imaging examination for chest pain [J]. *Chinese Circulation Journal*, 2016, 31 (z2): 22-27.

[11] *Report on Cardiovascular Diseases in China 2015* [M]. Beijing: Encyclopedia of China Publishing House, 2016.

[12] Pope J H, Ruthazer R, Beshansky J R, et al. Clinical features of emergency department patients presenting with symptoms suggestive of acute cardiac ischemia: A multicenter study [J]. *J Thromb Thrombolys*, 1998, 6: 63-74.

[13] Fesmire F M, Percy R F, Bardoner J B, et al. Usefulness of automated serial 12-lead ECG monitoring during the initial emergency department evaluation of patients with chest pain [J]. *Ann Emerg Med*, 1998, 31: 3-11.

[14] de Araujo G P, Ferreira J, Aguiar C, et al. TIMI, PURSUIT, and GRACE risk scores: Sustained prognostic value and interaction with revascularization in NSTE-ACS [J]. *Eur Heart J*, 2005, 26: 865-872.

[15] Aragam K G, Tamhane U U, Kline-Rogers E, et al. Does simplicity compromise accuracy in ACS risk prediction? A retrospective analysis of the TIMI and GRACE risk scores [J]. *PLoS One*, 2009, 4: e7947.

[16] Meine T J, Roe M T, Chen A Y, et al. Association of intravenous morphine use and outcomes in acute coronary syndromes: Results from the crusade quality improvement initiative [J]. *Am Heart J*, 2005, 149: 1043-

1049.

[17] Kubica J, Adamski P, Ostrowska M, et al. Morphine delays and attenuates ticagrelor exposure and action in patients with myocardial infarction: The randomized, double-blind, placebo-controlled IMPRESSION trial [J]. *Eur Heart J*, 2016, 37: 245-252.

[18] Lindholm D, Varenhorst C, Cannon C P, et al. Ticagrelor vs. Clopidogrel in patients with non-ST-elevation acute coronary syndrome with or without revascularization: Results from the PLATO trial [J]. *Eur Heart J*, 2014, 35: 2083-2093.

[19] Goyal A, Spertus J A, Gosch K, et al. Serum potassium levels and mortality in acute myocardial infarction [J]. *JAMA*, 2012, 307: 157-164.

[20] Ge J B, Xu Y J. *Internal Medicine*. 8th Edition [M] Beijing: People's Medical Publishing House, 2013: 359-372.

[21] White H D, Thygesen K, Alpert J S, et al. Clinical implications of the third universal definition of myocardial infarction [J]. *Heart*, 2014, 100 (5): 424-432.

[22] Interventional Cardiology Group of Chinese Society of Cardiology, Thrombosis Prevention Professional Committee of Cardiovascular Physician Branch of Chinese Medical Doctor Association, Editorial Board of Chinese Journal of Cardiovascular Diseases. Chinese guidelines for percutaneous coronary intervention (2016) [J]. *Chinese Journal of Cardiovascular Diseases*, 2016, 44 (5): 382-400.

[23] Roffi M, Patrono C, Collet J P, et al. 2015 ESC Guidelines for the management of acute coronary syndromes in patients presenting without persistent ST-segment elevation: Task force for the management of acute coronary syndromes in patients presenting without persistent ST-segment elevation of the European Society of Cardiology (ESC) [J]. *Eur Heart J*, 2016, 37 (3): 267-315.

[24] Wallentin L, Becker R C, Budaj A, et al. Ticagrelor versus clopidogrel in patients with acute coronary syndromes [J]. *N Engl J Med*, 2009, 361: 1045-1057.

[25] Han Y, Guo J, Zheng Y, et al. Bivalirudin vs heparin with or without tirofiban during primary percutaneous coronary intervention in acute myocardial infarction: the BRIGHT randomized clinical trial [J]. *JAMA*, 2015, 313 (13): 1336-1346.

[26] Huber K, Gersh B J, Goldstein P, et al. The organization, function, and outcomes of ST-elevation myocardial infarction networks worldwide: current state, unmet needs and future directions [J]. *Eur Heart J*, 2014, 35 (23): 1526-1532.

[27] Steg P G, Bonnefoy E, Chabaud S, et al. Impact of time to treatment on mortality after prehospital fibrinolysis or primary angioplasty: Data from the CAPTIM randomized clinical trial [J]. *Circulation*, 2003, 108 (23): 2851-2856.

[28] Editorial Board of Chinese Society of Cardiology, Editorial Board of Chinese Journal of Cardiovascular Diseases. Guidelines for the diagnosis and treatment of acute ST-segment elevation myocardial infarction [J]. *Chinese Journal of Cardiovascular Diseases*, 2015, 43 (5): 380-393.

[29] ISIS-4 (Fourth International Study of Infarct Survival) Collaborative Group. ISIS-4: A randomised factorial trial assessing early oral captopril, oral mononitrate, and intravenous magnesium sulphate in 58, 050 patients with suspected acute myocardial infarction [J]. *Lancet*, 1995, 345 (8951): 669-685.

[30] Pfeffer M A, McMurray J J, Velazquez E J, et al. Valsartan, captopril, or both in myocardial infarction complicated by heart failure, left ventricular dysfunction, or both [J]. *N Engl J Med*, 2003, 349 (20): 1893-1906.

[31] Baigent C, Keech A, Kearney P M, et al. Efficacy and safety of cholesterol-lowering treatment: Prospective meta-analysis of data from 90, 056 participants in 14 randomised trials of statins [J]. *Lancet*, 2005, 366 (9493): 1267-1278.

[32] Goldberg R J, Spencer F A, Gore J M, et al. Thirty-year trends (1975 to 2005) in the magnitude of, management of, and hospital death rates associated with cardiogenic shock in patients with acute myocardial infarction: a population-based perspective [J]. *Circulation*, 2009, 119 (9): 1211-1219.

[33] Lim Z, Gibbs G, Potts J E, et al. A review of sudden unexpected death in the young in British Columbia [J]. *Can J Cardiol*, 2010, 26 (1): 22-26.

[34] Perkins G D, Cooke M W. Variability in cardiac arrest survival: The NHS Ambulance Service Quality Indicators [J]. *Emerg Med J*, 2012, 29 (1): 3-5.

[35] Meaney P A, Nadkarni V M, Kern K B, et al. Rhythms and outcomes of adult in-hospital cardiac arrest [J]. *Crit Care Med*, 2010, 38 (1): 101-108.

[36] Chugh S S, Reinier K, Teodorescu C, et al. Epidemiology of sudden cardiac death: Clinical and research implications [J]. *Prog Cardiovasc Dis*, 2008, 51 (3): 213-228.

[37] Peberdy M A, Kaye W, Ornato J P, et al. Cardiopulmonary resuscitation of adults in the hospital: A report of 14, 720 cardiac arrests from the National Registry of Cardiopulmonary Resuscitation [J]. *Resuscitation*, 2003, 58 (3): 297-308.

[38] Rozenbaum E A, Shenkman L. Predicting outcome of in-hospital cardiopulmonary resuscitation [J]. *Crit Care Med*, 1988, 16 (6): 583-586.

[39] Hodgetts T J, Kenward G, Vlaconikolis I, et al. Incidence, location and reasons for avoidable in-hospital cardiac arrest in a district general hospital [J]. *Resuscitation*, 2002, 54 (2): 115-123.

[40] Cooper S, Janghorbani M, Cooper G. A decade of in-hospital resuscitation: Outcomes and prediction of survival [J]. *Resuscitation*, 2006, 68 (2): 231-237.

[41] Herlitz J, Andreasson A C, Bang A, et al. Long-term prognosis among survivors after in-hospital cardiac arrest [J]. *Resuscitation*, 2000, 45 (3): 167-171.

[42] Fredriksson M, Aune S, Thorén A B, et al. In-hospital cardiac arrest: An Utstein style report of seven years experience from the Sahlgrenska University Hospital [J]. *Resuscitation*, 2006, 68 (3): 351-358.

[43] Sandroni C, Nolan J, Cavallaro F, et al. In-hospital cardiac arrest: Incidence, prognosis and possible measures to improve survival [J]. *Intensive Care Med*, 2007, 33 (2): 237-245.

[44] Neumar R W, Shuster M, Callaway C W, et al. (Part 1) Executive summary: 2015 American Heart Association guidelines update for cardiopulmonary resuscitation and emergency cardiovascular care [J]. *Circulation*, 2015, 132 (18 Suppl 2): S315-S367.

[45] Idris A H, Guffey D, Pepe P E, et al. Chest compression rates and survival following out-of-hospital cardiac arrest [J]. *Crit Care Med*, 2015, 43 (4): 840-848.

[46] Vadeboncoeur T, Stolz U, Panchal A, et al. Chest compression depth and survival in out-of-hospital cardiac arrest [J]. *Resuscitation*, 2014, 85 (2): 182-188.

[47] Cheskes S, Schmicker R H, Christenson J, et al. Perishock pause: an independent predictor of survival from out-of-hospital shockable cardiac arrest [J]. *Circulation*, 2011, 124 (1): 58-66.

[48] Kleinman M E, Brennan E E, Goldberger Z D, et al. (Part 5) Adult basic life support and cardiopulmonary resuscitation quality: 2015 American Heart Association guidelines update for cardiopulmonary resuscitation and emergency cardiovascular care [J]. *Circulation*, 2015, 132 (18 Suppl 2): S414-S435.

[49] Elam J O, Greene D G, Schneider M A, et al. Head-tilt method of oral resuscitation [J]. *J Am Med Assoc*, 1960, 172 (8): 812-815.

[50] Singletary E M, Zideman D A, De Buck E D, et al. (Part 9) First aid: 2015 international consensus on first aid science with treatment recommendations [J]. *Circulation*, 2015, 132 (16 Suppl 1): S269-S311.

[51] Berg R A, Hemphill R, Abella B S, et al. (Part 5) Adult basic life support: 2010 American Heart

Association guidelines for cardiopulmonary resuscitation and emergency cardiovascular care [J]. *Circulation*, 2010, 122 (18 Suppl 3): S685-S705.

[52] Dörges V, Ocker H, Hagelberg S, et al. Smaller tidal volumes with room-air are not sufficient to ensure adequate oxygenation during bag-valve-mask ventilation [J]. *Resuscitation*, 2000, 44 (1): 37-41.

[53] Hallstrom A P, Ornato J P, Weisfeldt M, et al. Public-access defibrillation and survival after out-of-hospital cardiac arrest [J]. *N Engl J Med*, 2004, 351 (7): 637-646.

[54] Larsen M P, Eisenberg M S, Cummins R O, et al. Predicting survival from out-of-hospital cardiac arrest: a graphic model [J]. *Ann Emerg Med*, 1993, 22 (11): 1652-1658.

[55] Eftestøl T, Wik L, Sunde K, et al. Effects of cardiopulmonary resuscitation on predictors of ventricular fibrillation defibrillation success during out-of-hospital cardiac arrest [J]. *Circulation*, 2004, 110 (1): 10-15.

[56] van Alem A P, Chapman F W, Lank P, et al. A prospective, randomised and blinded comparison of first shock success of monophasic and biphasic waveforms in out-of-hospital cardiac arrest [J]. *Resuscitation*, 2003, 58 (1): 17-24.

[57] Dorian P, Cass D, Schwartz B, et al. Amiodarone as compared with lidocaine for shock-resistant ventricular fibrillation [J]. *N Engl J Med*, 2002, 346 (12): 884-890.

[58] Kudenchuk P J, Brown S P, Daya M, et al. Amiodarone, lidocaine, or placebo in out-of-hospital cardiac arrest [J]. *N Engl J Med*, 2016, 374 (18): 1711-1722.

[59] Varon J, Acosta P. Norepinephrine and the kidneys after cardiopulmonary resuscitation: What is the fuzz all about [J]. *Am J Emerg Med*, 2011, 29 (8): 922-923.

[60] Dybvik T, Strand T, Steen P A. Buffer therapy during out-of-hospital cardiopulmonary resuscitation [J]. *Resuscitation*, 1995, 29 (2): 89-95.

[61] Vukmir R B, Katz L. Sodium bicarbonate improves outcome in prolonged prehospital cardiac arrest [J]. *Am J Emerg Med*, 2006, 24 (2): 156-161.

[62] Chinese Abdomen-to-CPR Collaborative Group. Expert consensus on abdomen-to-CPR [J]. *Chinese Journal of Emergency Medicine*, 2013, 22 (9): 957-959.

[63] Vallejo-Manzur F, Varon J, Fromm R Jr. , et al. Moritz Schiff and the history of open-chest cardiac massage [J]. *Resuscitation*, 2002, 53 (1): 3-5.

[64] Ewy G A, Zuercher M. Role of manual and mechanical chest compressions during resuscitation efforts throughout cardiac arrest [J]. *Future Cardiol*, 2013, 9 (6): 863-873.

[65] Couper K, Yeung J, Nicholson T, et al. Mechanical chest compression devices at in-hospital cardiac arrest: A systematic review and meta-analysis [J]. *Resuscitation*, 2016, 103: 24-31.

[66] Lavonas E J, Drennan I R, Gabrielli A, et al. (Part 10) Special circumstances of resuscitation: 2015 American Heart Association guidelines update for cardiopulmonary resuscitation and emergency cardiovascular care [J]. *Circulation*, 2015, 132 (18 Suppl 2): S501-S518.

[67] Wang L X, Cheng X S. Prolonged cardiopulmonary resuscitation should be emphasized [J]. *Chinese Critical Care and Emergency Medicine*, 2002, 14 (4): 195-196.

[68] Kim H K, Jeong M H, Ahn Y, et al. Clinical outcomes of the intra-aortic balloon pump for resuscitated patients with acute myocardial infarction complicated by cardiac arrest [J]. *J Cardiol*, 2016, 67 (1): 57-63.

[69] Thiagarajan R R, Brogan T V, Scheurer M A, et al. Extracorporeal membrane oxygenation to support cardiopulmonary resuscitation in adults [J]. *Ann Thorac Surg*, 2009, 87 (3): 778-785.

[70] Callaway C W, Donnino M W, Fink E L, et al. (Part 8) Post-cardiac arrest care: 2015 American Heart Association guidelines update for cardiopulmonary resuscitation and emergency cardiovascular care [J]. *Circulation*, 2015, 132 (18 Suppl 2): S465-S482.

[71] Hollenbeck R D, McPherson J A, Mooney M R, et al. Early cardiac catheterization is associated with improved survival in comatose survivors of cardiac arrest without STEMI [J]. *Resuscitation*, 2014, 85 (1): 88-95.

[72] Sabahi M, Fanaei S A, Ziaee S A, et al. Efficacy of a rapid response team on reducing the incidence and mortality of unexpected cardiac arrests [J]. *Trauma Mon*, 2012, 17 (2): 270-274.

[73] Kronick S L, Kurz M C, Lin S, et al. (Part 4) Systems of care and continuous quality improvement: 2015 American Heart Association guidelines update for cardiopulmonary resuscitation and emergency cardiovascular care [J]. *Circulation*, 2015, 132 (18 Suppl 2): S397-S413.

[74] Vivekanandan S, Swaminathan R. Clinically effective CK-MB reporting: How to do it [J]. *J Postgrad Med*, 2010, 56: 226-228.

[75] Chen J Y, Shi Y L, Li L H, et al. Comparative analysis of serum CK-MB mass and activity detection results [J]. *Journal of Southern Medical University*, 2010, 6: 455-456.

[76] Strobel E S, Fritschka E, Schimke E, et al. Differential diagnosis macro/CK type 1 in thoracic pain syndrome and increased CK-MB [J]. *Med Klin* (Munich), 2003, 98: 583-586.

[77] Feng L, Ma X G, Sun Y Z, et al. Analysis of causes of false increase in serum CK-MB activity and its clinical significance [J]. *Chinese Journal of Experimental Diagnostics*, 2007, 11: 1041-1043.

[78] Sun G H. Discussion on the application of CK-MB mass and CK-MB activity in acute myocardial infarction and traumatic brain diseases [J]. *Journal of Dalian Medical University*, 2009, 4: 335-337.

[79] Navin T R, Hager W D. Creatine kinase MB isoenzyme in the evaluation of myocardial infarction [J]. *Curr Probl Cardiol*, 1979, 3: 1-32.

[80] Sadoh W E, Eregie C O, Nwaneri D U, et al. The diagnostic value of both troponin T and creatinine kinase isoenzyme (CK-MB) in detecting combined renal and myocardial injuries in asphyxiated infants [J]. *PLoS One*, 2014, 9 (3): e91338.

[81] Nakanishi R, Rajani R, Ishikawa Y, et al. Myocardial bridging on coronary CTA: An innocent bystander or a culprit in myocardial infarction [J]. *J Cardiovasc Comput Tomogr*, 2012, 6 (1): 3-13.

[82] Liu S H, Yang Q, Chen J H, et al. Myocardial bridging on dual-source computed tomography: Degree of systolic compression of mural coronary artery correlating with length and depth of the myocardial bridge [J]. *Clin Imaging*, 2010, 34 (2): 83.

[83] Alegria J R, Herrmann J, Holmes D J, et al. Myocardial bridging [J]. *Eur Heart J*, 2005, 26 (12): 1159-1168.

[84] Angelini P. Coronary myocardial bridges: Pathophysiology and clinical relevance [J]. *J Am Coll Cardiol*, 2014, 64 (20): 2178.

[85] Tremmel J A, Schnittger I. Myocardial bridging [J]. *J Am Coll Cardiol*, 2014, 64 (20): 2178-2179.

[86] Schwarz E R, Gupta R, Haager P K, et al. Myocardial bridging in absence of coronary artery disease: Proposal of a new classification based on clinical-angiographic data and long-term follow-up [J]. *Cardiology*, 2009, 112 (1): 13-21.

[87] Alessandri N, Giudici A D, De Angelis S, et al. Efficacy of calcium channel blockers in the treatment of the Myocardial Bridging: A pilot study [J]. *Eur Rev Med Pharmacol Sci*, 2012, 16 (6): 829-834.

[88] Ishikawa Y, Akasaka Y, Suzuki K, et al. Anatomic properties of myocardial bridge predisposing to myocardial infarction [J]. *Circulation*, 2009, 120 (5): 376-383.

[89] Jy Q, Zhang F, Dong M, et al. Prevalence and characteristics of myocardial bridging in coronary angiogram—data from consecutive 5, 525 patients [J]. *Chin Med J* (Engl), 2009, 122 (6): 632-635.

[90] Ferreira A G, Trotter S E, Knig B, et al. Myocardial bridges: morphological and functional aspects [J]. *Br Heart J*, 1991, 66 (5): 364-367.

[91] Ural E, Bildirici U, Celikyurt U, et al. Long-term prognosis of noninterventionally followed patients with isolated myocardial bridge and severe systolic compression of the left anterior descending coronary artery [J]. *Clin Cardiol*, 2009, 32 (8): 454-457.

[92] Noble J, Bourassa M G, Petitclerc R, et al. Myocardial bridging and milking effect of the left anterior descending coronary artery: Normal variant or obstruction [J]. *Am J Cardiol*, 1976, 37 (7): 993-999.

[93] Ge J, Erbel R, Gdrge G, et al. High wall shear stress proximal to myocardial bridging and atherosclerosis: Intracoronary ultrasound and pressure measurements [J]. *Br Heart*, 1995, 73 (5): 462-465.

[94] Bourassa M G, Butnaru A, Lespérance J, et al. Symptomatic myocardial bridges: Overview of ischemic mechanisms and current diagnostic and treatment strategies [J]. *J Am Coll Cardiol*, 2003, 41 (3): 351-359.

[95] Esteves V, Barbosa R R, Costa J R, et al. Acute myocardial infarction associated to myocardial bridging [J]. *Rev Bras Cardiol Invasiva*, 2010, 18 (4): 468-472.

[96] Rujic D, Nielsen M L. Nitroglycerine induced acute myocardial infarction in a patient with myocardial bridging [J]. *Case Rep Cardiol*, 2014, 2014: 289-879.

[97] Derkacz A, Nowieki P, Protasiewicz M, et al. Multiple percutaneous coronary stent implantation due to myocardial bridging—a case report [J]. *Kardiol Pol*, 2007, 65: 684-687.

[98] Tandar A, Whisenant B K, Michaels A D. Stent fracture following stenting of a myocardial bridge: Report of two cases [J]. *Catheter Cardio Inte*, 2008, 71: 191-196.

[99] Attaran S, Moscarelli M, Athanasiou T, et al. Is coronary artery bypass grafting an acceptable alternative to myotomy for the treatment of myocardial bridging? [J]. *Interact Cardiov Th*, 2013, 16 (3): 347-349.

[100] Yang L, Zhao L F, Li Y, et al. Diagnosis of myocardial bridge and wall coronary artery by multi-slice spiral CT and its clinical significance [J]. *Chinese Medical Journal*, 2006, 86 (40): 2858-2862.

[101] Greenland P, Alpert J S, Beller G A, et al. 2010 ACCF/AHA guideline for assessment of cardiovascular risk in asymptomatic adults: A report of the American College of Cardiology Foundation / American Heart Association Task Force on Practice Guidelines [J]. *J Am Cardiol*, 2010, 56: 50-103.

[102] Chobanian A V, Bakris G L, Black H R, et al. The Seventh Report of the Joint National Committee on Prevention, Detection, Evaluation, and Treatment of High Blood Pressure: the JNC 7 report [J]. *JAMA*, 2003, 289: 2560-2572.

[103] National Institute for Health and Clinical Excellence-Hypertension-Clinical management of primary hypertension in adults [EB/OL]. 2011.

[104] Graham I, Atar D, Borch-Johnsen K, et al. European guidelines on cardiovascular disease prevention in clinical practice: Full text—Fourth Joint Task Force of the European Society of Cardiology and other societies on cardiovascular disease prevention in clinical practice [J]. *Eur J Cardiovasc Prev Rehabil*, 2007, 14: S1-113.

[105] Erhardt L. Cigarette smoking: An undertreated risk factor for cardiovascular disease [J]. *Atherosclerosis*, 2009, 205: 23-32.

[106] Roger V L, Go A S, Lioyd-Jones D M, et al. Heart disease and stroke statistics-2011 update: A report from the American Heart Association [J]. *Circulation*, 2011, 123: 218-209.

[107] Schinkel A F, Bax J J, Geleijnse M L, et al. Noninvasive evaluation of ischaemic heart disease: Myocardial perfusion imaging or stress echocardiography [J]. *Eur Heart J*, 2003, 24: 789-800.

[108] Neefjes L A, Ten Kate G J, Rossi A, et al. CT coronary plaque burden in asymptomatic patients with familial hypercholesterolaemia [J]. *Heart*, 2011, 32: 1865-1874.

[109] Hadamitzky M, Meyer T, Hein F, et al. Prognostic value of coronary computed tomographic angiography in asymptomatic patients [J]. *Am J Cardiol*, 2010, 105: 1764-1851.

[110] Smith S C Jr, Allen J, Blair S N, et al. AHA/ACC guidelines for secondary prevention for patients with

coronary and atherosclerotic vascular disease: 2006 update: endorsed by the National Heart, Lung, and Blood institute [J]. *Circulation*, 2006, 113: 2363-2372.

[111] US Preventive Services Task Force. Aspirin for prevention of cardiovascular disease: U. S Prevention Services Task Force recommendation statement [J]. *Ann Inter Med*, 2009, 150: 396-404.

[112] Becker R C, Gurbel P A. Platelet P2Y12 receptor antagonist pharmacokinetics and pharmacodynamics: A foundation for distinguishing mechanisms of bleeding and anticipated risk for platelet-directed therapies [J]. *Thromb Haemost*, 2010, 103 (3): 535-544.

[113] Wallentin L, James S, Storey R F, et al. Effect of CYP2C19 and ABCB1 single nucleotide polymorphisms on outcomes of treatment with ticagrelor versus clopidogrel for acute coronary syndromes: A genetic substudy of the PLATO trial [J]. *Lancet*, 2010, 376 (9749): 1320-1328.

[114] Stapleton M P. Sir James Black and propranolol. The role of the basic sciences in the history of cardiovascular pharmacology [J]. *Tex Heart Inst J*, 1997, 24 (4): 336-342.

[115] Hamm C W, Bassand J P, Agewall S, et al. ESC Guidelines for the management of acute coronary syndromes in patients presenting without persistent ST-segment elevation: The task force for the management of acute coronary syndromes in patients presenting without persistent ST-segment elevation of the ESC [J]. *Eur Heart J*, 2011, 32: 2999-3054.

[116] Morrow D A, Givertz M M. Modulation of myocardial energetics: Emerging evidence for a therapeutic target in cardiovascular disease [J]. *Circulation*, 2005, 112: 3218-3221.

[117] Chazov E I, Lepakchin V K, Zharova E A, et al. Trimetazidine in angina combination therapy-the TACT study: Trimetazidine versus conventional treatment in patients with stable angina pectoris in a randomized, placebo-controlled, multicenter study [J]. *Am J Ther*, 2005, 12: 35-42.

[118] Walker A, McMurray J, Stewart S, et al. Economic evaluation of the impact of nicorandil in angina (IONA) trial [J]. *Heart*, 2006, 92: 619-624.

[119] Patel M R, Dehmer G J, Hirshfeld J W, et al. ACCF/SCAI/STS/AATS/AHA/ASNC/HFSA/SCCT 2012 Appropriate use criteria for coronary revascularization focused update: A report of the American College of Cardiology Foundation Appropriate Use Criteria Task Force, Society for Cardiovascular Angiography and Interventions, Society of Thoracic Surgeons, American Association for Thoracic Surgery, American Heart Association, American Society of Nuclear Cardiology, and the Society of Cardiovascular Computed Tomography [J]. *JAm CollCardiol*, 2012, 59 (9): 857-881.

[120] Windecker S, Kolh P, Alfonso F, et al. 2014 ESC/EACTS Guidelines on myocardial revascularization: The Task Force on Myocardial Revascularization of the European Society of Cardiology (ESC) and the European Association for Cardio-Thoracic Surgery (EACTS) developed with the special contribution of the European Association of Percutaneous Cardiovascular Interventions (EAPCI) [J]. *Eur Heart J*, 2014, 35 (37): 2541-2619.

[121] Nashef S A, Roques F, Sharples L D, et al. EuroSCORE Ⅱ [J]. *Eur J Cardiothorac Surg*, 2012, 41 (4): 734-745.

[122] Sianos G, Morel M A, Kappetein A P, et al. The SYNTAX Score: An angiographic tool grading the complexity of coronary artery disease [J]. *EuroIntervention*, 2005, 1 (2): 219-227.

[123] Farooq V, van Klaveren D, Steyerberg E W, et al. Anatomical and clinical characteristics to guide decision making between coronary artery bypass surgery and percutaneous coronary intervention for individual patients: Development and validation of SYNTAX score Ⅱ [J]. *Lancet*, 2013, 381 (9867): 639-650.

[124] Interventional Cardiology Group of Chinese Society of Cardiology, Editorial Board of Chinese Journal of Cardiovascular Diseases. Chinese guidelines for percutaneous coronary intervention 2016 [J]. *Chinese Journal of Cardiovascular Diseases*, 2016, 44 (5): 382-400.

[125] Fihn S D, Gardin J M, Abrams J, et al. 2012 ACCF/AHA/ACP/AATS/PCNA/SCAI/STS guideline for the diagnosis and management of patients with stable ischemic heart disease: A report of the American College of Cardiology Foundation/American Heart Association Task Force on Practice Guidelines, and the American College of Physicians, American Association for Thoracic Surgery, Preventive Cardiovascular Nurses Association, Society for Cardiovascular Angiography and Interventions, and Society of Thoracic Surgeons [J]. *J Am Coll Cardiol*, 2012, 60: e44-e164.

[126] Task Force on Myocardial Revascularization of the European Society of Cardiology (ESC) and the European Association for Cardio-Thoracic Surgery (EACTS), European Association for Percutaneous Cardiovascular Interventions (EAPCI), Wijns W, et al. Guidelines on myocardial revascularization [J]. *Eur Heart J*, 2010, 31: 2501-2555.

[127] Baber U, Mehran R, Sharma S K, et al. Impact of the everolimus-eluting stent on stent thrombosis: A meta-analysis of 13 randomized trials [J]. *J Am Coll Cardiol*, 2011, 58: 1569-1577.

[128] Bangalore S, Kumar S, Fusaro M, et al. Short-term and long-term outcomes with drug-eluting and bare-metal coronary stents: A mixed-treatment comparison analysis of 117, 762 patient-years of follow-up from randomized trials [J]. *Circulation*, 2012, 125: 2873-2891.

[129] Scirica B M, Morrow D A, Budaj A, et al. Ischemia detected on continuous electrocardiography after acute coronary syndrome: Observations from the MERLIN-TIMI 36 (metabolic efficiency with ranolazine for less ischemia in non-ST-elevation acute coronary syndrome-thrombolysis in myocardial infarction 36) trial [J]. *J Am Coll Cardiol*, 2009, 53 (16): 1411-1421.

[130] Akkerhuis K M, Klootwijk P A, Lindeboom W, et al. Recurrent ischaemia during continuous multilead ST-segment monitoring identifies patients with acute coronary syndromes at high risk of adverse cardiac events: Meta-analysis of three studies involving 995 patients [J]. *Eur Heart J*, 2001, 22 (21): 1997-2006.

[131] Amsterdam E A, Kirk J D, Diercks D B, et al. Immediate exercise testing to evaluate low-risk patients presenting to the emergency department with chest pain [J]. *J Am Coll Cardiol*, 2002, 40 (2): 251-256.

[132] El Mahalawy N, Abdel-Salam Z, Samir A, et al. Left ventricular transient ischemic dilation during dobutamine stress echocardiography predicts multi-vessel coronary artery disease [J]. *J Cardiol*, 2009, 54: 255-261.

[133] Viu K, Mitriagina S N, Syrkin A L, et al. Cost-effect clinical analysis in choice of coronary heart disease diagnosis [J]. *Ter Arkh*, 2008, 80: 8-11.

[134] Nucifora G, Schuijf J D, van Werkhoven J M, et al. Relation between Framingham risk categories and the presence of functionally relevant coronary lesions as determined on multislice computed tomography and stress testing [J]. *Am J Cardiol*, 2009, 104: 758-763.

[135] Muller J E, Abela G S, Nesto R W, et al. Triggers, acute risk factors and vulnerable plaques: The lexicon of a new frontier [J]. *J Am Coll Cardiol*, 1994, 23 (3): 809-813.

[136] Glaser R, Selzer F, Faxon D P, et al. Clinical progression of incidental, asymptomatic lesions discovered during culprit vessel coronary intervention [J]. *Circulation*, 2005, 111 (2): 143-149.

[137] Farb A, Burke A P, Tang A L, et al. Coronary plaque erosion without rupture into a lipid core: A frequent cause of coronary thrombosis in sudden coronary death [J]. *Circulation*, 1996, 93 (7): 1354-1363.

[138] Valentin F, Fayad Z A, Moreno P R, et al. Atherothrombosis and high-risk plaque: (Part Ⅱ) Approaches by noninvasive computed tomographic/magnetic resonance imaging [J]. *J Am Coll Cardiol*, 2005, 46 (7): 1209-1218.

[139] Interventional Cardiology Group of Chinese Society of Cardiology, Thrombosis Prevention Professional Committee of Cardiovascular Physician Branch of Chinese Medical Doctor Association, Editorial

Board of Chinese Journal of Cardiovascular Diseases Expert Group. 2016 Chinese guidelines for percutaneous coronary intervention [J]. *Chinese Journal of Cardiovascular Diseases*, 2016, 44 (5): 382-400.

[140] Di S G, Patti G, Pasceri V, et al. Effectiveness of in-laboratory high-dose clopidogrel loading versus routine pre-load in patients undergoing percutaneous coronary intervention: Results of the ARMYDA-5 PRELOAD (antiplatelet therapy for reduction of myocardial damage during angioplasty) randomized trial [J]. *J Am Coll Cardiol*, 2010, 56 (7): 550-557.

[141] Widimsky P, Motovská Z, Simek S, et al. Clopidogrel pre-treatment in stable angina: For all patients >6 h before elective coronary angiography or only for angiographically selected patients a few minutes before PCI? A randomized multicentre trial PRAGUE-8 [J]. *Eur Heart J*, 2008, 29 (12): 1495-1503.

[142] Baigent C, Blackwell L, Collins R, et al. Aspirin in the primary and secondary prevention of vascular disease: Collaborative meta-analysis of individual participant data from randomised trials [J]. *Lancet*, 2009, 373 (9678): 1849-1860.

[143] Steinhubl S R, Berger P B, Mann J T, et al. Early and sustained dual oral antiplatelet therapy following percutaneous coronary intervention: A randomized controlled trial [J]. *JAMA*, 2002, 288 (19): 2411-2420.

[144] Valgimigli M, Campo G, Monti M, et al. Short- versus long-term duration of dual-antiplatelet therapy after coronary stenting: A randomized multicenter trial [J]. *Circulation*, 2012, 125 (16): 2015-2026.

[145] Gwon H C, Hahn J Y, Park K W, et al. Six-month versus 12-month dual antiplatelet therapy after implantation of drug-eluting stents: The Efficacy of Xience/Promus Versus Cypher to Reduce Late Loss After Stenting (EXCELLENT) randomized, multicenter study [J]. *Circulation*, 2012, 125 (3): 505-513.

[146] Han Y, Jing Q, Li Y, et al. Sustained clinical safety and efficacy of a biodegradable-polymer coated sirolimus-eluting stent in "real-world" practice: Three-year outcomes of the CREATE (multi-center registry of EXCEL biodegradable polymer drug eluting stents) study [J]. *Catheter Cardiovasc Interv*, 2012, 79 (2): 211-216.

[147] Feres F, Costa R A, Abizaid A, et al. Three vs twelve months of dual antiplatelet therapy after zotarolimus-eluting stents: The OPTIMIZE randomized trial [J]. *JAMA*, 2013, 310 (23): 2510-2522.

[148] Kim B K, Hong M K, Shin D H, et al. A new strategy for discontinuation of dual antiplatelet therapy: The RESET Trial (REal safety and efficacy of 3-month dual antiplatelet therapy following endeavor zotarolimus-eluting stent implantation) [J]. *J Am Coll Cardiol*, 2012, 60 (15): 1340-1348.

[149] Collaborative meta-analysis of randomised trials of antiplatelet therapy for prevention of death, myocardial infarction, and stroke in high risk patients [J]. *BMJ*, 2002, 324 (7329): 71-86.

[150] Patrono C, Andreotti F, Arnesen H, et al. Antiplatelet agents for the treatment and prevention of atherothrombosis [J]. *Eur Heart J*, 2011, 32 (23): 2922-2932.

[151] Dewilde W J, Oirbans T, Verheugt F W, et al. WOEST study investigators—Use of clopidogrel with or without aspirin in patients taking oral anticoagulant therapy and undergoing percutaneous coronary intervention: An open-label, randomised, controlled trial [J]. *Lancet*, 2013, 381 (9872): 1107-1115.

[152] European Heart Rhythm Association, et al. Guidelines for the management of atrial fibrillation: The Task Force for the Management of Atrial Fibrillation of the European Society of Cardiology (ESC) [J]. *Eur Heart J*, 2010, 31 (19): 2369-2429.

[153] January C T, Wann L S, Alpert J S, et al. American College of Cardiology/American Heart Association Task Force on Practice Guidelines. 2014 AHA/ACC/HRS guideline for the management of patients with atrial fibrillation: A report of the American College of Cardiology/American Heart Association Task Force on Practice Guidelines and the Heart Rhythm Society [J]. *J Am Coll Cardiol*, 2014, 64 (21): e1-e76.

[154] Lip G Y, Windecker S, Huber K, et al. Management of antithrombotic therapy in atrial fibrillation patients presenting with acute coronary syndrome and/or undergoing percutaneous coronary or valve

interventions: A joint consensus document of the European Society of Cardiology Working Group on Thrombosis, European Heart Rhythm Association (EHRA), European Association of Percutaneous Cardiovascular Interventions (EAPCI) and European Association of Acute Cardiac Care (ACCA) endorsed by the Heart Rhythm Society (HRS) and Asia-Pacific Heart Rhythm Society (APHRS) [J]. *Eur Heart J*, 2014, 35 (45): 3155-3179.

[155] Kirchhof P, Benussi S, Kotecha D, et al. 2016 ESC Guidelines for the management of atrial fibrillation developed in collaboration with EACTS [J]. *Eur Heart J*, 2016, 37 (38): 2893-2962.

[156] Subherwal S, Bach R G, Chen A Y, et al. Baseline risk of major bleeding in non-ST-segment-elevation myocardial infarction: The CRUSADE (Can rapid risk stratification of unstable angina patients suppress adverse outcomes with early implementation of the ACC/AHA guidelines) bleeding score [J]. *Circulation*, 2009, 119: 1873-1882.

[157] Ma Y T. Relationship between bleeding after percutaneous coronary intervention and selection and dosage of anticoagulant drugs [J]. *Chinese Journal of Cardiovascular Diseases*, 2016, 44 (2): 96-99.

[158] Stone G W, Witzenbichler B, Guagliumi G, et al. Bivalirudin during primary PCI in acute myocardial infarction [J]. *N Engl J Med*, 2008, 358 (21): 2218-2230.

[159] Steg P G, van't Hof A, Hamm C W, et al. Bivalirudin started during emergency transport for primary PCI [J]. *N Engl J Med*, 2013, 369 (23): 2207-2217.

[160] Bangalore S, Toklu B, Kotwal A, et al. Anticoagulant therapy during primary percutaneous coronary intervention for acute myocardial infarction: A meta-analysis of randomized trials in the era of stents and P2Y12 inhibitors [J]. *BMJ*, 2014, 349: g6419.

[161] Han Y, Guo J, Zheng Y, et al. Bivalirudin vs heparin with or without tirofiban during primary percutaneous coronary intervention in acute myocardial infarction: The BRIGHT randomized clinical trial [J]. *JAMA*, 2015, 313 (13): 1336-1346.

[162] Mehran R, Rao S V, Bhatt D L, et al. Standardized bleeding definitions for cardiovascular clinical trials: A consensus report from the Bleeding Academic Research Consortium [J]. *Circulation*, 2011, 123: 2736-2747.

[163] Cardiovascular Physician Branch of Chinese Medical Doctor Association, Thrombosis Prevention Professional Committee of Cardiovascular Physician Branch of Chinese Medical Doctor Association, Digestive Endoscopy Branch of Chinese Medical Association, Beijing Neurology Association, Multidisciplinary Expert Consensus Group on Prevention and Treatment of Bleeding during Antithrombotic Therapy for Acute Coronary Syndromes. Multidisciplinary expert consensus on prevention and treatment of bleeding during antithrombotic therapy for acute coronary syndromes [J]. *Chinese Journal of Internal Medicine*, 2016, 55 (10): 813-824.

[164] Baigent C, Keech A, Kearney P M, et al. Efficacy and safety of cholesterol-lowering treatment: Prospective meta-analysis of data from 90, 056 participants in 14 randomised trials of statins [J]. *Lancet*, 2005, 366 (9493): 1267-1278.

[165] Zhao D, Liu J, Xie W, et al. Cardiovascular risk assessment: A global perspective [J]. *Nat Rev Cardiol*, 2015, 12 (5): 301-311.

[166] Reiner Z, Catapano A L, De Backer G, et al. ESC/EAS guidelines for the management of dyslipidaemias: The Task Force for the management of dyslipidaemias of the European Society of Cardiology (ESC) and the European Atherosclerosis Society (EAS) [J]. *Eur Heart J*, 2011, 32 (14): 1769-1818.

[167] Rabar S, Harker M, O'Flynn N, et al. Lipid modification and cardiovascular risk assessment for the primary and secondary prevention of cardiovascular disease: Summary of updated NICE guidance [J]. *BMJ*, 2014, 349: g4356.

[168] Joint Committee for Revision of Chinese Guidelines on Prevention and Treatment of Dyslipidemia

in Adults. Chinese guidelines on prevention and treatment of dyslipidemia in adults (2016 revision) [J]. *Chinese Journal of Cardiovascular Diseases*, 2016, 44 (10): 833-853.

[169] Wang Y, Liu J, Wang W, et al. Lifetime risk for cardiovascular disease in a Chinese population: The Chinese multi-provincial cohort study [J]. *Eur J Prev Cardiol*, 2015, 22 (3): 380-388.

[170] Joint Committee for Formulation of Chinese Guidelines on Prevention and Treatment of Dyslipidemia in Adults. Chinese guidelines on prevention and treatment of dyslipidemia in adults [J]. *Chinese Journal of Cardiovascular Diseases*, 2007, 35 (5): 390-419.

[171] Expert Dyslipidemia Panel of the International Atherosclerosis Society Panel members. An International Atherosclerosis Society Position Paper—global recommendations for the management of dyslipidemia: Full report [J]. *J Clin Lipidol*, 2014, 8 (1): 29-60.

[172] Organ Transplantation Branch of Chinese Medical Association, Physician Branch of Organ Transplantation of Chinese Medical Doctor Association. Chinese guidelines for lipid management in organ transplant recipients (2016 edition) [J]. *Organ Transplantation*, 2016, 7 (4): 243-254.

[173] Statin Safety Evaluation Working Group. Expert consensus on statin safety evaluation [J]. *Chinese Journal of Cardiovascular Diseases*, 2014, 42 (11): 890-894.

[174] Expert Consensus Group on Use of Statins in Elderly with Dyslipidemia in China. Expert consensus on use of statins in elderly with dyslipidemia in China [J]. *Chinese Journal of Internal Medicine*, 2016, 55 (5): 467-477.

[175] Organ Transplantation Branch of Chinese Medical Association. *Clinical Practice Guidelines* (Organ Transplantation Volume) (2010 Edition) [M]. Beijing: People's Medical Publishing House, 2010.

[176] Costanzo M R, Dipchand A, Starling R, et al. The International Society of Heart and Lung Transplantation Guidelines for the care of heart transplantations [J]. *J Heart Lung Transplant*, 2010, 29 (8): 914-956.

[177] Rational Drug Use Expert Committee of National Health and Family Planning Commission, Chinese Pharmacists Association. Rational drug use guidelines for thrombolytic therapy in acute ST-segment elevation myocardial infarction [J]. *Chinese Journal of Frontiers of Medical Science*, 2016, 8 (8): 25-41.

[178] Chen H Z, Lin G W, Wang J Y. *Practical Internal Medicine* [M]. Beijing: People's Medical Publishing House, 2014: 1483-1495.

[179] Lu Z Y. *Internal Medicine*. 7th Edition. [M] Beijing: People's Medical Publishing House, 2008: 217-225.

[180] Cardiovascular Disease Branch of Chinese Medical Association, Editorial Board of Chinese Journal of Cardiovascular Diseases. Guidelines for the diagnosis and treatment of acute ST-segment elevation myocardial infarction [J]. *Chinese Journal of Cardiovascular Diseases*, 2015, 43 (5): 380-393.

[181] O'Gara P T, Kushner F G, Ascheim D D, et al. 2013 ACCF/AHA guideline for the management of ST-elevation myocardial infarction: executive summary: A report of the American College of Cardiology Foundation/American Heart Association Task Force on Practice Guidelines [J]. *J Am Coll Cardiol*, 2013, 61 (4): 485-510.

[182] Steg P G, James S K, Atar D, et al. ESC Guidelines for the management of acute myocardial infarction in patients presenting with ST-segment elevation [J]. *Eur Heart J*, 2012, 33 (20): 2569-2619.

[183] Harper R W. Pre-hospital thrombolysis rather than primary percutaneous intervention is the treatment of choice for patients with ST-segment elevation myocardial infarction presenting early after the onset of symptoms [J]. *JACC Cardiovasc Interv*, 2010, 3 (10): 1093-1094; author reply 1094-1095.

[184] An Y L, Liu J N, Jing Q M, et al. The efficacy and safety of pharmacoinvasive therapy with prourokinase for acute ST-segment elevation myocardial infarction patients with expected long percutaneous

coronary intervention-related delay [J]. *Cardiovasc Ther*, 2013, 31 (5): 285-290.

[185] Acute Myocardial Infarction Reperfusion Therapy Research Collaborative Group. Randomized multicenter clinical trial of recombinant streptokinase and recombinant tissue-type plasminogen activator for the treatment of acute myocardial infarction [J]. *Chinese Journal of Cardiovascular Diseases*, 2007, 35 (8): 691-696.

[186] Kasanuki H, Honda T, Haze K, et al. A large scale prospective cohort study on the current status of therapeutic modalities for acute myocardial infarction in Japan: rationale and initial results of the HIJAMI Registry [J]. *Am Heart J*, 2005, 150: 411-418.

[187] Ikeda N, Yasu T, Kubo N, et al. Effect of reperfusion therapy on cardiac rupture after myocardial infarction in Japanese [J]. *Circ J*, 2004, 68: 422-426.

[188] Chevalier P, Burri H, Fahrat F, et al. Perioperative outcome and long-term survival of surgery for acute postinfarction mitral regurgitation [J]. *Eur J Cardiothorac Surg*, 2004, 26: 330-335.

[189] Tavakoli R, Weber A, Vogt P, et al. Surgical management of acute mitral valve regurgitation due to postinfarction papillary muscle rupture [J]. *Heart Valve Dis*, 2002, 11: 20-25.

[190] Expert Consensus on Diagnosis, Assessment and Management of Dyspnea. Expert consensus on diagnosis, assessment and management of dyspnea [J]. *Chinese Journal of Internal Medicine*, 2014, 53 (4): 337-341.

[191] Zhang J, Gan T Y. Diagnosis and differential diagnosis of dyspnea [J]. *Chinese Circulation Journal*, 2014, 29 (3): 164-166.

[192] Cardiovascular Disease Branch of Chinese Medical Association, Editorial Board of Chinese Journal of Cardiovascular Diseases. Chinese guidelines for the diagnosis and treatment of heart failure 2014 [J]. *Chinese Journal of Cardiovascular Diseases*, 2014, 42 (2): 98-122.

[193] Zhang K Z, Tian Y. *Clinical Heart Failure* [M]. Changsha: Hunan Science and Technology Press, 2014: 392-401.

[194] Chen H Z, Lin G W. *Practical Internal Medicine* (14th Edition) [M]. Beijing: People's Medical Publishing House, 2013: 1341-1352.

[195] Eshaghian S, Horwich T B, Fonarow G C. Relation of loop diuretic dose to mortality in advanced heart failure [J]. *Am J Cardiol*, 2006, 97: 1759-1764.

[196] Sharma K, Kass D A. Heart failure with preserved ejection fraction: mechanisms, clinical features, and therapies [J]. *Circ Res*, 2014, 115 (1): 79-96.

[197] Borlaug B A. The pathophysiology of heart failure with preserved ejection fraction [J]. *Nat Rev Cardiol*, 2014, 11 (9): 507-515.

[198] Mosterd A, Hoes A W. Clinical epidemiology of heart failure [J]. *Heart*, 2007, 93: 1137-1146.

[199] Rational Drug Use Expert Committee of National Health and Family Planning Commission, Chinese Pharmacists Association. Rational drug use guidelines for heart failure [J]. *Chinese Journal of Frontiers of Medical Science* (Electronic Edition), 2016, 8 (9): 19-66.

[200] Eshaghian S, Horwich T B, Fonarow G C. Relation of loop diuretic dose to mortality in advanced heart failure [J]. *Am J Cardiol*, 2006, 97: 1759-1764.

[201] Lau Y C, Lane D A, Lip G Y. Atrial fibrillation and heart failure: A bad combination [J]. *Am J Cardiol*, 2014, 113: 1196-1197.

[202] Rewiuk K, Wizner B, Fedyk-Lukasik M, et al. Epidemiology and management of coexisting heart failure and atrial fibrillation in an outpatient setting [J]. *Pol Arch Med Wewn*, 2011, 121: 392-399.

[203] Komajda M, Isnard R, Cohen-Solal A, et al. Effect of ivabradine in patients with heart failure with preserved ejection fraction: The EDIFY randomized placebo-controlled trial [J]. *Eur J Heart Fail*, 2017, 19 (4):

1-9.

[204] Traditional Chinese and Western Medicine Clinical Research Alliance for Coronary Heart Disease, Professional Committee of Cardiovascular Diseases of China Association of Integrative Medicine, Cardiac Disease Branch of China Association of Chinese Medicine. Expert consensus on traditional Chinese medicine diagnosis and treatment of chronic heart failure [J]. *Chinese Journal of Traditional Chinese Medicine*, 2014, 55 (14): 1258-1260.

[205] Professional Committee of Cardiovascular Diseases of China Association of Integrative Medicine, Expert Committee of Cardiovascular Diseases of Integrative Medicine Physician Branch of Chinese Medical Association. Expert consensus on integrated traditional Chinese and Western medicine diagnosis and treatment of chronic heart failure [J]. *Journal of Traditional Chinese Medicine Combined with Western Medicine*, 2016, 36: 133-141.

[206] You T, Huang J, Chen J C. Research progress in mechanical circulatory support for the treatment of heart failure [J]. *Advances in Cardiovascular Diseases*, 2014, 35 (3): 346-350.

[207] Werdan K, Russ M, Buerke M. Intra-aortic balloon counter pulsation in cardiogenic Shock [J]. *Springer New York*, 2010, 6 (1): 93-98.

[208] Gattinoni L, Carlesso E, Langer T. Clinical review: Extracorporeal membrane oxygenation [J]. *Crit Care*, 2011, 15 (6): 243-258.

[209] Ouyang Q. *Clinical Diagnostics* 2nd Edition [M]. Beijing: People's Medical Publishing House, 2012: 14-16.

[210] Liu C J. Causes and differential diagnosis of lower limb edema [J]. *Chinese Journal of Practical Surgery*, 2010, 30 (12): 1072-1074.

[211] Messerli F. Vasodilatory edema: A common side of antihypertensive therapy [J]. *Am J Hypertens*, 2001, 14 (10): 978-979.

[212] Makani H, Bangalore S, Romero J, et al. Effect of renin-angiotensin system blockade on calcium channel blocker-associated peripheral edema [J]. *Am J Med*, 2011, 124 (2): 128-135.

[213] Goldberg R J, Spencer F A, Gore J M, et al. Thirty-year trends (1975 to 2005) in the magnitude of, management of, and hospital death rates associated with cardiogenic shock in patients with acute myocardial infarction: A population-based perspective [J]. *Circulation*, 2009, 119 (9): 1211-1219.

[214] Wang L X, Xie J. Analysis of integrated traditional Chinese and Western medicine nursing for acute myocardial infarction complicated with cardiogenic shock [J]. *Journal of Cardiovascular Disease Combined with Traditional Chinese and Western Medicine* (Electronic Edition), 2015, 19: 117-118.

[215] Jeger R V, Radovanovic D, Hunziker P R, et al. Ten-year trends in the incidence and treatment of cardiogenic shock [J]. *Ann Intern Med*, 2008, 149 (9): 618-626.

[216] Smedira N G, Moazami N, Golding C M, et al. Cosgrove DM 3rd. Clinical experience with 202 adults receiving extracorporeal membrane oxygenation for cardiac failure: Survival at five years [J]. *J Thorac Cardiovasc Surg*, 2001, 122: 92-102.

[217] Rastan A J, Dege A, Mohr M, et al. Early and late outcomes of 517 consecutive adult patients treated with extracorporeal membrane oxygenation for refractory postcardiotomy cardiogenic shock [J]. *J Thorac Cardiovasc Surg*, 2010, 139: 302-311.

[218] Sylvin E, Stern D, Goldstein D. Mechanical support for postcarditomy cardiogenic shock: Has progress been made? [J] *J Card Surg*, 2010, 25: 442-454.

[219] Musiał R, Darocha T, Kosiński S, et al. Application of V-A ECMO therapies for short-term mechanical circulatory support in patients with cardiogenic shock [J]. *Anaesthesiol Intensive Ther*, 2015, 47: 324-327.

[220] Wheeler T M, Baker J N, Chad D A, et al. Case records of the Massachusetts General Hospital. Case 30-2015: A 50-year-old man with cardiogenic shock [J]. *N Engl J Med*, 2015, 373: 1251-1261.

[221] Garratti A, Colombo T, Russo C, et al. Different applications for the left ventricular mechanical support with the Impella Recover 100 microaxial blood pump [J]. *J Heart Lung Transplant*, 2005, 24: 481-485.

[222] Floras J S. Sympathetic activation in human heart failure: Diverse mechanisms, therapeutic opportunities [J]. *Acta Physiol Scand*, 2003, 177: 391.

[223] Davie P, Francis C M, Caruana L, et al. Assessing diagnosis in heart failure: Which features are any use [J]. *QJM*, 1997, 90: 335-339.

[224] Chen H Z. *Cardiovascular Disease* 9th Edition [M]. Beijing: People's Medical Publishing House, 2016: 523.

[225] Ahmed A, Allman R M, Aronow W S, et al. Diagnosis of heart failure in older adults: Predictive value of dyspnea at rest [J]. *Arch Gerontol Geriatr*, 2004, 238: 297.

[226] BC Guidelines. Chronic Heart Failure—Diagnosis and Management. 2015: 1.

[227] Chakko S, Woska D, Martinez H, et al. Clinical, radiographic, and hemodynamic correlations in chronic congestive heart failure: Conflicting results may lead to inappropriate care [J]. *Am J Med*, 1991, 90: 353.

[228] Van Riet E E S, Hoes A W, Limburg A, et al. Prevalence of unrecognized heart failure in older persons with shortness of breath on exertion [J]. *Eur J Heart Fail*, 2014, 16: 772-777.

[229] Mant J, Doust J, Roalfe A, et al. Systematic review and individual patient data meta-analysis of diagnosis of heart failure, with modelling of implications of different diagnostic strategies in primary care [J]. *Health Technol Assess*, 2009, 13: 201-207.

[230] Faris R, Flather M, Purcell H, et al. Current evidence supporting the role of diuretics in heart failure: A meta analysis of randomised controlled trials [J]. *Int J Cardiol*, 2002, 82: 149-158.

[231] Chen X, Jiang H, Ma J, et al. *Pathophysiology, Diagnosis and Treatment of Congestive Heart Failure* [M]. Beijing: Science Press, 2004: 355-356.

[232] Karl S, John C W, Olson S, et al. Guidelines for the diagnosis and treatment of chronic heart failure: Executive summary [J]. *Eur Heart J*, 2005, 26 (6): 1115-1140.

[233] Zhang Z L. Factors to consider when interpreting B-type natriuretic peptide and N-terminal pro-B-type natriuretic peptide test results [J]. *Chinese Journal of Laboratory Medicine*, 2012, 35 (2): 134-136.

[234] Ellison D H. Diuretic therapy and resistance in congestive heart failure [J]. *Cardiology*, 2001, 96: 132.

[235] Desai A S. Hyperkalemia in patients with heart failure: Incidence, prevalence, and management [J]. *Curr Heart Fail Rep*, 2009, 6: 272-280.

[236] Filippatos G, Farmakis D, Parissis J. Renal dysfunction and heart failure: Things are seldom what they seem [J]. *Eur Heart J*, 2014, 35: 416-418.

[237] O'Connor C M, Whellan D J, Lee K L, et al. HF-ACTION Investigators. Efficacy and safety of exercise training in patients with chronic heart failure: HF-ACTION randomized controlled trial [J]. *JAMA*, 2009, 301: 1439-1450.

[238] Gaggin H K, Mohammed A A, Bhardwaj A, et al. Heart failure outcomes and benefits of NT-proBNP-guided management in the elderly: Results from the prospective, randomized proBNP outpatient tailored chronic heart failure therapy (PROTECT) study [J]. *J Card Fail*, 2012, 18 (8): 626-634.

[239] Schuuring M J, van Riel A C, Vis J C, et al. New predictors of mortality in adults with congenital heart disease and pulmonary hypertension: Midterm outcome of a prospective study [J]. *Int J Cardiol*, 2015, 181: 270-276.

[240] van Veldhuisen D J, Linssen G C, Jaarsma T, et al. B-type natriuretic peptide and prognosis in heart

failure patients with preserved and reduced ejection fraction [J]. *J Am Coll Cardiol*, 2013, 61 (14): 1498-1506.

[241] AbouEzzeddine O F, McKie P M, Scott C G, et al. Biomarker-based risk prediction in the community [J]. *Eur J Heart Fail*, 2016, 18 (11): 1342-1350.

[242] Januzzi J L, Troughton R. Are serial BNP measurements useful in heart failure management? Serial natriuretic peptide measurements are useful in heart failure management [J]. *Circulation*, 2013, 127 (4): 500-507.

[243] Wieczorek S J, Wu A H, Christenson R, et al. A rapid B-type natriuretic peptide assay accurately diagnoses left ventricular dysfunction and heart failure: A multicenter evaluation [J]. *Am Heart J*, 2002, 144 (5): 834-839.

[244] Guo H F, Guo Z H. Effects of Shengjin Decoction combined with Danshen Drink on cardiac function and plasma BNP and NT-proBNP levels in chronic heart failure [J]. *Journal of Traditional Chinese Medicine*, 2013, 19 (7): 44-45.

[245] Cheng H, Fan W Z, Wang S C, et al. N-terminal pro-brain natriuretic peptide and cardiac troponin I for the prognostic utility in elderly patients with severe sepsis or septic shock in intensive care unit: A retrospective study [J]. *J Crit Care*, 2015, 30 (3): 654. e9-14.

[246] Jourdain P, Jondeau G, Funck F, et al. Plasma brain natriuretic peptide-guided therapy to improve outcome in heart failure: The STARS-BNP Multicenter Study [J]. *J Am Coll Cardiol*, 2007, 49 (16): 1733-1739.

[247] Zhao Y, Chen Q Q, Guo F, et al. Predictive value of serum cTnI and NT-proBNP in stable chronic heart failure patients [J]. *Journal of Cardiovascular Rehabilitation Medicine*, 2014, 8 (4): 401-404.

[248] Santhanakrishnan R, Chong J P, Ng T P, et al. Growth differentiation factor 15, ST2, high-sensitivity troponin T, and N-terminal pro brain natriuretic peptide in heart failure with preserved vs. reduced ejection fraction [J]. *Eur J Heart Fail*, 2012, 14 (12): 1338-1347.

[249] Solberg O G, Ueland T, Wergeland R, et al. High-sensitive troponin T and N-terminal-brain-natriuretic-peptide predict outcome in symptomatic aortic stenosis [J]. *Scand Cardiovasc J*, 2012, 46 (5): 278-285.

[250] Luo Y J, Tan Z H, Li X J, et al. Role of combined detection of serum cTnI, CK-MB, and NT-proBNP in pediatric sepsis patients [J]. *Chinese Modern Doctor*, 2016, 54 (11): 107-109.

[251] Ma G, Hong G L, Zhao G J, et al. Changes and significance of plasma B-type natriuretic peptide and cardiac troponin Ⅰ in sepsis patients [J]. *Journal of Integrated Traditional Chinese and Western Medicine in Intensive and Critical Cases*, 2014, 21 (2): 99-103.

[252] Xiao Z H, Liu J, Lu X L, et al. Clinical diagnostic value of plasma N-terminal pro-B-type natriuretic peptide level in pediatric sepsis patients with myocardial injury [J]. *Chinese Journal of Pediatric Emergency Medicine*, 2014, 21 (12): 782-785.

[253] Wang W Q, Qiu Z H. Relationship between plasma brain natriuretic peptide concentration and risk stratification of stroke caused by atrial fibrillation [J]. *Journal of Lingnan Cardiovascular Disease*, 2015, 21 (2): 211-213.

[254] Tuxun T, Aierken A, Xie X, et al. Association study of plasma NT-proBNP levels and severity of acute coronary syndrome [J]. *Genet Mol Res*, 2014, 13 (3): 5754-5757.

[255] Goyal B M, Sharma S M, Walia M. B-type natriuretic peptide levels predict extent and severity of coronary artery disease in non-ST elevation acute coronary syndrome and normal left ventricular function [J]. *Indian Heart J*, 2014, 66 (2): 183-187.

[256] Wei P, Wang H B, Fu Q, et al. Levels of BNP and stress blood glucose in acute coronary syndrome patients and their relationship with the severity of coronary artery lesion [J]. *Cell Biochem Biophys*, 2014, 68 (3): 535-539.

[257] Niu J M, Ma Z L, Xie C, et al. Association of plasma B-type natriuretic peptide concentration with

myocardial infarct size in patients with acute myocardial infarction [J]. *Genet Mol Res*, 2014, 13 (3): 6177-6183.

[258] Kajimoto K, Madeen K, Nakayama T, et al. Rapid evaluation by lung-cardiac-inferior vena cava (LCI) integrated ultrasound for differentiating heart failure from pulmonary disease as the cause of acute dyspnea in the emergency setting [J]. *Cardiovasc Ultrasound*, 2012, 10 (1): 49.

[259] Ding X D, Liu D J. Observation of plasma cTnT, NT-proBNP and myocardial enzyme levels in patients with acute pulmonary embolism [J]. *Journal of Aerospace Medicine*, 2015, 26 (5): 585-587.

[260] Vamsidhar A, Rajasekhar D, Vanaja V, et al. Comparison of PESI, echocardiogram, CTPA, and NT-proBNP as risk stratification tools in patients with acute pulmonary embolism [J]. *Indian Heart J*, 2017, 69 (1): 68-74.

[261] Heit J A. The epidemiology of venous thromboembolism in the community [J]. *Arterioscler Thromb Vasc Biol*, 2008, 28 (3): 370-372.

[262] Cohen A T, Agnelli G, Anderson F A, et al. Venous thromboembolism (VTE) in Europe. The number of VTE events and associated morbidity and mortality [J]. *Thromb Haemost*, 2007, 98 (4): 756-764.

[263] Lankeit M, Konstantinides S. Mortality risk assessment and the role of thrombolysis in pulmonary embolism [J]. *Crit Care Clin*, 2011, 27 (4): 953-967.

[264] Jia W B, Zhang C X, Zhen Z M. Analysis of literature on misdiagnosis of pulmonary embolism in China in recent four years [J]. *Chinese Journal of Cardiovascular Diseases*, 2006, 34 (3): 277-280.

[265] Minges K E, Bikdeli B, Wang Y, et al. National trends in pulmonary embolism hospitalization rates and outcomes for adults aged ≥65 years in the United States (1999 to 2010) [J]. *Am J Cardiol*, 2015, 116 (9): 1436-1442.

[266] Konstantinides S V. 2014 ESC Guidelines on the diagnosis and management of acute pulmonary embolism [J]. *Eur Heart J*, 2014, 35 (45): 3145-3146.

[267] Kurzyna M, Dabrowski M, Bielecki D, et al. Atrial septostomy in treatment of end-stage right heart failure in patients with pulmonary hypertension [J]. *Chest*, 2007, 131: 977-983.

[268] Pulmonary Vascular Disease Group of Chinese Society of Cardiology. Chinese expert consensus on diagnosis and treatment of acute pulmonary embolism (2015) [J]. *Chinese Journal of Cardiovascular Diseases*, 2016, 44 (3): 197-211.

[269] Editorial Board of Chinese Journal of Cardiovascular Diseases, Working Group on Myocarditis and Cardiomyopathy. Opinions on adopting the diagnostic reference criteria for acute viral myocarditis in adults and the definition and classification of cardiomyopathies by the WHO/ISFC Task Force [J]. *Chinese Journal of Cardiovascular Diseases*, 1999, 27 (6): 405-407.

[270] Editorial Board of Chinese Journal of Internal Medicine. Summary of National Symposium on Myocarditis and Cardiomyopathy [J]. *Chinese Journal of Internal Medicine*, 1987, 26: 597-601.

[271] Chen H Z. *Practical Internal Medicine* (12th Edition) [M]. Beijing: People's Medical Publishing House, 2005: 1571-1585.

[272] Organizing Committee of National Symposium on Myocarditis and Cardiomyopathy. Summary of National Symposium on Myocarditis and Cardiomyopathy [J]. *Clinical Journal of Cardiovascular Diseases*, 1995, 11: 324-326.

[273] Liu Y L. *Analysis of Diagnostic Thinking in Echocardiography* (2010 Edition) [M]. Beijing: Beijing Science and Technology Press, 2010: 589-621.

[274] Halliday B, Gulati A, Ali A, et al. Association between midwall late gadolinium enhancement and sudden cardiac death in patients with dilated cardiomyopathy and mild and moderate left ventricular systolic dysfunction [J]. *Circulation*, 2017, 135 (22): 2106-2115.

[275] Bozkurt B, Colvin M, Cook J, et al. Current diagnostic and treatment strategies for specific dilated cardiomyopathies: A scientific statement from the American Heart Association [J]. *Circulation*, 2016, 134 (23): e579-e646.

[276] Di Marco A, Schmitt M, Anguera I. (Reply) Risk stratification in dilated cardiomyopathy: Is the arrhythmogenic substrate stable over time? [J] *JACC Heart Fail*, 2017, 5 (5): 394-395.

[277] Levy W C. Should non-ischemic CRT candidates receive CRT-P or CRT-D? [J] *J Am Coll Cardiol*, 2017, 69 (13): 1679-1682.

[278] Zhu S H, Li Y, Huang W, et al. Feasibility of the 2014 European guidelines risk prediction model for sudden cardiac death in hypertrophic cardiomyopathy in Chinese patients [J]. *Zhonghua Xinxueguan Bing Za Zhi*, 2017, 45 (5): 404-408.

[279] Rowin E J, Maron B J, Haas T S, et al. Hypertrophic cardiomyopathy with left ventricular apical aneurysm: Implications for risk stratification and management [J]. *J Am Coll Cardiol*, 2017, 69 (7): 761-773.

[280] Maron B J, Maron M S. A discussion of contemporary nomenclature, diagnosis, imaging, and management of patients with hypertrophic cardiomyopathy [J]. *Am J Cardiol*, 2016, 118 (12): 1897-1907.

[281] Webb J, Villa A, Bekri I, et al. Usefulness of cardiac magnetic resonance imaging to measure left ventricular wall thickness for determining risk scores for sudden cardiac death in patients with hypertrophic cardiomyopathy [J]. *Am J Cardiol*, 2017, 119 (9): 1450-1455.

[282] Weissler-Snir A, Chan R H, Adler A, et al. Usefulness of 14-day holter for detection of nonsustained ventricular tachycardia in patients with hypertrophic cardiomyopathy [J]. *Am J Cardiol*, 2016, 118 (8): 1258-1263.

[283] Weissler-Snir A, Adler A, Williams L, et al. Prevention of sudden death in hypertrophic cardiomyopathy: Bridging the gaps in knowledge [J]. *Eur Heart J*, 2017, 38 (22): 1728-1737.

[284] Ruiz-Hurtado G, García-Prieto C F, Pulido-Olmo H, et al. Mild and short-term caloric restriction prevents obesity-induced cardiomyopathy in young zucker rats without changing in metabolites and fatty acids cardiac profile [J]. *Front Physiol*, 2017, 8: 42.

[285] Glaveckaitė S, Šerpytis P, Pečiūraitė D, et al. Clinical features and three-year outcomes of Tako-Tsubo (stress) cardiomyopathy: Observational data from one center [J]. *Hellenic J Cardiol*, 2016, 57 (6): 428-434.

[286] Olshansky B, Sullivan R M. Inappropriate sinus tachycardia [J]. *J Am Coll Cardiol*, 2013, 61 (8): 793-801.

[287] Huang Y Z, Zou J G. *Diagnosis and Differential Diagnosis of Wide QRS Complex and Narrow QRS Complex Tachycardia* [M]. Beijing: People's Medical Publishing House, 2016: 216-218.

[288] Al-Khatib S M, Arshad A, Balk E M, et al. Risk stratification for arrhythmic events in patients with asymptomatic pre-excitation: A systematic review for the 2015 ACC/AHA/HRS Guideline for the management of adult patients with supraventricular tachycardia: A report of the American College of Cardiology/American Heart Association Task Force on Clinical Practice Guidelines and the Heart Rhythm Society [J]. *Circulation*, 2016, 133 (14): e575-586.

[289] Chen X. Huang W. *Electrocardiography* 6th Edition [M]. Beijing: People's Medical Publishing House, 2015: 183-189, 361-373.

[290] Kalbfleisch S J, El-Atassi R, Calkins H, et al. Differentiation of paroxysmal narrow QRS complex tachycardias using the 12-lead electrocardiogram [J]. *J Am Coll Cardiol*, 1993, 21 (1): 85-89.

[291] Kim Y N, Sousa J, El-Atassi R, et al. Magnitude of ST segment depression during paroxysmal supraventricular tachycardia [J]. *Am Heart J*, 1991, 122 (5): 1486-1487.

[292] Olshansky B, Sullivan R M. Inappropriate sinus tachycardia [J]. *J Am Coll Cardiol*, 2013, 61 (8): 793-

801.

[293] Patel A, Markowitz S M. Atrial tachycardia: Mechanisms and management [J]. *Expert Rev Cardiovasc Ther*, 2008, 6 (6): 811-822.

[294] Oh S, Choi Y S, Sohn D W, et al. Differential diagnosis of slow/slow atrioventricular nodal reentrant tachycardia from atrioventricular reentrant tachycardia using concealed posteroseptal accessory pathway by 12-lead electrocardiography [J]. *Pacing Clin Electrophysiol*, 2003, 26 (12): 2296-2300.

[295] Lickfett L, Mittmann-Braun E, Weiss C, et al. Differences in clinical and echocardiographic parameters between paroxysmal and persistent atrial flutter in the AURUM 8 study: Targets for prevention of persistent arrhythmia [J]. *Pacing Clin Electrophysiol*, 2013, 36 (2): 194-202.

[296] Kirchhof P, Benussi S, Kotecha D, et al. 2016 ESC Guidelines for the management of atrial fibrillation developed in collaboration with EACTS [J]. *Eur Heart J*, 2016, 37 (38): 2893-2962.

[297] Durham D, Worthley L I. Cardiac arrhythmias: Diagnosis and management. The tachycardias [J]. *Crit Care Resusc*, 2002, 4 (1): 35-53.

[298] Chen X. *Clinical Arrhythmology* 2nd Edition [M]. Beijing: People's Medical Publishing House, 2009: 725-788.

[299] Al-Zaiti S S, Magdic K S. Paroxysmal supraventricular tachycardia: Pathophysiology, diagnosis, and management [J]. *Crit Care Nurs Clin North Am*, 2016, 28 (3): 309-316.

[300] Vereckei A. Current algorithms for the diagnosis of wide QRS complex tachycardias [J]. *Curr Cardiol Rev*, 2014, 10 (3): 262-276.

[301] Reising S, Kusumoto F, Goldschlager N. Life-threatening arrhythmias in the intensive care unit [J]. *J Intensive Care Med*, 2007, 22 (1): 3-13.

[302] Zhu J. Cardiovascular emergency treatment: Diagnosis and treatment of wide QRS complex tachycardia [J]. *Chinese Circulation Journal*, 2014, 29 (2): 84-86.

[303] Kireyev D, Gupta V, Arkhipov M V, et al. Approach to the differentiation of wide QRS complex tachycardias [J]. *Am Heart Hosp J*, 2011, 9 (1): E33-36.

[304] Brugada P, Brugada J, Mont L, et al. A new approach to the differential diagnosis of a regular tachycardia with a wide QRS complex [J]. *Circulation*, 1991, 83 (5): 1649-1659.

[305] Vereckei A, Duray G, Szénási G, et al. Application of a new algorithm in the differential diagnosis of wide QRS complex tachycardia [J]. *Eur Heart J*, 2007, 28 (5): 589-600.

[306] Vereckei A, Duray G, Szénási G, et al. New algorithm using only lead aVR for differential diagnosis of wide QRS complex tachycardia [J]. *Heart Rhythm*, 2008, 5 (1): 89-98.

[307] Arrhythmia Group of Cardiovascular Disease Branch of Chinese Medical Association, Editorial Board of Chinese Journal of Cardiovascular Diseases, Editorial Board of Chinese Journal of Cardiac Pacing and Electrophysiology. Recommendations for the prevention and treatment of acquired long QT syndrome [J]. *Chinese Journal of Cardiovascular Diseases*, 2010, 38 (11): 961-969.

[308] Evidence-based Working Group on Arrhythmia of Editorial Board of Chinese Journal of Cardiovascular Diseases. Chinese expert consensus on diagnosis and treatment of hereditary primary arrhythmia syndromes [J]. *Chinese Journal of Cardiovascular Diseases*, 2015, 43 (1): 5-20.

[309] Priori S G, Wilde A A, Horie M, et al. HRS/EHRA/APHRS expert consensus statement on the diagnosis and management of patients with inherited primary arrhythmia syndromes: document endorsed by HRS, EHRA, and APHRS in May 2013 and by ACCF, AHA, PACES, and AEPC in June 2013 [J]. *Heart Rhythm*, 2013, 10 (12): 1932-1963.

[310] Schwartz P J, Moss A J, Vincent G M, et al. Diagnostic criteria for the long QT syndrome [J]. *An*

update. Circulation, 1993, 88 (2): 782-784.

[311] Wang R R, Li N, Zhang Y H, et al. Novel compound heterozygous mutations T2C and 1149insT in the KCNQ1 gene cause Jervell and Lange-Nielsen syndrome [J]. *Int J Mol Med*, 2011, 28 (1): 41-46.

[312] Gao Y, Li C, Liu W, et al. Genotype-phenotype analysis of three Chinese families with Jervell and Lange-Nielsen syndrome [J]. *Cardiovasc Dis Res*, 2012, 3 (2): 67-75.

[313] Yang Y, Yang Y, Liang B, et al. Identification of a Kir3.4 mutation in congenital long QT syndrome [J]. *Am J Hum Genet*, 2010, 86 (6): 872-880.

[314] Chockalingam P, Crotti L, Girardengo G, et al. Not all beta-blockers are equal in the management of long QT syndrome types 1 and 2: Higher recurrence of events under metoprolol [J]. *J Am Coll Cardiol*, 2012, 60 (20): 2092-2099.

[315] Li J, Liu Y, Yang F, et al. Video-assisted thoracoscopic left cardiac sympathetic denervation: A reliable minimally invasive approach for congenital long QT syndrome [J]. *Ann Thorac Surg*, 2008, 86 (6): 1955-1958.

[316] Gao Y, Xue X, Hu D, et al. Inhibition of late sodium current by mexiletine: A novel pharmotherapeutical approach in timothy syndrome [J]. *Circ Arrhythm Electrophysiol*, 2013, 6 (3): 614-622.

[317] Li C L, Zhang L, Hu D Y, et al. Clinical features and research status of related gene mutations in 85 Chinese probands with long QT syndrome [J]. *Chinese Journal of Arrhythmia*, 2004, (86): 328-334.

[318] Li C L, Hu D Y, Wang J Y, et al. Follow-up observation of 11 cases of long QT syndrome treated with left cardiac sympathetic denervation [J]. *Chinese Journal of Cardiac Pacing and Electrophysiology*, 2006, 20 (1): 21-24.

[319] Hong K, Hu J, Yu J, et al. Concomitant Brugada-like and short QT electrocardiogram linked to SCN5A mutation [J]. *Eur J Hum Genet*, 2012, 20 (11): 1189-1192.

[320] Wilde A A, Antzelevitch C, Borggrefe M, et al. Proposed diagnostic criteria for the Brugada syndrome: Consensus report [J]. *Circulation*, 2002, 106 (19): 2514-2519.

[321] Eckardt L, Probst V, Smits J P, et al. Long-term prognosis of individuals with right precordial ST-segment-elevation Brugada syndrome [J]. *Circulation*, 2005, 111 (3): 257-263.

[322] Priori S G, Gasparini M, Napolitano C, et al. Risk stratification in Brugada syndrome: Results of the PRELUDE (Programmed Electrical stimUlation preDictive valuE) registry [J]. *J Am Coll Cardiol*, 2012, 59 (1): 37-45.

[323] Antzelevitch C, Brugada P, Brugada J, et al. Brugada syndrome: 1992—2002, A historical perspective [J]. *J Am Coll Cardiol*, 2003, 41: 1665.

[324] Brugada J, Brugada R, Antzelevitch C, et al. Long-term follow-up of individuals with the electrocardiographic pattern of right bundle-branch block and ST-segment elevation in precordial leads V1 to V3 [J]. *Circulation*, 2002, 105 (11): 73.

[325] Brugada J, Brugada R, Brugada P. Determinants of sudden cardiac death in individuals with the electrocardiographic pattern of Brugada syndrome and no previous cardiac arrest [J]. *Circulation*, 2003, 108 (25): 3092-3096.

[326] Sarkozy A, Boussy T, Kourgiannides G, et al. Long-term follow-up of primary implantable cardioverter-defibrillator therapy in Brugada syndrome [J]. *Eur Heart J*, 2007, 28 (3): 334-344.

[327] Task Force for the Diagnosis and Management of Syncope, European Society of Cardiology (ESC), European Heart Rhythm Association (EHRA), et al. Guidelines for the diagnosis and management of syncope (version 2009) [J]. *Eur Heart J*, 2009, 30: 2631-2671.

[328] Brignole M, Alboni P, Benditt D G, et al. Guidelines on management (diagnosis and treatment) of syncope-update 2004 [J]. *Europace*, 2004, 6: 467-537.

[329] Wisten A, Forsberg H, Krantz P, et al. Sudden cardiac death in 15-35-year olds in Sweden during 1992—1999 [J]. *J Intern Med*, 2002, 6: 529-536.

[330] Del Rosso A, Alboni P, Brignole M, et al. Relation of clinical presentation of syncope to the age of patients [J]. *Am J Cardiol*, 2005, 10: 1431-1435.

[331] Strickberger S A, Benson D W, Biaggioni I, et al. AHA/ACCF Scientific Statement on the evaluation of syncope [J]. *Circulation*, 2006, 113: 316-327.

[332] Parry S W, Steen I N, Baptist M, et al. Amnesia for loss of consciousness in carotid sinus syndrome [J]. *J Am Coll Cardiol*, 2005, 11: 1840-1843.

[333] Grubb B P. Neurocardiogenic syncope and related disorders of orthostatic intolerance [J]. *Circulation*, 2005, 115: 2997-3006.

[334] Benditt D G, Sutton R. Tilt-table testing in the evaluation of syncope [J]. *J Cardiovasc Electrophysiol*, 2005, 16: 356-340.

[335] Wolf P A, Abbott R D, Kannel W B. Atrial fibrillation as an independent risk factor for stroke: The Framingham Study [J]. *Stroke*, 1991, 22: 983-988.

[336] Wattigney W A, Mensah G A, Croft J B. Increasing trends in hospitalization for atrial fibrillation in the United States, 1985 through 1999: Implications for primary prevention [J]. *Circulation*, 2003, 108: 711-716.

[337] Gage B F, Waterman A D, Shannon W, et al. Validation of clinical classification schemes for predicting stroke: Results from the National Registry of Atrial Fibrillation [J]. *JAMA*, 2001, 285: 2864-2870.

[338] Lip G Y, Nieuwlaat R, Pisters R, et al. Refining clinical risk stratification for predicting stroke and thromboembolism in atrial fibrillation using a novel risk factor-based approach: The euro heart survey on atrial fibrillation [J]. *Chest*, 2010, 137: 263-272.

[339] Pisters R, Lane D A, Nieuwlaat R, et al. A novel user-friendly score (HAS-BLED) to assess 1-year risk of major bleeding in patients with atrial fibrillation: the Euro Heart Survey [J]. *Chest*, 2010, 138: 1093-1100.

[340] van Spall H G C, Wallentin L, Yusuf S, et al. Variation in warfarin dose adjustment practice is responsible for differences in the quality of anticoagulation control between centers and countries: An analysis of patients receiving warfarin in the randomized evaluation of long-term anticoagulation therapy (RE-LY) Trial [J]. *Circulation*, 2012, 126: 2309-2316.

[341] Miller V T, Rothrock J F, Pearce L A, et al. Ischemic stroke in patients with atrial fibrillation: Effect of aspirin according to stroke mechanism. Stroke Prevention in Atrial Fibrillation Investigators [J]. *Neurology*, 1993, 43: 32-36.

[342] McBride R, Chesebro J H, Wiebers D O, et al. Warfarin versus aspirin for prevention of thromboembolism in atrial fibrillation: Stroke Prevention in Atrial Fibrillation Ⅱ Study [J]. *Lancet*, 1994, 343: 687-691.

[343] Collins L J, Silverman D I, Douglas P S, et al. Cardioversion of nonrheumatic atrial fibrillation: Reduced thromboembolic complications with 4 weeks of precardioversion anticoagulation are related to atrial thrombus resolution [J]. *Circulation*, 1995, 92: 160-163.

[344] Klein A L, Grimm R A, Murray R D, et al. Use of transesophageal echocardiography to guide cardioversion in patients with atrial fibrillation [J]. *N Engl J Med*, 2001, 344: 1411-1420.

[345] Khan I A. Transient atrial mechanical dysfunction (stunning) after cardioversion of atrial fibrillation and flutter [J]. *Am Heart J*, 2002, 144: 11-22.

[346] Giugliano R P, Ruff C T, Braunwald E, et al. Edoxaban versus warfarin in patients with atrial fibrillation [J]. *N Engl J Med*, 2013, 369: 2093-2104.

[347] Patel M R, Mahaffey K W, Garg J, et al. Rivaroxaban versus warfarin in nonvalvular atrial fibrillation

[J]. *N Engl J Med*, 2011, 365: 883-891.

[348] Granger C B, Alexander J H, McMurray J J, et al. Apixaban versus warfarin in patients with atrial fibrillation [J]. *N Engl J Med*, 2011, 365: 981-992.

[349] Connolly S J, Ezekowitz M D, Yusuf S, et al. Dabigatran versus warfarin in patients with atrial fibrillation [J]. *N Engl J Med*, 2009, 361: 1139-1151.

[350] Lip G Y, Windecker S, Huber K, et al. Management of antithrombotic therapy in atrial fibrillation patients presenting with acute coronary syndrome and/or undergoing percutaneous coronary or valve interventions: A joint consensus document of the European Society of Cardiology Working Group on Thrombosis, European Heart Rhythm Association (EHRA), European Association of Percutaneous Cardiovascular Interventions (EAPCI) and European Association of Acute Cardiac Care (ACCA) endorsed by the Heart Rhythm Society (HRS) and Asia-Pacific Heart Rhythm Society (APHRS) [J]. *Eur Heart J*, 2014, 35: 3155-3179.

[351] January C, Wann L, Alpert J, et al. AHA/ACC/HRS guideline for the management of patients with atrial fibrillation: A report of the American College of Cardiology/American Heart Association Task Force on Practice Guidelines. Developed in Collaboration With the Society of Thoracic Surgeons [J]. *J Am Coll Cardiol*, 2014, 1097: 01740-01749.

[352] Maeda K, Koga M, Okada Y, et al. Nationwide survey of neurospecialists' opinions on anticoagulant therapy after intracerebral hemorrhage in patients with atrial fibrillation [J]. *J Neurol Sci*, 2012, 312: 82-85.

[353] Abrams J, Allen J, Allin D, et al. Efficacy and safety of esmolol vs propranolol in the treatment of supraventricular tachyarrhythmias: A multicenter double-blind clinical trial [J]. *Am Heart J*, 1985, 110: 913-922.

[354] Ellenbogen K A, Dias V C, Plumb V J, et al. A placebo-controlled trial of continuous intravenous diltiazem infusion for 24-hour heart rate control during atrial fibrillation and atrial flutter: A multicenter study [J]. *J Am Coll Cardiol*, 1991, 18: 891-897.

[355] Siu C W, Lau C P, Lee W L, et al. Intravenous diltiazem is superior to intravenous amiodarone or digoxin for achieving ventricular rate control in patients with acute uncomplicated atrial fibrillation [J]. *Crit Care Med*, 2009, 37: 2174-2179.

[356] Ahmed I, Gertner E, Nelson W B, et al. Continuing warfarin therapy is superior to interrupting warfarin with or without bridging anticoagulation therapy in patients undergoing pacemaker and defibrillator implantation [J]. *Heart Rhythm*, 2010, 7: 745-749.

[357] Di Biase L, Burkhardt J D, Mohanty P, et al. Peri-procedural stroke and management of major bleeding complications in patients undergoing catheter ablation of atrial fibrillation [J]. *Circulation*, 2010, 121: 2550-2556.

[358] Di Biase L, Burkhardt J D, Santangeli P, et al. Periprocedural stroke and bleeding complications in patients undergoing catheter ablation of atrial fibrillation with different anticoagulation management: Results from the role of coumadin in preventing thromboembolism in atrial fibrillation (AF) patients undergoing catheter ablation (COMPARE) randomized trial [J]. *Circulation*, 2014, 129: 2638-2644.

[359] Wang H J, Zhu P X, Huang Z J, et al. Application of temporary cardiac pacing in emergency rescue [J]. *Chinese General Practice*, 2004, (19): 1417-1418.

[360] Hu Y Z, Lu J H, He Z Y, et al. Analysis of the application of temporary pacing in acute viral myocarditis complicated with third-degree atrioventricular block [J]. *Chinese Journal of Cardiovascular Research*, 2005, 6: 450-451.

[361] Huang Y, Yang X J, Zhang J J, et al. Effects of protective temporary pacing during emergency percutaneous coronary intervention for acute inferior myocardial infarction on hemodynamics and in-hospital cardiovascular events [J]. *Journal of Practical Medicine*, 2015, 18: 2972-2975.

[362] Wang Z P, Shen X L, Liu T S, et al. Application of bedside temporary pacing in emergency rescue for

acute myocardial infarction [J]. *Journal of Clinical Electrocardiology*, 2010, 3: 210-212.

[363] Gu L D, Wu Z, Qu M Y, et al. Rehabilitation of patients with temporary epicardial pacing wires after extracorporeal circulation in cardiac surgery [J]. *Chinese Journal of Cardiovascular Surgery*, 2017, 4: 321-323.

[364] Yang G M. Bedside temporary pacing for rescuing cardiac arrest and severe bradyarrhythmia [J]. *System Medicine*, 2017, 1: 23-26.

[365] Zhang L, Yue X Y, Chen J J, et al. Discussion on temporary pacing at different sites of the right ventricle via different approaches [J]. *Chinese Journal of Cardiac Pacing and Electrophysiology*, 2016, 6: 539-542.

[366] Lai Q, Guang X F, Jing S N, et al. Discussion on the surgical method of temporary pacing for acute inferior myocardial infarction complicated with high-degree atrioventricular block [J]. *Journal of Kunming Medical University*, 2013, 9: 110-112.

[367] Lin J F, Chen X S, Zhang J H, et al. Discussion on the venous approach and catheter placement method for emergency bedside temporary cardiac pacing using a conventional temporary pacing catheter [J]. *Zhejiang Practical Medicine*, 2008, 3: 160-162, 165.

[368] Li X B, Li D, Guo J H, et al. Clinical observation of cardiac temporary pacing using a balloon flotation electrode catheter [J]. *Chinese Journal of Cardiac Arrhythmias*, 2003, 1: 29-32.

[369] Wang Z P, Shen X L, Liu T S, et al. Application of bedside temporary pacing in emergency rescue for acute myocardial infarction [J]. *Journal of Clinical Electrocardiology*, 2010, 3: 210-212.

[370] Chen H Z, Lin G W, Wang J Y, et al. *Practical Internal Medicine* (14th Edition) [M]. Beijing: People's Medical Publishing House, 2013: 1366-1369.

[371] Wan X H, Lu X F. *Diagnostics* 8th Edition [M]. Beijing: People's Medical Publishing House, 2013: 24.

[372] Latchamsetty R, Bogun F. Premature ventricular complexes and premature ventricular complex induced cardiomyopathy [J]. *Curr Probl Cardiol*, 2015, 40 (9): 379-422.

[373] Tran C T, Calkins H. Premature ventricular contraction-induced cardiomyopathy: An emerging entity [J]. *Expert Rev Cardiovasc Ther*, 2016, 14 (11): 1227-1234.

[374] Yang Y J, Hua W. *Fuwai Cardiovascular Medicine Handbook* 2nd Edition [M]. Beijing: People's Medical Publishing House, 2015: 404-414.

[375] Swan H. Investigation and treatment of premature beats [J]. *Duodecim*, 2013, 129 (6): 599-607.

[376] Adams J C, Srivathsan K, Shen W K, et al. Advances in management of premature ventricular contractions [J]. *J Interv Card Electrophysiol*, 2012, 35 (2): 137-149.

[377] Deng X M, Li W X. *Application of Cardiovascular Drugs in the Perioperative Period* [M]. Beijing: People's Medical Publishing House, 2002: 221-226.

[378] Revision Committee of Chinese Guidelines for Prevention and Treatment of Hypertension. Chinese guidelines for prevention and treatment of hypertension 2010 [J]. *Chinese Journal of Cardiovascular Diseases*, 2011, 39 (7): 579-616.

[379] Mancia G, De Backer G, Dominiczak A, et al. 2007 guidelines for the management of arterial hypertension: The Task Force for the management of arterial hypertension of the European Society of Hypertension (ESH) and of the European Society of Cardiology (ESC) [J]. *Eur Heart J*, 2007, 28 (12): 1462-1536.

[380] Sabina S, Olivera B M, Farid L, et al. Clinical presentation of hypertensive crises in emergency medical services [J]. *Mater Sociomed*, 2014, 26 (1): 12-16.

[381] Emergency Physician Branch of Chinese Medical Doctor Association. Chinese expert consensus on

diagnosis and treatment of emergency hypertension [J]. *Chinese Journal of Emergency Medicine*, 2010, 30 (10): 865-876.

[382] Christos V, Vasiliki K, Petros N, et al. Cardiovascular hypertensive crisis: recent evidence and review of the literature [J]. *Front Cardiovasc Med*, 2016, 3: 51.

[383] Joseph V, Paul E M. Clinical review: The management of hypertensive crises [J]. *Crit Care*, 2003, 7 (5): 374-384.

[384] Wityk R J. The management of blood pressure after stroke [J]. *Neurologist*, 2007, 13 (4): 171-181.

[385] Emergency Physician Branch of Chinese Medical Doctor Association. Chinese expert consensus on diagnosis and treatment of emergency hypertension [J]. *Chinese Journal of Emergency Medicine*, 2010, 30 (10): 865-876.

[386] Chen X J, Tan H B, Liu Z. Analysis of imaging features of hypertensive encephalopathy [J]. *Chinese Journal of Clinical Neurosurgery*, 2010, 15 (5): 281-282.

[387] Howard D P, Banerjee A, Fairhead J F, et al. Population-based study of incidence and outcome of acute aortic dissection and premorbid risk factor control: 10-year results from the Oxford Vascular Study [J]. *Circulation*, 2013, 127: 2031-2037.

[388] Erbel R, Aboyans V, Boileau C, et al. 2014 ESC Guidelines on the diagnosis and treatment of aortic diseases [J]. *Eur Heart J*, 2014, 72 (12): 1169-1252.

[389] Trimarchi S, Tolenaar J L, Tsai T T, et al. Influence of clinical presentation on the outcome of acute type B aortic dissection: Evidences from IRAD [J]. *J Cardiovasc Surg* (Torino), 2012, 53: 161-168.

[390] Klompas M. Does this patient have an acute thoracic aortic dissection? [J]. *JAMA*, 2002, 287: 2262-2272.

[391] Erbel R, Alfonso F, Boileau C, et al. Task Force on Aortic Dissection, European Society of Cardiology. Diagnosis and management of aortic dissection [J]. *Eur Heart J*, 2001, 22: 1642-1681.

[392] Feldstein C. Management of hypertensive crises [J]. *Am J Ther*, 2007, 14: 135-139.

[393] Yin F C, Brin KP, Ting C T, et al. Arterial hemodynamics indexes in Marfan's syndrome [J]. *Circulation*, 1989, 79: 854-862.

[394] Golledge J, Eagle K A. Acute aortic dissection [J]. *Lancet*, 2008, 372: 55-66.

[395] Luo J L, Wu C K, Lin Y H, et al. Type A aortic dissection manifesting as acute myocardial infarction: Still a lesson to learn [J]. *Acta Cardiol*, 2009, 64 (4): 499-504.

[396] Spittell P C, Spittell J A J R, Joyce J W, et al. Clinical features and differential diagnosis of aortic dissection: Experience with 236 cases (1980 through 1990) [J]. *Mayo Clin Proc*, 1993, 68 (7): 642-651.

[397] Geriatric Medicine Branch of Chinese Medical Association, Hypertension Professional Committee of Chinese Medical Doctor Association. Expert recommendations on characteristics of hypertension in the elderly and clinical diagnosis and treatment process [J]. *Chinese Journal of Geriatric Medicine*, 2014, 33 (7): 689-701.

[398] Hypertension Branch of Chinese Geriatric Medicine Association. Chinese expert consensus on blood pressure management in very elderly [J]. *Chinese Journal of Cardiovascular Diseases*, 2015, 20 (6): 401-409.

[399] Revision Committee of Chinese Guidelines for Prevention and Treatment of Hypertension. Chinese guidelines for prevention and treatment of hypertension 2010 [J]. *Chinese Journal of Hypertension*, 2011, 19 (8): 701.

[400] Tian G X, Meng Q Y. Treatment of hypertensive emergencies: The rise of nicardipine [J]. *Chinese Evidence-Based Cardiovascular Medicine*, 2010, 2 (1): 6-8.

[401] Revision Committee of Chinese Guidelines for Prevention and Treatment of Hypertension. Chinese guidelines for prevention and treatment of hypertension 2010 [J]. *Chinese Journal of Hypertension*, 2011, 19:

701-743.

[402] Sun N L, Huo Y, Wang J G, et al. Chinese expert consensus on diagnosis and treatment of refractory hypertension [J]. *Chinese Journal of Interventional Cardiology*, 2013, 21 (2): 69-73.

[403] China Blood Pressure Measurement Working Group. Chinese guidelines for blood pressure measurement [J]. *Chinese Journal of Hypertension*, 2011, 19: 1101-1115.

[404] Laurent S, Schlaich M, Esler M. New drugs, procedures, and devices for hypertension [J]. *Lancet*, 2012, 380: 591-600.

[405] Potthoff S A, Vonend O. Multidisciplinary approach in the treatment of resistant hypertension [J]. *Curr Hypertens Rep*, 2017, 19 (1): 9.

[406] Ryan D H, Yockey S R. Weight loss and improvement in comorbidity: Differences at 5%, 10%, 15%, and over [J]. *Curr Obes Rep*, 2017, 6 (2): 187-194.

[407] Pajak A, Szafraniec K, Kubinova R, et al. Binge drinking and blood pressure: Cross-sectional results of the HAPIEE study [J]. *PLoS One*, 2013, 8 (6): e65856.

[408] Wang M, Moran A E, Liu J, et al. A Meta-analysis of effect of dietary salt restriction on blood pressure in Chinese adults [J]. *Glob Heart*, 2015, 10 (4): 291-299.

[409] Appel L J. The effects of dietary factors on blood pressure [J]. *Cardiol Clin*, 2017, 35 (2): 197-212.

[410] Whehon S P, Chin A, Xin X, et al. Effect of aerobic exercise on blood pressure: a meta-analysis of randomized, controlled trials [J]. *Ann Intern Med*, 2002, 136: 493-503.

[411] Jordan J, Yumuk V, Schlaich M, et al. Joint statement of the European Association for the Study of Obesity and the European Society of Hypertension: Obesity and difficult to treat arterial hypertension [J]. *J Hypertens*, 2012, 30: 1047-1055.

[412] Symplicity HTN-1 Investigators. Catheter-based renal sympathetic denervation for resistant hypertension: Durability of blood pressure reduction out to 24 months [J]. *Hypertension*, 2011, 57: 911-917.

[413] Symplicity HTN-2 Investigators, Esler M D, Krum H, et al. Renal sympathetic denervation in patients with treatment-resistant hypertension (The Symplicity HTN-2 Trial): A randomised controlled trial [J]. *Lancet*, 2010, 376 (9756): 1903-1909.

[414] Coppolino G, Pisano A, Rivoli L, et al. Renal denervation for resistant hypertension [J]. *Cochrane Database SystRev*, 2017, 21: 2.

[415] Li N F, Lin L, Wang L, et al. Analysis of causes of hypertension in hospitalized patients in the hypertension specialty from 1999 to 2008 [J]. *Chinese Journal of Cardiovascular Diseases*, 2010, 38 (10): 939-942.

[416] Kalra P A. Renal-specific secondary hypertension [J]. *J Ren Care*, 2007, 23 (1): 4-10.

[417] Li Y, Feng X B, Zhang Q Y, et al. Study on abnormal circadian rhythm of blood pressure in patients with chronic kidney disease [J]. *Chinese Journal of Nephrology*, 2006, 22 (6): 328-331.

[418] Hao M. New progress in diagnosis and treatment of renal parenchymal hypertension [J]. *Medical Review*, 2013, 19 (16): 2953-2955.

[419] Samadian F, Dalili N, Jamalian A, et al. New insights into pathophysiology, diagnosis, and treatment of renovascular hypertension [J]. *Iran J Kidney Dis*, 2017, 11 (2): 79-89.

[420] Worthley S G, Wilkins G T, Webster M W, et al. Safety and performance of the second generation EnligHTN™ Renal Denervation System in patients with drug-resistant, uncontrolled hypertension [J]. *Atherosclerosis*, 2017, 262: 94-100.

[421] Tafur J D, White C J. Renal artery stenosis: When to revascularize in 2017 [J]. *Curr Probl Cardiol*. 2017, 42 (4): 110-135.

[422] Pappachan J M, Buch H N. Endocrine hypertension: A practical approach [J]. *Adv Exp Med Biol*, 2017, 956: 215-237.

[423] Gyamlani G, Headley C M, Naseer A, et al. Primary aldosteronism: Diagnosis and management [J]. *Am J Med Sci*, 2016, 352 (4): 391-398.

[424] Carey R M. Diagnosing and managing primary aldosteronism in hypertensive patients: A case-based approach [J]. *Curr Cardiol Rep*, 2016, 18 (10): 97.

[425] Steichen O, Amar L, Chaffanjon P, et al. SFE/SFHTA/AFCE consensus on primary aldosteronism, Part 6: Adrenal surgery [J]. *Ann Endocrinol* (Paris), 2016, 77 (3): 220-225.

[426] Azadeh N, Ramakrishna H, Bhatia N L, et al. Therapeutic goals in patients with pheochromocytoma: A guide to perioperative management [J]. *Ir J Med Sci*, 2016, 185 (1): 43-49.

[427] Kiernan C M, Solórzano C C. Pheochromocytoma and paraganglioma: Diagnosis, genetics, and treatment [J]. *Surg Oncol Clin N Am*, 2016, 25 (1): 119-138.

[428] Jain V. Clinical perspective of obstructive sleep apnea-induced cardiovascular complications [J]. *Antioxid Redox Signal*, 2007, 9 (6): 701-710.

[429] Sharabi Y, Rabin K, Grossman E. Sleep apnea-induced hypertension: Mechanisms of vascular changes [J]. *Expert Rev Cardiovasc Ther*, 2005, 3 (5): 937-940.

[430] Bradley T D, Phillipson E A. Pathogenesis and pathophysiology of the obstructive sleep apnea syndrome [J]. *Med Clin North Am*, 1985, 69 (6): 1169-1185.

[431] Hu P J, Xie C M. *Differential Diagnosis of Internal Medicine Diseases* 6th Edition [M]. Beijing: People's Medical Publishing House, 2014: 344-355.

[432] Douglas L, Mann Douglas P, Zipes, et al. *Braunwald's heart disease* (version 10) [M]. Philadelphia: Elsevier Saunders, 2015: 1640-1646.

[433] Richard A, Walsh James C, Fang, et al. *Hurst's the Heart Disease* (13th Edition) [M]. States: The McGraw-Hill Companies, Inc. 2013: 491-494.

[434] Ge J B, Xu Y J. *Internal Medicine* 8th Edition [M]. Beijing: People's Medical Publishing House, 2014: 315-319.

[435] European Society of Cardiology. Current state of knowledge on aetiology, diagnosis, management, and therapy of myocarditis: A position statement of the European Society of Cardiology Working Group on Myocardial and Pericardial Diseases [J]. *Eur Heart J*, 2013, 34: 2636-2648.

[436] Gould F K, Denning D W, Elliott T S, et al. Guidelines for the diagnosis and antibiotic treatment of endocarditis in adults: A report of the Working Party of the British Society for Antimicrobial Chemotherapy [J]. *J Antimicrob Chemother*, 2012, 67: 269-289.

[437] Perez de Isla L, Zamorano J, Lennie V, et al. Negative blood culture infective endocarditis in the elderly: Long-term follow-up [J]. *Gerontology*, 2007, 53: 245-249.

[438] Raoult D, Casalta J P, Richet H, et al. Contribution of systematic serological testing in diagnosis of infective endocarditis [J]. *J Clin Microbiol*, 2005, 43: 5238-5242.

[439] Lamas C C, Eykyn S J. Blood culture negative endocarditis: Analysis of 63 cases presenting over 25 years [J]. *Heart*, 2003, 89: 258-262.

[440] Brouqui P, Raoult D. New insight into the diagnosis of fastidious bacterial endocarditis [J]. *FEMS Immunol Med Microbiol*, 2006, 27: 1-13.

[441] Li J S, Sexton D J, Mick N, et al. Proposed modifications to the Duke criteria for the diagnosis of infective endocarditis [J]. *Clin Infect Dis*, 2000, 30: 633-638.

[442] Regitz-Zagrosek V, Blomstrom Lundqvist C, Borghi C, et al. ESC Guidelines on the management of

cardiovascular diseases during pregnancy: The Task Force on the Management of Cardiovascular Diseases during Pregnancy of the European Society of Cardiology (ESC) [J]. *Eur Heart J*, 2011, 32: 3147-3197.

[443] Nishimura R A, Otto C M, Bonow R O, et al. 2017 AHA/ACC focused update of valvular heart disease guideline [J]. *Circulation*, 2017, 135 (25): e1159-e1195.

[444] Rick A, Catherine M, Robert O, et al. 2014 AHA/ACC Valvular Heart Disease Guideline [J]. *Circulation*, 2014, 63 (22): 157-185.

[445] Rubin L J. Primary pulmonary hypertension [J]. *N Engl J Med*, 1997, 336: 111-117.

[446] Humbert M, Khaltaev N, Bousquet J, et al. Pulmonary hypertension: From an orphan disease to a public health problem [J]. *Chest*, 2007, 132: 365-367.

[447] Simonneau G, Robbins I M, Beghetti M, et al. Updated clinical classification of pulmonary hypertension [J]. *J Am Coll Cardiol*, 2009, 54 (1 Suppl): S43-54.

[448] Chung L, Liu J, Parsons L, et al. Characterization of connective tissue disease-associated pulmonary arterial hypertension from REVEAL: Identifying systemic sclerosis as a unique phenotype [J]. *Chest*, 2010, 138 (6): 1383-1394.

[449] Galié N, Hoeper M M, Humbert M, et al. Guidelines for the diagnosis and treatment of pulmonary hypertension [J]. *J Am Coll Cardiol*, 2009, 53: 1573-1619.

[450] Arcasoy S M, Christie J D, Ferrari V A, et al. Echocardiographic assessment of pulmonary hypertension in patients with advanced lung disease [J]. *Am J Respir Crit Care Med*, 2003, 167: 735-740.

[451] Lu W X, Wang C. *Pulmonary Circulatory Disease* [M]. Beijing: People's Medical Publishing House, 2007: 304.

[452] Pengo V, Lensing A W, Prins M H, et al. Incidence of chronic thromboembolic pulmonary hypertension after pulmonary embolism [J]. *N Engl J Med*, 2004, 350: 2257-2264.

[453] Ferris A, Jacobs T, Widlitz A, et al. Pulmonary arterial hypertension and thyroid disease [J]. *Chest*, 2001, 119 (6): 1980-1981.

[454] Scicchitano P, Dentamaro I, Tunzi F, et al. Pulmonary hypertension in thyroid diseases [J]. *Endocrine*, 2016, 54 (3): 578-587.

[455] Zhu X Y, Zhang R Z. 2015 Chinese expert consensus on diagnosis and treatment of pulmonary arterial hypertension associated with congenital heart disease [J]. *Chinese Journal of Interventional Cardiology*, 2015, 23 (2): 61-69.

[456] McLaughlin V V, Archer S L, Badesch D B, et al. ACCF/AHA 2009 Expert Consensus Document on Pulmonary Hypertension [J]. *J Am Coll Cardiol*, 2009, 53: 1573-1619.

[457] Xu X Q, Jing Z C. Pulmonary hypertension associated with hemolytic anemia [J]. *Internal Medicine Theory and Practice*, 2008, 3 (6): 436-438.

[458] Hachulla E, Gressin V, Guillevin L, et al. Early detection of pulmonary arterial hypertension in systemic sclerosis: A French nationwide prospective multicenter study [J]. *Arthritis Rheum*, 2005, 52: 3792-3800.

[459] Paulus W J, Tschope C, Sanderson J E, et al. How to diagnose diastolic heart failure: A consensus statement on the diagnosis of heart failure with normal left ventricular ejection fraction by the Heart Failure and Echocardiography Associations of the European Society of Cardiology [J]. *Eur Heart J*, 2007, 28: 2539-2550.

[460] Sitbon O, Humbert M, Jais X, et al. Long-term response to calcium channel blockers in idiopathic pulmonary arterial hypertension [J]. *Circulation*, 2005, 111: 3105-3111.

[461] Jing Z C, Xu X Q, Jiang X, et al. Feasibility study of right heart catheterization and pulmonary arteriography via antecubital venous approach [J]. *Chinese Journal of Cardiovascular Diseases*, 2009, 37: 142-144.

[462] Ross R M. ATS/ACCP statement on cardiopulmonary exercise testing [J]. *Am J Respir Crit Care Med*, 2003, 167: 1451.

[463] Jing Z C. Clinical application of 6-minute walk distance [J]. *Chinese Journal of Cardiovascular Diseases*, 2006, 34: 183-186.

[464] Olschewski H, Hoeper M M, Behr J, et al. Long-term therapy with inhaled iloprost in patients with pulmonary hypertension [J]. *Respir Med*, 2010, 104: 731-740.

[465] Hoeper M M, Gall H, Seyfarth H J, et al. Long-term outcome with intravenous iloprost in pulmonary arterial hypertension [J]. *Eur Respir J*, 2009, 34: 132-137.

[466] Higenbottam T, Butt A Y, McMahon A, et al. Long-term intravenous prostaglandin (epoprostenol or iloprost) for treatment of severe pulmonary hypertension [J]. *Heart*, 1998, 80: 151-155.

[467] Barst R J, McGoon M, McLaughlin V V, et al. Beraprost therapy for pulmonary arterial hypertension [J]. *J Am Coll Cardiol*, 2003, 41: 2119-2125.

[468] Galié N, Humbert M, Vachiéry J L, et al. Effects of beraprost sodium, an oral prostacyclin analogue, in patients with pulmonary arterial hypertension: A randomized, double-blind, placebo-controlled trial [J]. *J Am Coll Cardiol*, 2002, 39: 1496-1502.

[469] Jing Z C, Strange G, Zhu X Y, et al. An open-label, multicenter study to assess the efficacy, safety and tolerability of bosentan in Chinese patients with pulmonary arterial hypertension [J]. *Heart and Lung Transplantation*, 2010, 29: 150-156.

[470] Barst R J, Langleben D, Frost A, et al. Sitaxsentan therapy for pulmonary arterial hypertension [J]. *Am J Respir Crit Care Med*, 2004, 169: 441-447.

[471] Barst R J, Langleben D, Badesch D, et al. Treatment of pulmonary arterial hypertension with the selective endothelin-A receptor antagonist sitaxsentan [J]. *J Am Coll Cardiol*, 2006, 47: 2049-2056.

[472] Galié N, Olschewski H, Oudiz R J, et al. Ambrisentan for the treatment of pulmonary arterial hypertension: Results of the Ambrisentan in Pulmonary Arterial Hypertension, Randomized, Double-Blind, Placebo-Controlled, Multicenter, Efficacy (ARIES) Study 1 and 2 [J]. *Circulation*, 2008, 117: 3010-3019.

[473] Leon M B, Smith C R, Mack M J, et al. PARTNER 2 Investigators. Transcatheter or surgical aortic-valve replacement in intermediate-risk patients [J]. *N Engl J Med*, 2016, 374 (17): 1609-2036.

[474] Pan W Z, Zhou D X, Zhang L, et al. A case of transcatheter aortic valve replacement via carotid artery approach [J]. *Chinese Journal of Cardiovascular Diseases*, 2016, 44 (4): 348-349.

[475] Mylotte D, Sudre A, Teiger E, et al. Transcarotid Transcatheter aortic valve replacement: Feasibility and safety [J]. *JACC Cardiovasc Interv*, 2016, 9 (5): 472-480.

[476] EuroPCR 2016: Half of transcatheter heart valves show degeneration within 10 years of TAVI [EQ/OL].

[477] Peter R M, Flack J M. Hypertensive disorders of pregnancy [J]. *J Obstet Gynecol*, 2004, 33 (2): 209-220.

[478] Duley L. The global impact of pre-eclampsia and eclampsia, 2009, 33 (3): 130-137.

[479] National Preeclampsia Research Collaborative Group. Epidemiological survey of preeclampsia in China [J]. *Chinese Journal of Obstetrics and Gynecology*, 1991, 2: 67-71.

[480] Shanghai Pregnancy Hypertension Syndrome Survey Collaborative Group. A 10-year study on the incidence of pregnancy hypertension syndrome in Shanghai [J]. *Chinese Journal of Obstetrics and Gynecology*, 2001, 36 (3): 137-139.

[481] American College of Obstetricians and Gynecologists Task Force on Hypertension in Pregnancy. Hypertension in pregnancy: Report of the American College of Obstetricians and Gynecologists' Task Force on

Hypertension in Pregnancy [J]. *Obstet Gynecol*, 2013, 122 (5): 1122-1131.

[482] Broekhuijsen K, van Baaren G J, van Pampus M G, et al. Immediate delivery versus expectant monitoring for hypertensive disorders of pregnancy between 34 and 37 weeks of gestation (HYPITAT- Ⅱ): An open-label, randomised controlled trial [J]. *Lancet*, 2015, 385 (9986): 2492-2501.

[483] Wang H Y, Sun N L. Introduction and interpretation of guidelines for rational use of antihypertensive drugs [J]. *Chinese Journal of Hypertension*, 2016, 24 (6): 515-518.

[484] Schmidt M I, Duncan B B, Castilhos C, et al. Lifestyle intervention for diabetes prevention after pregnancy (LINDA-Brasil): Study protocol for a multicenter randomized controlled trial [J]. *BMC Pregnancy Childbirth*, 2016, 16 (68): 1-12.

[485] Molvi S N, Mir S, Rana V S, et al. Role of antihypertensive therapy in mild to moderate pregnancy-induced hypertension: A prospective randomized study comparing labetalol with alpha methyldopa [J]. *Arch Gynecol Obstet*, 2012, 285 (6): 1553-1562.

[486] Collins R, Yusuf S, Peto R. Overview of randomised trials of diuretics in pregnancy [J]. *Br Med J* (Clin Res Ed.), 1985, 290 (6461): 17-23.

[487] Shrout T, Rudy D W, Piascik M T. Hypertension update: JNC8 and beyond [J]. *Curr Opin Pharmacol*, 2017, 33: 41-46.

[488] Rocheleau C M, Bertke S J, Lawson C C, et al. Factors associated with employment status before and during pregnancy: Implications for studies of pregnancy outcomes. National Birth Defects Prevention Study [J]. *Am J Ind Med*, 2017, 60 (4): 329-341.

[489] European Society of Gynecology (ESG), Association for European Paediatric Cardiology (AEPC), German Society for Gender Medicine (DGesGM), et al. ESC Guidelines on the management of cardiovascular diseases during pregnancy: The Task Force on the Management of Cardiovascular Diseases during Pregnancy of the European Society of Cardiology (ESC) [J]. *Eur Heart J*, 2011, 32 (24): 3147-3197.

[490] Fuller B S, Voeltz M D. Clinical updates in women's health care summary: arrhythmias: Primary and preventive care review [J]. *Obstet Gynecol*, 2017, 129 (5): 969.

[491] Tse G. Mechanisms of cardiac arrhythmias [J]. *J Arrhythm*, 2016, 32 (2): 75-81.

[492] Metz T D, Khanna A. Evaluation and management of maternal cardiac arrhythmias [J]. *Obstet Gynecol Clin North Am*, 2016, 43 (4): 729-745.

[493] Lewey J, Haythe J. Cardiomyopathy in pregnancy [J]. *Semin Perinatol*, 2014, 38 (5): 309-317.

[494] Moghbeli N, Pare E, Webb G. Practical assessment of maternal cardiovascular risk in pregnancy [J]. *Congenit Heart Dis*, 2008, 3 (5): 308-316.

[495] Priori S G, Blomström-Lundqvist C, Mazzanti A, et al. 2015 ESC Guidelines for the management of patients with ventricular arrhythmias and the prevention of sudden cardiac death: The Task Force for the management of patients with ventricular arrhythmias and the prevention of sudden cardiac death of the European Society of Cardiology (ESC). Endorsed by: Association for European Paediatric and Congenital Cardiology (AEPC) [J]. *Eur Heart J*, 2015, 36 (41): 2793-2867.

[496] Bates S M, Greer I A, Middeldorp S, et al. VTE, thrombophilia, antithrombotic therapy, and pregnancy: Antithrombotic therapy and prevention of thrombosis. 9th ed. American College of Chest Physicians evidence-based clinical practice guidelines [J]. *Chest*, 2012, 141 (2 Suppl): e691S-e736S.

[497] Saw J. Pregnancy-Associated spontaneous coronary artery dissection represents an exceptionally high-risk spontaneous coronary artery dissection cohort [J]. *Circ Cardiovasc Interv*, 2017, 10 (3): e004941.

[498] Havakuk O, Goland S, Mehra A, et al. Pregnancy and the risk of spontaneous coronary artery dissection: An analysis of 120 contemporary cases [J]. *Circ Cardiovasc Interv*, 2017, 10 (3): e004941.

[499] Bitting C P, Zumwalt R E. Repeat coronary artery dissection in pregnancy: A case report and review of the literature [J]. *J Forensic Sci*, 2017, 62 (5): 1389-1394.

[500] Gong Y. Clinical treatment of cardiovascular diseases complicating pregnancy [J]. *Journal of Qiqihar Medical University*, 2011, 32 (10): 1584-1585.

[501] Liu Q Z, Liu M L. Interpretation of the 2011 ESC Guidelines on the Management of Cardiovascular Diseases During Pregnancy [J]. *Chinese Journal of Cardiovascular Diseases*, 2012, 40 (9): 807-808.

[502] ESC issued the first Guidelines on the Management of Cardiovascular Diseases During Pregnancy [J]. *Pharmacy and Clinical Research*, 2011, 19 (5): 416.

[503] Taylor J. The first ESC Guidelines on the management of cardiovascular diseases during pregnancy [J]. *Eur Heart J*, 2011, 32 (24): 3055-3056.

[504] Hagan P G, Nienaber C A, Isselbacher E M, et al. The international registry of acute aortic dissection (IRAD): New insights into an old disease [J]. *JAMA*, 2002, 283: 897-903.

[505] Yang Z H, Hong T, Wang C S. Surgical treatment of 2 cases of acute aortic dissection complicating pregnancy [J]. *Fudan University Journal of Medical Sciences*, 2010, 37: 755-756.

[506] Collins D. aetiology and management of acute cardiac tamponade [J]. *Crit Care Resusc*, 2004, 6: 54-58.

[507] Goland S, Elkayam U. Cardiovascular problems in pregnant women with marfan syndrome [J]. *Circulation*, 2009, 119: 619-623.

[508] Yu L, Ding Y L. Early recognition and management of aortic aneurysm complicating pregnancy [J]. *Chinese Journal of Practical Gynecology and Obstetrics*, 2017, 33 (3): 272-276.

[509] Pagni S, Ganzel B L, Tabb T. Hemiarch aortic replacement for acute type A dissection in a Marfan patient with twin pregnancy [J]. *Interact Cardiovasc Thorac Surg*, 2008, 7: 740-741.

[510] Yan C L, Gao C Q, Xiao C S, et al. Clinical features of young patients with Stanford type A aortic dissection [J]. *Chinese Journal of Cardiovascular Surgery*, 2012, 19: 251-253.

[511] Yuan D H, Liu H Y, Liu Y Q. Ultrasonic diagnosis of aortic dissection [J]. *Chinese Circulation Journal*, 1994, 12: 757-759.

[512] Le Jie. *Obstetrics and Gynecology* 7th Edition [M]. Beijing: People's Medical Publishing House, 2008: 134.

[513] Qiu Y H, Wang F, Wang L Y. Clinical analysis of 58 cases of pregnancy complicated with heart disease [J]. *Chinese Journal of Practical Gynecology and Obstetrics*, 2006, 22 (12): 937-938.

[514] Zhang Y S, Ma D J, Xu M, et al. Observation on the efficacy of simultaneous transcatheter treatment of complex congenital heart disease [J]. *Chinese Journal of Interventional Cardiology*, 2005, 13 (3): 146-148.

[515] Xie A L, Yang A S, Yan L Z, et al. Perinatal outcomes of patients with pregnancy complicated with pulmonary hypertension and heart failure [J]. *Chinese Journal of Emergency Medicine*, 2011, 20 (6): 650-653.

[516] Wang X X. Clinical analysis of 120 cases of pregnancy complicated with heart disease [J]. *Chinese Continuing Medical Education*, 2016, 9: 72-73.

[517] Liu H, Huang T T, Zhao W X, et al. Pregnancy outcomes and relative risk factors among Chinese women with congenital heart disease [J]. *International Journal of Gynecology & Obstetrics*, 2013, 120 (3): 245-248.

[518] Haynes A B, Weiser T G, Berry W R, et al. A surgical safety checklist to reduce morbidity and mortality in a global population [J]. *N Engl J Med*, 2009, 360 (5): 491-499.

[519] Devereaux P J, Chan M T, Alonso-Coello P, et al. Association between postoperative troponin levels and 30-day mortality among patients undergoing noncardiac surgery [J]. *JAMA*, 2012, 307 (21): 2295-304.

[520] Wirthlin D J, Cambria R P. Surgery-specific considerations in the cardiac patient undergoing noncardiac surgery [J]. *Prog Cardiovasc Dis*, 1998, 40 (5): 453-468.

[521] Guay J, Choi P, Suresh S, et al. Neuraxial blockade for the prevention of post-operative mortality and major morbidity: An overview of Cochrane systematic reviews [J]. *Cochrane Database Syst Rev*, 2014, 1: CD010108.

[522] Kristensen S D, Knuuti J, Saraste A, et al. 2014 ESC/ESA Guidelines on non-cardiac surgery: Cardiovascular assessment and management: The Joint Task Force on non-cardiac surgery: Cardiovascular assessment and management of the European Society of Cardiology (ESC) and the European Society of Anaesthesiology (ESA) [J]. *Eur Heart J*, 2014, 35 (35): 2383-2431.

[523] Poldermans D, Bax J J, Boersma E, et al. Guidelines for pre-operative cardiac risk assessment and perioperative cardiac management in non-cardiac surgery [J]. *Eur Heart J*, 2009, 30 (22): 2769-2812.

[524] Gupta P K, Gupta H, Sundaram A, et al. Development and validation of a risk calculator for prediction of cardiac risk after surgery [J]. *Circulation*, 2011, 124 (4): 381-387.

[525] Myers J, Bader D, Madhavan R, et al. Validation of a specific activity questionnaire to estimate exercise tolerance in patients referred for exercise testing [J]. *Am Heart J*, 2001, 142 (6): 1041-1046.

[526] Velasco A, Reyes E, Hage F G. Guidelines in review: Comparison of the 2014 ACC/AHA guidelines on perioperative cardiovascular evaluation and management of patients undergoing noncardiac surgery and the 2014 ESC/ESA guidelines on noncardiac surgery—Cardiovascular assessment and management [J]. *J Nucl Cardiol*, 2017, 24 (1): 165-170.

[527] Wijns W, Kolh P, Danchin N, et al. Guidelines on myocardial revascularization [J]. *Eur Heart J*, 2010, 31 (20): 2501-2555.

[528] Upshaw J, Kiernan M S. Preoperative cardiac risk assessment for noncardiac surgery in patients with heart failure [J]. *Curr Heart Fail Rep*, 2013, 10 (2): 147-156.

[529] Leung J M, Voskanian A, Bellows W H, et al. Automated electrocardiograph ST segment trending monitors: Accuracy in detecting myocardial ischemia [J]. *Anesth Analg*, 1998, 87 (1): 4-10.

[530] Rohde L E, Polanczyk C A, Goldman L, et al. Usefulness of transthoracic echocardiography as a tool for risk stratification of patients undergoing major noncardiac surgery [J]. *Am J Cardiol*, 2001, 87 (5): 505-509.

[531] Schulmeyer C, Farías J, Rajdl E, et al. Utility of transesophageal echocardiography during severe hypotension in non-cardiac surgery [J]. *Rev Bras Anestesiol*, 2010, 60 (5): 513-521.

[532] Mark D B, Berman D S, Budoff M J, et al. ACCF/ACR/AHA/NASCI/SAIP/SCAI/SCCT 2010 expert consensus document on coronary computed tomographic angiography: A report of the American College of Cardiology Foundation Task Force on Expert Consensus Documents [J]. *J Am Coll Cardiol*, 2010, 55 (23): 2663-2699.

[533] Weber M, Luchner A, Seeberger M, et al. Incremental value of high-sensitive troponin T in addition to the revised cardiac index for peri-operative risk stratification in non-cardiac surgery [J]. *Eur Heart J*, 2013, 34 (11): 853-862.

[534] Wang T J, Larson M G, Levy D, et al. Plasma natriuretic peptide levels and the risk of cardiovascular events and death [J]. *N Engl J Med*, 2004, 350 (7): 655-663.

[535] Ponikowski P, Voors A A, Anker S D, et al. 2016 ESC Guidelines for the diagnosis and treatment of acute and chronic heart failure: The Task Force for the diagnosis and treatment of acute and chronic heart failure of the European Society of Cardiology (ESC) Developed with the special contribution of the Heart Failure Association (HFA) of the ESC [J]. *Eur Heart J*, 2016, 37 (27): 2129-2200.